Aphasia: Clinical Perspectives

Aphasia: Clinical Perspectives

Editor: Adlan Brooks

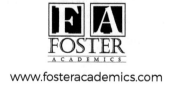

www.fosteracademics.com

www.fosteracademics.com

Cataloging-in-Publication Data

Aphasia : clinical perspectives / edited by Adlan Brooks.
     p. cm.
Includes bibliographical references and index.
ISBN 978-1-64646-611-5
1. Aphasia. 2. Aphasia--Diagnosis. 3. Aphasia--Treatment.
4. Brain--Diseases. 5. Language disorders. 6. Speech disorders.
I. Brooks, Adlan.
RC425 .A643 2023
616.855 2--dc23

Foster Academics,
118-35 Queens Blvd., Suite 400,
Forest Hills, NY 11375, USA

ISBN 978-1-64646-611-5 (Hardback)

Contents

Preface

Every book is initially just a concept; it takes months of research and hard work to give it the final shape in which the readers receive it. In its early stages, this book also went through rigorous reviewing. The notable contributions made by experts from across the globe were first molded into patterned chapters and then arranged in a sensibly sequential manner to bring out the best results.

Aphasia is a condition in which a person's ability to communicate is affected. It is caused by an impairment of specific brain regions responsible for language. It may affect both written as well as spoken language. Stroke (cerebral vascular accident) and head trauma are the most common causes for this condition. However, aphasia can also be caused due to brain tumors or progressive neurodegenerative damage. It usually indicates towards the presence of some other condition such as stroke. Auditory comprehension, vocal expression, reading and writing, and functional communication are the four modalities of communication. Diagnosis of aphasia requires determining if the brain damage was followed by problems in one or more communication modalities of a person's speech or language. The risk of aphasia can be lowered by taking few precautions such as regular exercise, nutritious diet, no alcohol and tobacco consumption, and controlling blood pressure levels. Various types of speech and language therapies such as visual communication therapy (VIC), functional communication therapy (FCT), and melodic intonation therapy (MIT) are helpful in managing aphasia. The extensive content of this book provides the readers with a thorough understanding of clinical perspectives with reference to aphasia. It aims to serve as a resource guide for students and medical practitioners alike.

It has been my immense pleasure to be a part of this project and to contribute my years of learning in such a meaningful form. I would like to take this opportunity to thank all the people who have been associated with the completion of this book at any step.

Editor

Different Cognitive Profiles of Patients with Severe Aphasia

Chiara Valeria Marinelli,[1,2] **Simona Spaccavento,**[3] **Angela Craca,**[3] **Paola Marangolo,**[2,4] **and Paola Angelelli**[1]

[1]*Lab of Applied Psychology and Intervention, Department of History Society and Human Studies, University of Salento, Lecce, Italy*
[2]*IRCCS Foundation Santa Lucia, Rome, Italy*
[3]*Neurorehabilitation Unit, Department of Humanities Studies, ICS Maugeri SPA SB, IRCCS Institute of Cassano Murge, Bari, Italy*
[4]*Department of Humanities Studies, University of Napoli Federico II, Napoli, Italy*

Correspondence should be addressed to Chiara Valeria Marinelli; chiaravaleria.marinelli@unisalento.it

Academic Editor: Rufus Akinyemi

Cognitive dysfunction frequently occurs in aphasic patients and primarily compromises linguistic skills. However, patients suffering from severe aphasia show heterogeneous performance in basic cognition. Our aim was to characterize the cognitive profiles of patients with severe aphasia and to determine whether they also differ as to residual linguistic abilities. We examined 189 patients with severe aphasia with standard language tests and with the CoBaGA (Cognitive Test Battery for Global Aphasia), a battery of nonverbal tests that assesses a wide range of cognitive domains such as attention, executive functions, intelligence, memory, visual-auditory recognition, and visual-spatial abilities. Twenty patients were also followed longitudinally in order to assess their improvement in cognitive skills after speech therapy. Three different subgroups of patients with different types and severity of cognitive impairment were evidenced. Subgroups differed as to residual linguistic skills, in particular comprehension and reading-writing abilities. Attention, reasoning, and executive functions improved after language rehabilitation. This study highlights the importance of an extensive evaluation of cognitive functions in patients with severe aphasia.

1. Introduction

Formerly, aphasia was considered exclusively as a linguistic deficit [1]. However, it is difficult to explain the variability of patients with aphasia if only linguistic factors are considered [2, 3]. McNeil and Kimelman [4] suggested that other cognitive impairments in addition to linguistic deficits might compromise the communicative skills of aphasic patients. As the association between language function and cognition is stronger in more severe aphasic conditions [5], there is now greater interest in studying the neuropsychological deficits associated with linguistic impairment in severe aphasics.

Cognitive impairments have frequently been observed in patients with aphasia [6]. A recent review by Fonseca et al. [7] of 47 studies (with a total of 1710 aphasic patients) found that 61.3% of studies showed that patients with aphasia following a stroke tend to obtain lower scores than healthy subjects on most nonverbal cognitive tests. Several studies highlighted the presence of memory deficits (e.g., [8]), attention (e.g., [9]), recognition abilities (e.g., [10]), logic skills (e.g., [11]), and executive functions (e.g., [12]) in aphasic patients.

According to some authors, the occurrence of other cognitive deficits in association with language impairment can seriously worsen the symptomatology of aphasia [13] and may influence the efficacy of rehabilitative training [13, 14]. In fact, it has been found that patients with aphasia and concomitant cognitive deficits benefit less from speech therapy than patients without cognitive deficits [15, 16]. On the other hand, a high level of cognitive abilities predicts better and faster recovery of linguistic abilities [17]. Furthermore, patients with persisting aphasia were found to be more cognitively impaired and severe cognitive impairment is associated with poor functional outcome [18]. Many studies investigating patients with aphasia examined the integrity of a single cognitive function and its relationship to linguistic abilities; by contrast, studies investigating a wider range of cognitive domains (thus providing a profile of the cognitive impairment) are rare. Recently, some studies (e.g., [5, 19, 20]) tried to examine the cognitive deficit in aphasia; however, the question was largely unresolved because of the small number of subjects in the sample, the heterogeneity of clinical types of aphasia, and the need for verbal responses in most nonlinguistic cognitive tests. In fact, it is not easy to test the cognitive abilities of aphasic individuals because neuropsychological tests have a linguistic mediation and are therefore inappropriate for use with this population. Moreover, many tests are too complex; thus, patients with severe aphasia show an invariant profile with very low accuracy (floor effect).

For this reason, some authors have introduced simple nonverbal test batteries for assessing the cognitive abilities of aphasic patients. For example, Kalbe et al. [13] developed the Aphasia Check List (ACL). This nonverbal test battery allows assessing linguistic abilities as well as visual memory, selective attention, and logical reasoning. The authors found that 94% of the 154 patients examined (with moderate to severe aphasia) presented a deficit in at least one of the cognitive functions investigated. According to this study, linguistic performance correlates with memory, attention, and reasoning. El Hachioui et al. [18] used a nonlinguistic cognitive examination to test 147 aphasic patients. It included abstract reasoning, visual memory, visual perception and construction, and executive functioning. The authors found that 88% of the patients were impaired in at least one nonlinguistic cognitive domain after three months and 80% after one year. Impairment of visual memory was most frequent at three months and one year. Impairment of visual perception and construction was least common, and performance on this task was adequate after one year. Similarly, Kauhanen et al. [21] investigated visual memory, problem solving, and visual-constructive abilities in 31 aphasic patients (with different types of aphasia) using some nonverbal tests derived from standard neuropsychological batteries. The authors found that the aphasic patients' performance (but not that of left brain-damaged patients without aphasia) was impaired in all functions investigated also when patients with severe comprehension deficits (global, Wernicke's and transcortical sensory aphasia) were excluded from the sample. This finding was replicated three and 12 months after the stroke. Moreover, all patients suffering from moderate/severe aphasia obtained lower scores on all of the nonverbal cognitive tests compared to patients with mild aphasia.

Helm-Estabrooks [6] also examined the cognitive profile of 13 patients with moderate to severe aphasia using the Cognitive Linguistic Quick Test (CLQT; [22]), which assesses the integrity of language as well as executive functions, attention, memory, and visual-spatial abilities. The author found that the patients' performances were extremely different on the various cognitive tests. Helm-Estabrooks also found that the level of the cognitive deficit is not usually linked to the severity of aphasia. The absence of a correlation between linguistic deficit and cognitive impairment was also demonstrated in a preliminary study [23] of 34 aphasic patients, none of whom had global aphasia. Helm-Estabrooks' studies demonstrate the importance of carrying out a comprehensive cognitive assessment, because the

integrity of nonlinguistic abilities cannot be estimated according to the severity of aphasia.

Van Mourik et al. [24] studied the cognitive abilities of patients with global aphasia. The authors examined the performance of 17 patients with global aphasia using the GANBA (Global Aphasic Neuropsychological Battery), which includes nonverbal tests aimed at assessing auditory comprehension and the following cognitive functions: attention/concentration, memory, intelligence, and visual and auditory nonverbal recognition. The authors reported that the three subgroups of patients could be separated into those with global aphasia who had different cognitive profiles: (i) the first group had almost spared cognitive functions and thus required a neurolinguistic treatment; (ii) the second group suffered from a selective deficit in attention and visual-auditory recognition; (iii) and the third group displayed severe cognitive impairments that made the rehabilitative treatment impossible. Patients belonging to the last group had no possibility of communicating and could only express their emotions with facial expressions. Also in this study, the degree of cognitive impairment was independent from the language dysfunction, at least regarding auditory comprehension.

Hinckley and Nash [25] replicated the study of Van Mourik et al. [24] using the GANBA in four patients with mild aphasia, 21 patients with moderate aphasia, and four patients with severe aphasia. The authors found that selective attention, auditory recognition, and memory abilities were related to the severity of aphasia. This finding is in contrast with the results of Van Mourik et al. [24] and Helm-Estabrooks et al. [22, 23].

In summary, according to the studies mentioned above, most patients with aphasia also suffer from other neuropsychological disorders [13]. Moreover, the population of patients with aphasia seems to be extremely heterogeneous as to type and severity of cognitive dysfunctions [6, 24]. However, only one study [24] extended the investigation to a wider range of cognitive domains and identified different subgroups of patients on the basis of their cognitive profile. Unfortunately, this latter study was based exclusively on a qualitative evaluation of cognitive test performances. On the basis of our knowledge, no studies have investigated whether different cognitive profiles are associated with a deficit in a specific linguistic domain. Moreover, the above-mentioned studies reported discordant results about the relationship between cognitive and linguistic dysfunctions. Some studies declared that cognitive and linguistic impairments were independent, and others found that cognitive deficits depended on the severity of the linguistic disorder. These discordant results might also be due to the selection of a small sample with different aphasic disturbances. The extreme variability of cognitive abilities among patients with aphasia necessarily requires the use of large samples [25] to allow the generalization of results.

The first aim of the present study was to evaluate the existence of different profiles of cognitive impairment in a large sample of patients with severe aphasia based on the severity and type of cognitive deficits (study 1). The cognitive abilities studied were attention, executive functions, logical reasoning, visual-spatial ability, memory, and visual and auditory recognition. The integrity of these functions was evaluated with a battery of simple tests that do not require verbal responses and are, thus, suitable for patients with severe aphasia. We were also interested in verifying whether patients with different profiles of cognitive deficits also differ in terms of their residual linguistic skills.

The second aim of the present study was to examine whether speech therapy also improves cognitive skills and which cognitive skill is predictive of greater language recovery (study 2). For this purpose, we examined a group of patients longitudinally pre and post treatment.

2. Study 1

In this study, we assessed the existence of different profiles of cognitive impairment in patients with severe aphasia and the relationship between cognitive and linguistic skills. The linguistic skills investigated were oral and written comprehension, naming, reading-spelling, and repetition.

3. Participants

One hundred eighty-nine patients (111 males and 78 females), mean age 66 years (SD: ±11.6), were examined 126 days (SD: ±180) after a stroke. Mean educational level was 6.3 years (SD: ±4). The inclusion criteria were the presence of a selective lesion of the left cerebral hemisphere and severe aphasia. In particular, only patients with a score on the Token Test ([26]; see 2.2a) less than 15 (mean accuracy = 6.4; SD: ±4.8) were included. All subjects were Italian and have global aphasia. Patients were excluded if they had bilateral lesions, previous stroke, previous drug abuse, and a positive history of psychiatric disorders or dementia (OMS, 1994).

The performance of patients with aphasia was compared to the performance of healthy subjects paired for educational level with the aphasic individuals. Two control groups were included: the first one included 43 subjects (22 males and 21 females, mean age: 53.4) with moderate–high school attendance (>6 years, mean school attendance: 10.4), and the second group included 33 subjects (21 males and 12 females; mean age: 67.9) with low school attendance (≤5 years mean school attendance: 4.5). Subjects with a history of neurological impairment and developmental linguistic disorders were not included in the control sample.

The study was conducted in accordance with the Declaration of Helsinki (1964) and was approved by the Ethical Committee.

4. Analysis of Lesions

Lesion sites were classified on the basis of neuroradiological and clinical evidence of the cerebral arterial territory involved. In particular, the Oxford Community Stroke Project (OCSP; [27]) classification was adopted. Most of the patients (69%) presented partial anterior circulation infarcts (PACI), 8% had posterior circulation infarcts (POCI), 6% had total anterior circulation infarcts (TACI), and very few (1%) had lacunar lesions (LACI). Note that neuroimaging exams were performed to identify lesion location, but further information such as lesion volumes could not be established.

5. Materials

The CoBaGa (Cognitive Test Battery for Global Aphasia; [28, 29]) was used to assess cognitive functions. This is a test battery that is suitable for patients with severe aphasia because it requires only manipulative answers and not verbal responses. The CoBaGa is made up of five subtests that evaluate the following cognitive functions: attention, executive functions, logical reasoning, memory, visual-auditory recognition, and visual-spatial ability. The score of each subtest is the sum of the scores obtained on the various items. There is no time limit. A more detailed description of the items included in each subtest can be found in Appendix A.

The CoBaGa is a reliable battery; it has a good test-retest correlation one month after it has been administered ($r = 0.71$) and good internal consistency (Cronbach's α is 0.80 in all tests and 0.73 and 0.9 in different subsets) and discriminant validity (i.e., it can discriminate patients with aphasia from healthy subjects, $p < 0.0001$, and patients with aphasia from neurological patients without aphasia, $p < 0.05$). Moreover, the CoBaGa has good convergent validity with other etero-valutative instruments (with cognitive scores of Functional Independence Measure (FIM; [30]): r Pearson (Pearson's r) = 0.72, $p < 0.001$) as well as good divergent validity (with FIM motor score: r Pearson (Pearson's r) = 0.32, p = ns). The CoBaGa also has proven sensitive in detecting follow-up changes in performance (at least $p < 0.05$).

Patients' cognitive ability was tested with the CoBaGa (see Appendix A) and with two different linguistic tests to ensure the generalization of results. In particular, 63 patients were examined with the Aachener Aphasia Test (AAT; [31]) and 111 patients with the Examination of Language Test [32]. The Token Test [26] was used to analyze severity of aphasia. Only 15 patients were administered another language test; due to the small sample, these data were not analyzed. The following language abilities were investigated: repetition, reading-spelling, naming, and oral and written comprehension. A more complete description of the subtests used in the two language batteries can be found in Appendix B.

6. Procedure

All patients consecutively admitted to the Neuropsychological Unit of the Department of Neurological Rehabilitation, Salvatore Maugeri IRCCS Foundation, Cassano delle Murge (Bari, Italy), from 2005 to 2010 participated in the study. Patients and their caregivers were informed about the aims of the study and gave their consent to participate. To avoid distraction, patients were evaluated individually in a quiet room. Testing was interrupted if a patient showed any sign of tiredness. Before the tests were administered, information was gathered concerning patients' clinical history and previous abilities. Any human data included in this manuscript was obtained in compliance with the Declaration of Helsinki.

7. Data Analysis

A cluster analysis was performed on accuracy scores of the different subtests of the CoBaGa. A hierarchical cluster analysis was performed preliminarily to determine the number of clusters in the examined population. Subsequently, a K-means cluster analysis was performed to optimize the assignment of patients to the clusters.

A one-way analysis of variance (ANOVA) was performed to determine whether the clusters of the patients identified differed as to sociodemographic and clinical variables such as age (in months), time from stroke, and years of schooling. Significant differences were examined with the post hoc Tukey test. Analysis of χ^2 was performed to verify gender distribution in the groups.

An ANCOVA analysis was used to determine whether the groups performed differently on the CoBaGa subsets. The dependent variable was the accuracy percentage on each CoBaGa subset. The independent variable was the cluster membership of the subjects. Significant sociodemographic variables that emerged from previous analyses were used as covariates in the ANCOVA.

Moreover, to better characterize the cognitive impairment in each group, an ANOVA was performed with the type of subset (i.e., five levels, corresponding to the five cognitive functions examined) as independent variable and the subset mean percentages of accuracy for each cluster as dependent variables. The significant effects were explored with a post hoc Tukey test.

Finally, for each group, the number of patients who performed pathologically was computed for each subset. Severity of impairment was also evaluated. In particular, performances 2 SD lower than the mean of the control groups paired for school attendance (low or high school attendance) were considered pathological. In patients who performed pathologically, the severity of the deficit was evaluated on the basis of the performance of the whole group of patients [13] with comparable amount of school attendance (high versus low). In particular, according to Kalbe et al. [13], patients who performed below the 30th percentile of the whole group distribution scores had a severe deficit, patients with performances ranging from the 31st to the 60th percentile had moderate impairment, and patients whose performances were higher than the 61st percentile had mild deficits. In each group identified by cluster analysis, the prevalence of severe, moderate, and mild deficits or normal performance on each cognitive function was explored by the χ^2 tests.

An ANCOVA was performed on the accuracy scores of both the EoL and the AAT tests to verify whether subjects who belonged to the three clusters differed as to accuracy on the linguistic tests. Significant sociodemographic variables were used as covariates. Interactions were explored by planned comparisons.

Furthermore, the linguistic skills able to predict the total score on the CoBaGA were also examined separately for the AAT and the EoL score. In particular, regression analyses were performed with the total score on the CoBaGa as dependent variable and oral and written comprehension, naming, reading-spelling, and repetition as independent variables. Analyses were replicated also controlling for the effect of significant sociodemographic variables. In this case, the significant sociodemographic variables were entered first as predictors and after the other language scores.

8. Results

8.1. Profiles of Cognitive Deficits in Aphasic Patients. The cluster analysis showed that there were three subgroups of patients with different cognitive profiles. The first group included 34% of the patients (65 patients), the second group 40% (75 patients), and the third group 26% (49 patients). Demographic and clinical characteristics of the three groups are presented in Table 1.

The analysis of variance revealed that the three groups of patients were comparable for mean age and time from stroke but differed for years of schooling ($F_{(2,182)} = 8.52$, $p < 0.0001$). In particular, the first group had a significantly higher educational level than the second ($p < 0.001$) and the third ($p < 0.001$) groups. No gender differences were observed in the three groups (all χ^2 n.s.).

Figure 1 shows mean percentages of accuracy for each subset in the three subgroups of patients. According to the ANCOVA, the three groups had significantly different performances in all subsets of the CoBaGa ($p < 0.0001$ in all comparisons) also when the level of school attendance of the patients was taken into account. The first group had higher percentages of accuracy than the second and the third groups for all cognitive functions. The second group had intermediate percentages of accuracy, and the third group had the lowest percentages of accuracy in all subtests, suggesting severe cognitive impairment.

In each group, a significant difference emerged for subtest accuracy (group 1: $F_{(4,256)} = 40.7$, $p < 0.0001$; group 2: $F_{(4,296)} = 135.3$, $p < 0.0001$; group 3: $F_{(4,192)} = 27$, $p < 0.0001$). An examination of subtest means showed that the first group had the highest percentages of accuracy in the memory test (93%, $p < 0.01$ compared with other subsets) and the lowest percentages of accuracy in the executive functions and logical reasoning subsets (61%, $p < 0.0001$ compared with other subsets). The accuracy of this group in attention, visual-spatial ability, and visual-auditory recognition tests was comparable, with 80% accuracy. Subtest comparisons were also significant in the second (at least $p < 0.05$) and in the third group ($p < 0.05$). The second group was characterized by high performance in the memory test (82% of accuracy), moderate performance in visual-auditory recognition (59%), and low performance in visual-spatial ability (38%), attention (27%), and executive functions-logical reasoning (20%). The third group was characterized by generally low percentages of accuracy, that is, 7% for attention and executive functions-logical reasoning, 16% for visual-spatial ability, 25% for memory, and 33% for visual-auditory recognition.

Figure 2 and Table 2 present for each group the percentages of patients with severe, moderate, and mild pathology in each subtest. As observed in Figure 2, the three profiles

TABLE 1: Demographic and clinical variables of the three groups of patients with different cognitive profiles.

Group	Number of subjects	Sex	Age (years)	School attendance (years)	Time from disease (months)	Token test accuracy ($N = 36$)
1	65 (34%)	23 F, 42 M	63.8 (SD: 10.9)	7.9 (SD: 4.6)	127 (SD: 157)	8.8 (SD: 4.7)
2	75 (40%)	35 F, 40 M	65.7 (SD: 11.5)	5.5 (SD: 3.2)	121 (SD: 190)	5.9 (SD: 4.3)
3	49 (26%)	20 F, 29 M	68.7 (SD: 12.3)	5.2 (SD: 3.9)	135 (SD: 196)	4 (SD: 4.1)

F: female; M: male; for the age variable, school attendance, time from disease, and Token test accuracy, means and standard deviations (SD) of each group are reported.

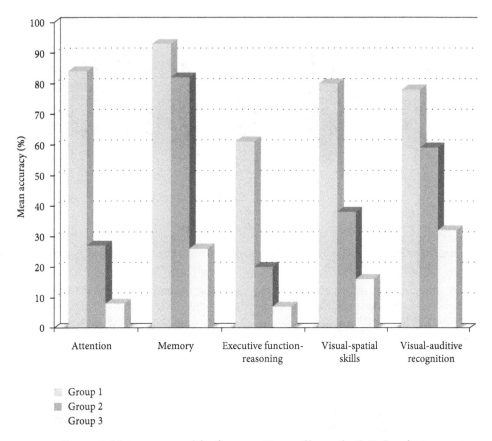

FIGURE 1: Mean accuracy of the three cognitive profiles on the CoBaGa subsets.

differed progressively for severity of cognitive impairment. In fact, for all cognitive functions studied, the percentage of impaired patients was lower in the first group than in the second (at least $p < 0.01$) and the third (at least $p < 0.0001$) groups. Conversely, the percentage of patients with severe cognitive deficits increased progressively from the first to the third group (at least $p < 0.01$) in each subtest, with the exception of visual-spatial impairment (patients with this deficit were not observed in the first and the second group).

In particular, in the first group, the percentages of patients with nonpathological conditions were significantly higher than those of patients with mild, moderate, and severe deficits (at least $p < 0.05$ for all comparisons). The percentages of nonpathological patients were 67% for attention, 78% for memory, 56% for executive functions-logical reasoning, and 72% for visual-spatial ability. The percentages of nonpathological patients were 35.4% only for the visual-auditory recognition subset; in fact, 43.1% and 20% of patients had mild or

moderate deficits, respectively. The percentages of patients with severe deficits in the first group were very low (1.5% for attention, executive functions-logical reasoning, and visuo-acoustic recognition) or zero (in memory and visual-spatial ability) and were significantly lower than the percentages of patients with mild and moderate deficits (at least $p < 0.05$ for all comparisons). Regarding the comparison between moderate and mild deficits in the first group, moderate impairment of memory ($p < 0.001$) and mild deficits in executive functions and logical reasoning ($p < 0.05$) were those most frequently observed. No significant differences were observed between patients with mild and moderate impairments of attention and visual-spatial ability.

The second group of patients showed heterogeneous performances. A moderate deficit of visual-spatial ability (for 70.7% of patients; at least $p < 0.0001$), executive functions-logical reasoning (for 47% of patients; at least $p < 0.001$), and visual-auditory recognition (for 45% of patients; at least

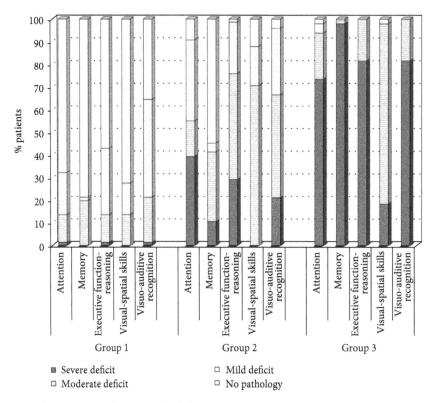

FIGURE 2: Percentage of patients in each group with deficits in cognitive functions differentiated by severity of impairment.

$p < 0.001$) prevailed in this group. Memory abilities were normal in 55% of the patients and moderately impaired in 31% of patients; 40% and 36% of patients in this group demonstrated, respectively, severe and mild impairment of attention.

According to Figure 2, in the third group, most patients had severe deficits in all subtests (from 73.5% to 98% of patients; $p < 0.0001$ in all comparisons) except for visual-spatial ability. Moderate deficits were less frequently observed (from 2% to 20.4%; $p < 0.001$ in all comparisons) in this group. Moderate impairments were frequently observed only for visual-spatial ability (79.6%), and severe deficits were rare (18.4%; $\chi^2 = 18.8$; $p < 0.0001$). The percentage of patients who performed normally or had mild impairments was low (from 0% to 4.1%).

8.2. Brief Summary of Results. Patients with severe aphasia can be divided into three groups according to their cognitive profile. In the first group, most patients' intellectual functions were spared and a high percentage of patients had no pathology. The second group was more heterogeneous and performances were generally worse than in the first group. The third group primarily included patients with severely impaired performance in all cognitive functions investigated.

In particular, the first group showed high mean accuracy for all cognitive functions studied. In fact, this group consisted mainly of patients without cognitive impairment who had visual-auditory recognition abilities. One-third of the patients in this group had no recognition deficits, but two-thirds showed mild–moderate impairment.

The second group of patients was the most heterogeneous. The best mean performance of this group was observed on the memory subtest. In fact, a large percentage of patients in this group displayed no memory deficits. Two-thirds of the patients showed moderately impaired visual-spatial ability, but none suffered from a severe deficit. Almost all patients in this group had deficits in executive functions-logical reasoning and visual-auditory recognition. In particular, half of the patients demonstrated moderate deficits of these functions and the rest showed mild or severe impairment. The attention deficit of this group was mostly severe or mild.

The third group had very low mean accuracy in all subtest of the CoBaGa. This group was composed mainly by patients with severe deficits in all cognitive functions except for visual-spatial ability. In fact, most aphasic patients in this group had moderately impaired visual-spatial skills.

These three subpopulations of patients did not differ for mean age and time from stroke. Therefore, it seems that these variables do not influence cognitive functioning. The three groups were different regarding level of school attendance. In particular, the group with the best cognitive efficiency was characterized by the highest level of school attendance. We can suppose that a high level of school attendance served as a protective factor for cognitive functions. These results contradict the results reported by Helm-Estabrooks et al. [23]. According to these authors, cognitive functions were not influenced by age and level of school attendance.

8.3. Cognitive Deficits and Language Skills. The previous analysis revealed the presence of three different cognitive

TABLE 2: Percentage of patients in each group with a deficit in the cognitive function was investigated and computed for severity of the impairment.

Severity of cognitive deficit	Attention			Memory			Executive functions-logical reasoning			Visual-spatial ability			Visual-auditory recognition		
	Group 1	Group 2	Group 3	Group 1	Group 2	Group 3	Group 1	Group 2	Group 3	Group 1	Group 2	Group 3	Group 1	Group 2	Group 3
Severe	1.5%	39.7%	73.5%	0%	10.7%	98%	1.5%	29.3%	81.6%	0%	0%	18.4%	1.5%	21.3%	81.6%
Moderate	12.3%	16%	20.4%	20%	30.7%	2%	12.3%	46.7%	18.4%	13.8%	70.7%	79.6%	20%	45.3%	18.4%
Mild	18.5%	36%	4.1%	1.5%	3.9%	0%	29.2%	22.7%	0%	13.9%	17.3%	0%	43.1%	29.3%	0%
No deficit	67.7%	9.3%	2%	78.5%	54.7%	0%	56.9%	1.3%	0%	72.3%	12%	2%	35.4%	4%	0%

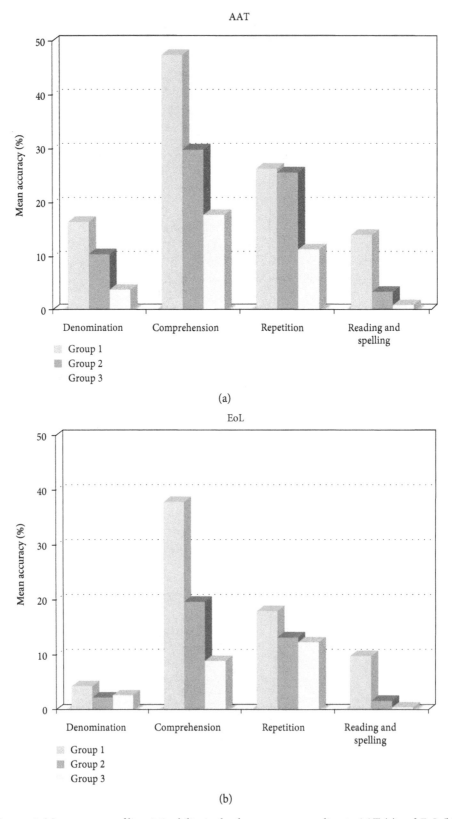

FIGURE 3: Mean accuracy of linguistic ability in the three groups according to AAT (a) and EoL (b).

profiles in patients with severe aphasia. The aim of this second set of analyses was to verify whether the groups clustered on the basis of different cognitive profiles were

characterized by different residual linguistic abilities. The performance of the three groups on the EoL and AAT is presented in Figure 3.

According to the ANCOVA, the groups were comparable for repetition and naming, but differed for reading-spelling abilities (AAT: $F_{(2,59)} = 14.98$, $p < 0.0001$; EoL: $F_{(2,106)} = 19.38$, $p < 0.0001$) and oral-written comprehension (AAT: $F_{(2,59)} = 4.4$, $p < 0.05$; EoL: $F_{(2,106)} = 22.9$, $p < 0.0001$). The first group was significantly more accurate in reading and spelling than the second (AAT: $F_{(2,59)} = 13.05$, $p < 0.001$; EoL: $F_{(2,106)} = 28.7$, $p < 0.0001$) and the third (AAT: $F_{(2,59)} = 26.17$, $p < 0.0001$; EoL: $F_{(2,106)} = 32.56$, $p < 0.0001$). In fact, the first group's reading-spelling accuracy was 14% on the AAT and 10% on the EoL, whereas the second (AAT: 3%, EoL: 1%) and third (AAT: 2%, EoL: 0%) groups were characterized by lower accuracy. The second and third groups were similar with regard to reading-spelling abilities. The three groups performed differently in oral and written comprehension (at least $p < 0.01$). In fact, in this test, the first group showed higher accuracy (AAT: 48%, EoL: 38%) compared to the second group (AAT: 30%, EoL: 20%) and especially the third group (AAT: 18%, EoL: 9%).

The regression analysis performed on the scores of the AAT showed that linguistic skills explain 43% of the variance in cognitive performance. Significant predictors were naming ($\beta = -0.41$, $t = -2.06$, $p < 0.05$), comprehension ($\beta = 0.65$, $t = 5.72$, $p < 0.0001$), and reading and spelling skills ($\beta = 0.27$, $t = 1.97$, $p < 0.05$). When years of school attendance were added to the analysis, the variance explained by the model was 45%. In this case, comprehension was a significant predictor ($\beta = 0.64$, $t = 5.43$, $p < 0.0001$) and reading and spelling approached significance ($\beta = 0.25$, $t = 1.76$, $p = 0.08$); however, naming was still not significant ($\beta = -0.35$, $t = 1.66$, $p = 0.10$). Years of school attendance was not significant. Repetition skill did not predict the CoBaGa performance in either analysis.

The regression analysis performed on the EoL scores demonstrated that language skills explain 60% of the variance on the CoBaGa test. Significant predictors were naming ($\beta = -0.27$, $t = -2.44$, $p < 0.05$), comprehension ($\beta = 0.72$, $t = 8.65$, $p < 0.0001$), and reading and spelling skills ($\beta = 0.19$, $t = 2.15$, $p < 0.05$). When years of school attendance were added to the analysis, the variance explained by the model was 63%. In this case, significant predictors were naming ($\beta = -0.24$, $t = -2.19$, $p < 0.01$) and comprehension ($\beta = 0.69$, $t = 8.58$, $p < 0.0001$) as well as years of school attendance ($\beta = 0.19$, $t = 3.10$, $p < 0.01$). Reading and spelling skills were still not significant ($\beta = -0.14$, $t = 1.66$, $p = 0.10$). Repetition skill did not predict the CoBaGa performance in either analysis.

8.4. Brief Summary of Results. The three groups identified on the basis of cognitive abilities also had different residual linguistic skills, in particular they differed for comprehension, reading, and spelling performance. The results were confirmed independently of the linguistic test used. Therefore, it seems that comprehension and reading-spelling skills were the linguistic abilities most linked to general cognitive functioning.

Regarding linguistic abilities that differed in the three groups, it seems that there were differences in severity of linguistic impairment between groups. Therefore, severity of the linguistic deficit seems to be connected to severity of the cognitive impairment. In fact, the group with mild cognitive deficits (group 1) demonstrated less marked difficulty in reading-spelling and comprehension than the second and especially the third group. In fact, the third group was characterized by the most severe deficits in both linguistic and cognitive abilities. We can suppose that linguistic difficulties and patients' general cognitive functioning were strictly related.

The present study also shows that it is possible to predict the cognitive profile of patients with severe aphasia on the basis of linguistic impairments, and in particular on the basis of naming, comprehension, and reading and spelling skills. This result is in accordance with the results of Kalbe et al. [13] and Hinckley and Nash [25], which support the existence of a relationship between cognitive and linguistic deficits. In fact, the present results do not support the hypothesis [6, 24] of total independence between the two impairments and the impossibility of predicting linguistic deficits on the basis of cognitive ability. The small number of subjects examined by Van Mourik et al. [24] and Helm-Estabrooks [6] may be responsible for the discordant results.

9. Study 2

Twenty patients were examined longitudinally pre and post speech therapy to investigate whether, by the end of therapy, language treatment also improves cognitive skills and which cognitive abilities are most likely to recover after speech therapy.

10. Participants

The 20 patients (11 females and 9 males) in study 1 also participated in study 2. They were tested at the end of speech therapy, which lasted about 4 months (SD = 2). They were all right handed and with global aphasia. The mean age of the sample was 65 years (SD: ±7.8) and the mean educational level was 6.6 (SD: ±3) years. The patients were examined 101 (SD: ±81) days after they had experienced a stroke. Almost all of them had partial anterior circulation infarcts (PACI), and two had total anterior circulation infarcts (TACI), following the Bamford et al. [27] classification. Among all of them, 11 patients belong to the 3rd group and 9 to the 2nd group in study 1. Language therapy was focused on both oral and written comprehension and production, as well as on rehabilitation of articulatory difficulty.

11. Materials

All participants performed the CoBaGa and EoL both pre and post test.

12. Procedure

Same as that in study 1.

13. Data Analysis

Preliminarily, we checked whether speech therapy led to improved language skills, as expected. In particular, an ANOVA was performed with treatment (pre- versus post-) and language skills (comprehension, naming, repetition, reading, and spelling) as repeated measures.

With respect to the specific aims of this study, a second ANOVA was performed on the CoBaGa scores to determine whether speech therapy also resulted in detectable improvements in cognitive performance. In particular, treatment (pre- versus post-) and type of subset (5 levels: corresponding to the five cognitive functions examined) were entered as repeated measures.

All analyses were replicated also controlling for years of education and duration of speech therapy (in days) to assess whether these variables mediated the relation between cognition and language. In particular, in the ANOVAs, these variables were entered as covariates.

14. Results

14.1. Effect of Speech Therapy on Language Skills. As expected, speech therapy led to improved language performance. In fact, the ANOVAs showed the significance of the main effects of the rehabilitation ($F_{(1,18)} = 10.16$, $p < 0.01$) and language domain ($F_{(3,54)} = 17.05$, $p < 0.0001$), indicating that accuracy improved from 13.5% to 20.0% and that comprehension and repetition skills were more impaired than naming and reading-spelling skills (5.1% and 7.2% versus 33.8% and 20.6%, resp., at least $p < 0.01$). Also, the rehabilitation by language domain interaction was significant ($F_{(3,54)} = 5.16$, $p < 0.01$), indicating a significant improvement in performance in the posttest respect to the pretest only for comprehension (reduction of errors of 12.3%, $p < 0.0001$) and repetition (reduction of errors of 6.1%, $p < 0.05$), but not for naming (3.3%) and reading and spelling skills (4.0%).

When education and speech therapy duration were added as covariates, only the main effect of rehabilitation was still significant ($F_{(1,16)} = 8.72$, $p < 0.01$); in fact, the language domain ($F_{(3,48)} = 1.50$, n.s.) and the rehabilitation by language domain ($F_{(3,48)} = 0.97$, n.s.) interactions were no longer significant, indicating that all areas of language improved with language rehabilitation if years of schooling and therapy duration were taken into account. Neither covariate was significant (Fs < 1).

14.2. Effect of Speech Therapy on Cognitive Skills. The ANOVAs on cognitive skills pre and post speech therapy revealed the significance of the main effect of rehabilitation ($F_{(1,24)} = 23.29$, $p < 0.0001$) and cognitive domain ($F_{(4,96)} = 36.29$, $p < 0.0001$), indicating that accuracy improved from 24.9% to 33.1% and that memory and visual-spatial skills were more impaired with respect to attention, executive function and visuo-acoustic recognition (5.9% and 15.0% versus 38.7%, 37.8% and 47.8%, resp., at least $p < 0.0001$). The rehabilitation by cognitive domain interaction was

also significant ($F_{(4,96)} = 7.93$, $p < 0.0001$), indicating a significant improvement in performance only for attention (improvement of 21.2%, $p < 0.0001$) and reasoning/executive function (improvement = 12.6%, $p < 0.01$) after speech therapy; memory (improvement = 0.9%), visual-spatial ability (improvement = 2.0%), and visuo-acoustic recognition (improvement = 4.3%) did not differ pre and post test.

When covariates were added to the analysis, the results did not change: both the main effect of rehabilitation ($F_{(1,24)} = 21.53$, $p < 0.0001$) and cognitive domain ($F_{(4,96)} = 33.90$, $p < 0.0001$) were still significant, as well as the rehabilitation by cognitive domain ($F_{(4,96)} = 6.58$, $p < 0.0001$) interaction. Both covariates were nonsignificant (Fs < 1).

14.3. Brief Summary of Results. As expected, speech therapy produced a significant improvement in each linguistic domain. It also improved cognitive skills and, in particular, attention and reasoning/executive functions.

15. General Discussion

The present study indicates that in subjects with severe aphasia, it is possible to identify subgroups of patients with different profiles of cognitive impairment. Here, three subgroups were identified. The first was characterized by relatively spared cognitive abilities but visual-auditory recognition deficits. These patients seemed to have no cognitive impairment but had linguistic and recognition difficulties. The second group of aphasic patients presented with spared memory and moderate deficits in other cognitive functions. This cognitive profile was accompanied by mild deficits of attention in some patients and very severe deficits in others. The third cognitive profile was characterized by the lowest percentages of accuracy in all subtests, indicating severe and diffuse cognitive deficits. Our finding of three different cognitive profiles in global aphasic patients confirms previous observations by Van Mourik et al. [24] in a large sample of patients. As Van Mourik et al. [24] suggested, groups with different profiles may have different outcomes in rehabilitation training. This hypothesis should be further investigated in subsequent studies.

The present study also showed that groups with different cognitive profiles also have different reading-spelling skills and oral-written comprehension abilities. In particular, according to previous studies [21, 25], patients with more severe cognitive impairment also have more severe linguistic deficits. Moreover, the link between language impairment and general cognitive functioning is also supported by the finding that it is possible to predict with a certain degree of accuracy the cognitive profile of patients with severe aphasia on the basis of their linguistic impairment. In this framework, reading and spelling abilities, naming, and oral-written comprehension skills have a crucial role. The latter language abilities are probably those most affected by cognitive impairment. The nature of this relationship, as well as the specific type of cognitive deficit that compromises reading-spelling and comprehension abilities, requires further investigation.

A strong relationship between linguistic deficits and cognitive skills was also found longitudinally in a study that examined patients' pre and post speech therapy. Note that speech therapy produces a nonspecific improvement in cognitive skills that goes beyond language recovery. In fact, we found that speech therapy not only improves language skills but also attention, reasoning, and executive functions. Thus, it seems that these abilities were involved in the speech therapy and were improved. On the other hand, most studies (e.g., [33]) agree about the importance of executive functions, working memory, and attention for the efficacy of language therapy. As suggested by Fonseca et al. [7], attention and nonverbal memory "are two abilities that might be systematically evaluated as baseline measures that might affect the success of speech rehabilitation." (p. 11)

In any case, the relationship between language and other cognitive domains is still controversial and different hypotheses have been proposed to explain it [34]. For example, in the 1800s, Finkelnburg [35] hypothesized that the disruption of preverbal symbolic activities caused the verbal and nonverbal cognitive disorders in aphasic patients. Trousseau [36] considered language very important for the development of thought and proposed that severe language disorders might lead to impairment of both verbal and nonverbal cognitive skills. Later, Goldstein [37] proposed that language is not only a means of communicating thoughts but is also important for its development. Davis [38] defined cognition as an information processing skill; specifically, because language uses information processing, it may be embedded in cognition.

In more recent years, Jefferies and Lambon Ralph [39] proposed the "semantic hub" hypothesis to explain the "unexpected brain-language relationships in aphasia" [40]. These authors assumed that the deficits of aphasic patients are due to a preverbal conceptual disorder which cannot be attributed to a loss of semantic representations but rather to a deficit in their controlled retrieval. The cognitive deficit is due to a control deficit involved in the selection and activation of conceptual representations: these mechanism of semantic control flexibility activate information by means of the underlying amodal concept and focus attention on particular features of concepts (while ignoring others) to produce task/context-appropriate behaviour. In this vein, aphasic patients have difficulty in controlling semantic representations appropriately and in working flexibly with the knowledge they have retained. This deficit in cognitive control is associated with executive function impairment (i.e., in the left inferior prefrontal cortex). In this vein, the relationship between language and cognition is mediated by executive functions.

Other hypotheses considered the role of executive functions [13, 41], short-term memory [42, 43], or attentional resources [9, 44] in negatively affecting language deficits. According to an attentional hypothesis, syntactic processing deficits in aphasia can be explained by a deficit of resource capacity or a reduced ability to allocate attentional resources [45]. McNeil et al. [3] also proposed an "integrated attention theory of aphasia." According to these authors, there is a relationship among attention, arousal, and language processing and individuals with aphasia have a deficit in allocating attentional resources.

Cahana-Amitay and Albert [46] incorporated nonlinguistic functions into language models and hypothesized the existence of "neural multifunctionality" in which a constant and dynamic interaction exists among neural networks subserving cognitive, affective, and praxic functions with neural networks specialized for lexical retrieval, sentence comprehension, and discourse processing, giving rise to language.

According to other authors, language and cognition are not strictly related. For example, Hauser et al. [47] argued that language is an abstract linguistic computational system which is independent of other systems it interacts with and establishes interfaces. In fact, the presence of aphasia does not necessarily produce other neuropsychological impairments [48] and cognitive deficits in aphasic patients are not always correlated with language impairment (e.g., [49, 50]). Recently, some authors [51] provided evidence from neuroimaging and neurological data that despite global aphasic patients' near-total loss of language, they are able to perform some nonlinguistic tasks such as arithmetic, storing information in working memory, inhibiting prepotent responses or listening music. The authors concluded that many aspects of cognition engage distinct brain regions which do not necessarily depend on language. On the other hand, Fonseca et al. [7] reported that patients with aphasia always perform similarly to patients with brain damage without aphasia. This indicates that some of the impairments of aphasic patients are not secondary to language impairment but to brain dysfunction per se. As highlighted by Seniów et al. [52], evidence of aphasia is not necessarily associated with impairment of other cognitive functions, suggesting that these deficits may be independent of one another.

The present study highlights that patients with severe aphasia are heterogeneous with regard to cognitive impairment, which ranges from spared to severely impaired cognitive function. In any case, in this study, we found a strong relationship between language impairment and general cognitive functioning: patients with more severe cognitive impairment also had more severe linguistic deficits. Note that in this study, the relationship between linguistic deficits and cognitive abilities was evaluated in a population of patients with severe aphasia. We do not know whether the present results can be generalized to the entire population of patients with aphasia. It might be interesting to repeat this study in a population of patients with less severe aphasia to examine the relationship between linguistic impairment and cognitive abilities and to identify cognitive profiles among these patients. Moreover, the population of the present study was characterized by severe aphasia and both language comprehension and production deficits. It would be interesting to know whether different profiles of cognitive impairment in patients with less severe aphasia are related to different syndromes of aphasia and selective deficits of linguistic comprehension/production. Moreover, we do not know the role of other variables that might affect patients' cognitive profile, such as premorbid IQ and other factors that might affect cognitive performance.

In light of the present results, we can affirm the importance of assessing cognitive functions as well as linguistic deficits in aphasic patients. A correct assessment of cognitive abilities and comprehension of lost and preserved functions might be useful in programming individualized rehabilitation training. Several studies [53–55] found a reduction of linguistic deficits after rehabilitative training for attention, memory, visual perception, or executive function-problem solving in aphasic patients who did not benefit from speech and language treatment. This suggests the greater advantage of combined rehabilitation for both language impairment and cognitive deficits in aphasic patients.

Appendix

A. Tests Included in Each Subtest of the CoBaGa [28]

1. Attention. This subset included letter cancellation [56], numbers [57], and the Toulouse-Pieron test [58].

In the first test, patients were asked to cross out all the "A's" in a series of letters arranged in 17 lines. The maximum score was 60 (1 point for each letter identified).

In the second test, the numbers from 0 to 9 were arranged in 13 lines. The patients were asked to cross out all the number "5's." The maximum score was 14, corresponding to the total number of target stimuli.

In the Toulouse-Pieron test, the patients were instructed to identify and cancel a specific symbol (one square and two segments oriented in a particular way inside this square). Different symbols were arranged in 10 lines. The maximum score was 13.

Accuracy on this subset was the total number of correct answers minus the number of false alarms.

2. Executive Functions and Logical Reasoning. This subset consisted of a modified version of Raven's Coloured Progressive Matrices [59] and some WAIS-R tests [60]. In particular, it included the construction of a human figure, drawing with cubes, association of symbols and numbers (reduced version), and two sequence ordering tests of the WAIS-R.

Raven's Coloured Progressive Matrices consist of 36 items of increasing difficulty. The subject has to choose the one item from 6 different alternatives that completes the figure according to an exact logic. In the present study, the alternatives were located one under the other on the left side of the page to limit the effects of difficulty with visual-spatial exploration. The score was calculated as the sum of correct answers. The maximum score was 36.

In the construction of a human figure test, a shape of the human body was presented on one page along with 5 cards showing a head, trunk, and four limbs. Patients had to recompose the dummy using the 5 cards and the shape of the human body. The maximum score was 5 and corresponded to the number of correct positions of the cards.

Drawing with cubes involved reproducing 6 figures presented on the pages using 4 colored cubes. The maximum

score was 24; it was the correct combination of cubes to construct the figure.

In the test of association of symbols and numbers, the patients were shown numbers from 1 to 9 that were associated with different symbols located under each number. Forty numbers were presented below in random order. The patients had to reproduce the correct symbol under each number, as demonstrated in the example. The maximum score (i.e., 40) corresponded to the correct number of associations.

In the sequence ordering test, the patients had to correctly order a series of cards based on the temporal sequence of events. Two different situations were used. The first sequence represented the blooming of a plant (from bud to flower, 3 cards). The second sequence represented the construction of a house (starting from bricks and arriving at a complete house in 4 cards). The score was the sum of the number of cards located correctly in each sequence. The maximum score was 7.

3. Memory. This subset consisted of a visual memory test of faces and objects.

The patients were shown four faces and were told to remember them. Subsequently, the same faces were shown to the patients in random order together with 4 distractors. The patients were asked to recognize the faces shown before. The score was the number of correct answers.

The same procedure and score calculation were used in the memory test for objects. This probe required recognizing 4 objects out of 8 figures.

4. Visual-Auditory Recognition. This subset consisted of the following tests: recognition of unknown faces [61], identification of complex figures [62], and identification of colors, association of colors, association of figures, association of objects and colors, association of objects and figures, association of visually different objects and figures, and recognition of sounds and noise. In all tasks, one point was given for each correct item.

The test of recognition of unknown faces consisted of two parts. First, patients had to recognize the target face out of 6 faces in different conditions of illumination. In the second part of the test, the target face was similar to 3 out of 6 alternative faces proposed.

In the identification of complex figures test (included in the left table), one complex shape without sense (target figure) was shown, and on the right three different complex shapes were shown. Patients had to recognize the target shape among the three figures shown in the tables on the right. The maximum score on this test was 4.

In the identification of colors test, one table was presented that showed six colors. The examiner named each color separately. The patients had to identify the named colors.

The association of colors test was presented in one table that showed six colors and six colored cards. The patients had to put the cards on the table by matching the corresponding colors.

The association of figures test was presented in two tables with 7 figures. One table was used by the examiner; another table was given to the patient. The examiner indicated one figure and the patient had to indicate the corresponding figure on the table.

The test of association of objects and colors was presented in one table containing six colors. The examiner demonstrated 6 objects to the patient, who had to associate each object with a corresponding color. The score was the number of correct answers.

The test of association of objects and figures consisted of one table that presented 6 figures and 6 corresponding objects. The patient had to associate each object with the corresponding figure.

The test of association of visually different objects and figures was presented in the same table described in the previous test and included 6 slightly different objects.

The patients listened to sounds registered on an audio-cassette in the recognition of sounds and noise test. Then, they had to indicate the correct answer out of three possibilities illustrated in three squares.

5. Visual-Spatial Ability. To evaluate visual-spatial ability, we used one test of line orientation judgment [63] and one test of recognizing objects shown in unusual perspectives.

In the judgment of line orientation test, 10 tables with lines drawn at different inclinations were shown to the patients. They had to compare the lines drawn in the table with a model consisting of lines of all possible inclinations. The score was the total number of lines whose orientation was correctly recognized. The maximum score was 20.

In the recognition of objects constructed in unusual per-spectives test, the patients had to identify a target object out of three alternative objects drawn in different perspectives.

B. Language Tests

1. Aachener Aphasia Test (AAT; [30]). Only subsets of repetition, written language, naming, and comprehension of AAT [30] were used in this study.

The repetition subtest consisted of repeating single sounds, words with progressively increasing difficulty and length, foreign words, composed words, and phrases. Each part included 10 items. From 0 to 3 points were assigned for each repeated item on the basis of the subject's perfor-mance. The complex score of the repetition subset varied from 0 to 150.

The evaluation of written language skills included three different probes: reading aloud, dictation for composition, and dictation by hand of words or phrases. In particular, in the dictation for composition patients had to compose printed words or parts of words to form the complex words and phrases pronounced by the examiner. Each part included 10 items. The score of each subset varied from 0 to 30 and the total score varied from 0 to 90.

The naming subtest consisted of four parts (i.e., naming of objects, colors, objects with names, and descriptions of simple figures). Each of the parts included 10 items. The score for each of the four parts varied from 0 to 30 and the total score varied from 0 to 120.

The comprehension subtest consisted of four parts. Each of the parts included 10 items examining, respectively, oral comprehension of isolated words, oral comprehension of phrases, comprehension of written words, and comprehen-sion of written phrases. Patients were required to identify the target figure out of the four alternatives presented. The score for each of the four parts varied from 0 to 30, and the total score varied from 0 to 120.

2. Examination of Language (EoL; [31]). Tests evaluating naming ability, oral and written comprehension, repetition, and reading-spelling of the EoL [31] were administered to the patients.

In the naming ability test, subjects had to indicate figures representing nouns and verbs and describe one figure or event (one day spent at the sea or in the mountains).

Comprehension ability was evaluated using tests of oral and written comprehension. The oral part consisted of one test of word comprehension and of semantically similar words and phrases. In the first two cases, 20 figures were presented to the patients and they had to indicate the specific figure named by the examiner. In the phrase comprehension test, patients had to carry out the examiner's orders. In the test of written comprehension, patients had to read semantically similar words and phrases and to indicate the corresponding figure or carry out the order they had read.

In the repetition test, patients had to repeat phonemes, words, nonwords, and phrases pronounced by the examiner.

Finally, reading-spelling ability was tested with the copying of written words and reading and spelling to dictation of words, nonwords, sounds, and phrases.

Mean percentages of accuracy were calculated for each subset.

Acknowledgments

The authors thank Dr. Elisabetta Cafforio, Fara Cellamare, Antonella Colucci, Marcella Colaprico, and Rosanna Falcone for the data collection and Claire Montagna for the style editing. This research has been supported by "Fondo di Sviluppo e Coesione 2007–2013"—APQ Ricerca Regione Puglia "Programma regionale a sostegno della specializzazione intelligente e della sostenibilità sociale ed ambientale—FutureInResearch."

References

[1] A. Caramazza and E. B. Zurif, "Dissociation of algorithmic and heuristic processes in language comprehension: evidence from aphasia," *Brain and Language*, vol. 3, no. 4, pp. 572–582, 1976.

[2] M. R. McNeil, "Auditory comprehension in aphasia: a language deficit or reduced efficiency of processes supporting language?" *Clinical Aphasiology*, vol. 10, pp. 342–345, 1981.

[3] M. R. McNeil, K. Odell, and C. H. Tseng, "Toward the integra-tion of resource allocation into a general theory of aphasia," *Clinical Aphasiology*, vol. 20, pp. 21–39, 1991.

[4] M. R. McNeil and M. D. Z. Kimelman, "Toward an integrative information processing structure of auditory comprehension and processing in adult aphasia," *Seminars in Speech and Language*, vol. 7, no. 02, pp. 123–146, 1986.

[5] E. K. Kang, H. S. Jeong, E. R. Moon, J. Y. Lee, and K. J. Lee, "Cognitive and language function in aphasic patients assessed with the Korean version of Mini-Mental Status Examination," *Annals of Rehabilitation Medicine*, vol. 40, no. 1, pp. 152–161, 2016.

[6] N. Helm-Estabrooks, "Cognition and aphasia: a discussion and a study," *Journal of Communication Disorders*, vol. 35, pp. 171–186, 2002.

[7] J. Fonseca, J. J. Ferreira, and I. P. Martins, "Cognitive performance in aphasia due to stroke: a systematic review," *International Journal on Disability and Human Development*, 2016.

[8] G. Gainotti, C. Caltagirone, and G. Miceli, "Immediate visual-spatial memory in hemisphere-damaged patients: impairment of verbal coding and of perceptual processing," *Neuropsychologia*, vol. 16, no. 4, pp. 501–507, 1978.

[9] L. L. Murray, "Attention and aphasia: theory, research and clinical implications," *Aphasiology*, vol. 13, no. 2, pp. 91–111, 1999.

[10] J. R. Duffy and L. B. Watkins, "The effect of response choice relatedness on pantomime and verbal recognition ability in aphasic patients," *Brain and Language*, vol. 21, no. 2, pp. 291–306, 2004.

[11] A. Kertesz and P. McCabe, "Intelligence and aphasia: Performance of aphasics on Raven's coloured progressive matrices (RCPM)," *Brain and Language*, vol. 2, no. 4, pp. 387–395, 1975.

[12] M. Purdy, "Executive function ability in persons with aphasia," *Aphasiology*, vol. 16, no. 4, pp. 549–557, 2002.

[13] E. Kalbe, N. Reinhold, M. Brand, and M. J. Kessler, "A new test battery to assess aphasic disturbances and associated cognitive dysfunctions - German normative data on the aphasia check list," *Journal of Clinical and Experimental Neuropsychology*, vol. 27, no. 7, pp. 779–794, 2005.

[14] M. L. Albert, "Treatment of aphasia," *Archives of Neurology*, vol. 55, no. 11, pp. 1417–1419, 1998.

[15] L. L. Murray, K. Ballard, and L. Karcher, "Linguistic specific treatment: just for Broca's aphasia?" *Aphasiology*, vol. 18, no. 9, pp. 785–809, 2004.

[16] G. Goldenberg, H. Dettmers, C. Grothe, and J. Spatt, "Influence of linguistic and nonlinguistic capacities on spontaneous recovery of aphasia and on success of language therapy," *Aphasiology*, vol. 8, no. 5, pp. 443–456, 1994.

[17] S. Bailey, G. Powell, and E. Clark, "A note on intelligence and recovery from aphasia: the relationship between Raven's Matrices Scores and change on the Schuell Aphasia Test," *British Journal of Disorders of Communication*, vol. 16, no. 3, pp. 193–203, 1981.

[18] H. El Hachioui, E. G. Visch-Brink, H. Lingsma et al., "Nonlinguistic cognitive impairment in poststroke aphasia: a prospective study," *Neurorehabilitation and Neural Repair*, vol. 28, no. 3, pp. 273–281, 2014.

[19] B. Lee and S. B. Pyun, "Characteristics of cognitive impairment in patients with post-stroke aphasia," *Annals of Rehabilitation Medicine*, vol. 38, no. 6, pp. 759–765, 2014.

[20] M. V. Bonini and M. Radanovic, "Cognitive deficits in post-stroke aphasia," *Arquivos de Neuro-Psiquiatria*, vol. 73, no. 10, pp. 840–847, 2015.

[21] M. L. Kauhanen, J. T. Korpelainen, P. Hiltunen et al., "Aphasia, depression, and non-verbal cognitive impairment in ischaemic stroke," *Cerebrovascular Diseases*, vol. 10, no. 6, pp. 455–461, 2000.

[22] N. Helm-Estabrooks, *Cognitive Linguistic Quick Test*, The Psychological Corporation, San Antonio, TX, 2001.

[23] N. Helm-Estabrooks, K. Bayles, A. Ramage, and S. Bryant, "Relation between cognitive deficit and aphasia severity, age, and education: female versus males," *Brain and Language*, vol. 51, no. 1, pp. 139–141, 1995.

[24] M. Van Mourik, M. Verschaeve, P. Boon, P. Paquier, and F. Van Harskamp, "Cognition in global aphasia: indicators for therapy," *Aphasiology*, vol. 6, no. 5, pp. 491–499, 1992.

[25] J. Hinckley and C. Nash, "Cognitive assessment and aphasia severity," *Brain and Language*, vol. 103, no. 1, pp. 8–249, 2007.

[26] E. De Renzi and P. Faglioni, "Normative data and the screening power of a shortened version of the Token test," *Cortex*, vol. 14, no. 1, pp. 41–49, 1978.

[27] J. Bamford, P. Sandercock, M. Dennis, J. Burn, and C. Warlow, "Classification and natural history of clinically identifiable subtypes of cerebral infarction," *Lancet*, vol. 337, no. 8756, pp. 1521–1526, 1991.

[28] C. V. Marinelli, A. Craca, A. Colucci et al., "Evaluation of cognitive deficit in global aphasia," *Neurological Sciences*, vol. 27, p. 235, 2006.

[29] C. V. Marinelli, A. Craca, C. Lograno, and P. Angelelli, "The influence of cognitive abilities on language deficits: a longitudinal study on patients with severe aphasia," *European Journal of Neurology*, vol. 16, p. 441, 2009.

[30] S. Forer and C. V. Granger, *Functional Independence Measure*, State University of New York at Buffalo, Buffalo General Hospital, Buffalo, 1987.

[31] C. Luzzatti, K. Willmes, and R. De Bleser, *Aachen Aphasie Test (AAT): Italian Version*, Organizzazioni Speciali, Firenze, 2th edition edition, 1996.

[32] P. Ciurli, P. Marangolo, and A. Basso, *Esame del linguaggio*, Organizzazioni Speciali, Firenze, 2nd edition edition, 1996.

[33] J. K. Fillingham, K. Sage, and M. Lambon Ralph, "The treatment of anomia using errorless learning to aphasic disorders: a review of theory and practice," *Neuropsychological Rehabilitation*, vol. 13, no. 2, pp. 337–363, 2006.

[34] G. Gainotti, "Old and recent approaches to the problem of non-verbal conceptual disorders in aphasic patients," *Cortex*, vol. 53, pp. 78–89, 2014.

[35] D. C. Finkelnburg, "Niederrhenische Gesellschaft, Sitzung vom 21 Marz 1870 in Bonn," *Berliner Klinische Wochenschrift*, vol. 7, pp. 448–450, 1870, 460-462.

[36] A. Trousseau, *Clinique Médicale de l'Hotel Dieu de Paris*, Baillière, Paris, 1865.

[37] K. Glodstein, *Language and Language Disturbances*, Grune & Stratton, New York, 1948.

[38] G. A. Davis, "The cognition of language and communication," in *Cognition and Acquired Language Disorders*, R. K. Peach and L. P. Shapiro, Eds., p. 1, Elsevier Mosby, 2012.

[39] E. Jefferies and M. A. Lambon Ralph, "Semantic impairment in stroke aphasia versus semantic dementia: a case-series comparison," *Brain*, vol. 129, no. Part 8, pp. 2132–2147, 2006.

[40] M. L. Berthier, "Unexpected brain-language relationships in aphasia: evidence from transcortical sensory aphasia

associated with frontal lobe lesions," *Aphasiology*, vol. 15, no. 2, pp. 99–130, 2001.

[41] J. C. Borod and M. CarperH. Goodglass, "WAIS performance IQ in aphasia as a function of auditory comprehension and constructional apraxia," *Cortex*, vol. 18, no. 2, pp. 199–210, 1982.

[42] P. M. Beeson, K. A. Bayles, A. B. Rubens, and A. W. Kaszniak, "Memory impairment and executive control in individuals with stroke-induced aphasia," *Brain and Language*, vol. 45, no. 2, pp. 253–275, 1993.

[43] S. C. Christensen and H. H. Wright, "Verbal and non-verbal working memory in aphasia: what three n-back tasks reveal," *Aphasiology*, vol. 24, no. 6–8, pp. 752–762, 2010.

[44] R. Fucetola, L. T. Connor, M. J. Strube, and M. Corbetta, "Unravelling non-verbal cognitive performance in acquired aphasia," *Aphasiology*, vol. 23, no. 12, pp. 1418–1426, 2009.

[45] L. L. Murray, A. L. Holland, and P. M. Beeson, "Auditory processing in individuals with mild aphasia: a study of resource allocation," *Journal of Speech, Language, and Hearing Research*, vol. 40, no. 4, pp. 792–808, 1997.

[46] D. Cahana-Amitay and M. L. Albert, "Brain and language: evidence for neural Multifunctionality," *Behavioural Neurology*, vol. 260381, pp. 1–16, 2014.

[47] M. C. Hauser, N. Chomsky, and T. Fitch, "The faculty of language: what is it, who has it, and how did it evolve?" *Science*, vol. 298, no. 5598, pp. 1569–1579, 2002.

[48] Z. M. Archibald, J. M. Wepman, and L. V. Jones, "Nonverbal cognitive performance in aphasic and nonaphasic brain-damaged patients," *Cortex*, vol. 3, no. 3, pp. 275–294, 1967.

[49] A. Basso, E. De Renzi, P. Faglioni, G. Scotti, and H. Spinnler, "Neuropsychological evidence for the existence of cerebral areas critical to the performance of intelligence tasks," *Brain*, vol. 96, no. 4, pp. 715–728, 1973.

[50] A. Basso, E. Capitani, C. Luzzatti, and H. Spinnler, "Intelligence and left hemisphere disease: the role of aphasia, apraxia and size of lesion," *Brain*, vol. 104, no. Part 4, pp. 721–734, 1981.

[51] E. Fedorenko and R. Varley, "Language and thought are not the same thing: evidence from neuroimaging and neurological patients," *Annals of new York Academy of Sciences*, vol. 1369, no. 1, pp. 132–153, 2016.

[52] J. Seniów, M. Litwin, and M. Leśniak, "The relationship between non-linguistic cognitve deficits and language recovery in patients with aphasia," *Journal of Neurological Sciences*, vol. 283, no. 1–2, pp. 91–94, 2009.

[53] N. Helm-Estabrooks, L. T. Connor, and M. L. Albert, "Treating attention to improve auditory comprehension in aphasia," *Brain and Language*, vol. 74, no. 3, pp. 469–472, 2000.

[54] K. Kohnert, "Cognitive and cognate-based treatments for bilingual aphasia: a case study," *Brain and Language*, vol. 91, no. 3, pp. 294–302, 2004.

[55] L. L. Murray, J. L. Keeton, and L. Karcher, "Treating attention in mild aphasia: evaluation of attention process training-II," *Journal of Communication Disorders*, vol. 39, no. 1, pp. 37–61, 2006.

[56] L. Diller, Y. Ben Yishai, L. J. Gerstman, R. Goodkin, W. Gordow, and J. Weinberger, *Studies in Recognition and Rehabiltation in Hemiplegia*, New York University Medical Center, New York, 1974.

[57] H. Spinnler and G. Tognoni, "Standardizzazione e taratura italiana di tests neuropsicologici," *Italian Journal of Neurological Sciences*, no. 8, pp. 8–120, 1987.

[58] E. Y. Toulouse and H. Pieron, *Toulouse-Pieron: prueba perceptiva y de atencion manual*, TEA, Madrid, 1972.

[59] J. C. Raven, J. H. Court, and J. Raven, *Coloured Progressive Matrices*, Lewis, London, 1977.

[60] D. Wechsler, *Wechsler Adult Intelligence Scale-Revised*, The Psychological, San Antonio, Texas, 1981.

[61] A. L. Benton, K. D. Hamsher, N. R. Varney, and O. Spreen, *Test di riconoscimento di volti ignoti- Italian version*, Organizzazioni Speciali, Firenze, 1992.

[62] R. Angelini and D. Grossi, *La terapia razionale dei disordini costruttivi (Te.Ra.Di.C.)*, IRCCS Santa Lucia, Roma, 1993.

[63] A. L. Benton, K. D. Hamsher, and N. R. Varney, *Test di giudizio di orientamento di linee- Italian version*, Organizzazioni Speciali, Firenze, 1990.

Conversational Therapy through Semi-Immersive Virtual Reality Environments for Language Recovery and Psychological Well-Being in Post Stroke Aphasia

A. Giachero,[1,2] M. Calati,[1] L. Pia ⓘ,[2] L. La Vista,[1] M. Molo,[1] C. Rugiero,[1] C. Fornaro,[1] and P. Marangolo ⓘ[1,3,4]

[1]*Aphasia Experimental Laboratory-Fondazione Carlo Molo Onlus, Turin, Italy*
[2]*Dipartimento di Psicologia, University of Turin, Italy*
[3]*Dipartimento di Studi Umanistici, University Federico II, Naples, Italy*
[4]*IRCCS Fondazione Santa Lucia, Rome, Italy*

Correspondence should be addressed to P. Marangolo; paola.marangolo@gmail.com

Academic Editor: Luigi Trojano

Aphasia is a highly disabling acquired language disorder generally caused by a left-lateralized brain damage. Even if traditional therapies have been shown to induce an adequate clinical improvement, a large percentage of patients are left with some degree of language impairments. Therefore, new approaches to common speech therapies are urgently needed in order to maximize the recovery from aphasia. The recent application of virtual reality (VR) to aphasia rehabilitation has already evidenced its usefulness in promoting a more pragmatically oriented treatment than conventional therapies (CT). In the present study, thirty-six chronic persons with aphasia (PWA) were randomly assigned to two groups. The VR group underwent conversational therapy during VR everyday life setting observation, while the control group was trained in a conventional setting without VR support. All patients were extensively tested through a neuropsychological battery which included not only measures for language skills and communication efficacy but also self-esteem and quality of life questionnaires. All patients were trained through a conversational approach by a speech therapist twice a week for six months (total 48 sessions). After the treatment, no significant differences among groups were found in the different measures. However, the amount of improvement in the different areas was distributed over far more cognitive and psychological aspects in the VR group than in the control group. Indeed, the within-group comparisons showed a significant enhancement in different language tasks (i.e., oral comprehension, repetition, and written language) only in the VR group. Significant gains, after the treatment, were also found, in the VR group, in different psychological dimensions (i.e., self-esteem and emotional and mood state). Given the importance of these aspects for aphasia recovery, we believe that our results add to previous evidence which points to the ecological validity and feasibility of VR treatment for language recovery and psychosocial well-being.

1. Introduction

Aphasia is one of the most socially disabling consequences post stroke [1–3] which manifests itself in about one-third of left brain-damaged people (30% of acute vs. 10-20% of chronic stroke patients [1]). The aphasic symptoms are heterogeneous varying in terms of severity and degree of involvement across the modalities of language, including the expression and comprehension of speech, reading, and writing [4]. Variation in the severity of expressive impairments, for example, may range from the patient's occasional inability to find the correct word to telegraphic and much reduced speech output [5]. Thus, persons with aphasia (PWA) experience frustration and depression since their exclusion from language-dependent activities has strong implications for many aspects of their emotional condition and social status. Indeed, language difficulties determine loss of autonomy with reduced opportunities for social exchanges with friends and for practising language skills in everyday life contexts [6]. Most aphasic patients show some degree of spontaneous recovery, most notably during the first 2–3 months following stroke onset; however, studies indicate that further improvements, even in chronic patients, are possible when they are provided with an intervention (see for review [7]). The impact and the consequential implications of having aphasia for the individuals themselves and their families highlight the importance of planning efficacious treatment methods [8, 9]. The traditional aphasia therapy approaches are largely based on compensatory strategies or repetitive training of lost functions [7]. However, although there is convincing evidence that those approaches are useful, over the last years, there has been a shift from impairment-oriented language therapy to functional approaches that train language skills in more realistic contexts. A central goal here is to facilitate the successful participation of the patients in authentic conversation by increasing communicative confidence, thus, empowering PWA to improve their quality of life [10, 11]. Accordingly, the latest Cochrane review on speech and language therapy following stroke concluded that therapy should enhance functional communication in ecological contexts [7]. Indeed, a common observation regarding PWA is that they can communicate much more than their linguistic abilities would suggest. Therefore, the hypothesis has been advanced that a more ecological approach aimed at restoring the patient's ability to communicate in different daily contexts would be proved useful in rehabilitation [12–15]. Within this approach, conversational therapy is one such treatment [12–16]. The main objective of this approach is to set up a natural conversation between the therapist and the PWA, a condition of communicative exchange, in which both speakers participate using their available communicative resources [14, 15]. Within this therapeutic approach, not only language but also any intentional action (e.g., gesturing, drawing) can be used to communicate. The therapeutic goal shifts from a purely analytic treatment aimed at the recovery of the damaged linguistic processes, still used in the traditional approach, to a global approach. The latter considers the ability of the PWA to communicate as a whole through strengthening his/her residual communicative functions [12–16].

In these last years, scientific advancements in language conceptualization and the progress of new technologies have made new tools available for professional therapists and educators. Digital technologies offer exciting opportunities to PWAs who live with long-term communication deficits (see for review [17]). Among these technologies, computer therapies deliver individually tailored exercises for training a range of language skills, including word retrieval [18, 19], sentence building [20, 21], and language comprehension [22]. The StepByStep (PLOS) computer program includes over 10,000 language exercises ranging from listening to writing words or producing sentences [17, 19]. It was shown that patients who received StepByStep training achieved greater improvement in naming ability compared with patients who received the standard speech and language therapy [19]. A study that investigated Multicue as a rehabilitation program demonstrated significant improvement in naming abilities mea-

sured through the Boston Naming Test in patients who received the training; however, no significant improvement was shown in verbal communication skills [18, 23, 24]. Overall, these studies suggested that independent computerized therapies can be as effective as clinician-guided therapies [24]. However, most of these studies exhibited a positive effect on word finding in picture naming tasks but not on communicative abilities [18, 23, 24]. Additionally, iPad-based aphasia rehabilitation treatments have been investigated but, as for computer therapies, most of the findings investigated the impact only on language functions [25–28].

Among the applied technologies, an area that particularly merits exploration is virtual reality (VR). Development of VR applications for rehabilitation of aphasia is still in its early stages ([29–32]; see for a review [17]). This involves a computer-generated simulation of 3D environments with which the user can experience a semi-immersive interaction that may encourage language practice in real context communication settings. Typically, an individual entering a virtual environment feels a part of this world and he/she has the opportunity to interact with it almost as he/she would do in the real world. Uses of VR in healthcare are widespread, ranging from the treatment of physical impairments [33, 34], post traumatic stress disorders [35], and anxiety [36, 37]. Virtual reality applications have been also explored on different communication disorders such a speaking phobias [38], stuttering [39], and autism [40, 41]. However, to date, the use of VR for language recovery in aphasia has been limited. Stark et al. [42] developed a virtual house to promote individual language practice. In Aphasia Script [43], therapy is based on the oral production of scripts, which are short functional dialogs structured around communication of everyday activities. Script treatment can be delivered by a virtual therapist (VT) through a computer or by a real therapist. A randomized controlled cross-over study using Aphasia Script was conducted to investigate the effect of high or low cuing on treatment outcomes over time [43]. Eight participants were recruited and randomized to receive intensive computer-based script training differing in the amount of high or low cuing provided during treatment. In the high cue treatment condition, participants could hear the virtual therapist (VT) during listening, choral reading, and reading aloud, with auditory cues (therapist speaking) and visual cues (therapist's mouth movements) available at the start, during, and after practice. In the low cue condition, they received visual and auditory cues when listening to the script being read aloud initially and after practice, but did not receive auditory and visual support during sentence practice.

Performance was measured by averaging the sentence level word accuracy of participants' production of ten sentences (ten words in length) during each assessment session. Accuracy of words were rated using a previously validated six-point scale, and the overall session score expressed on a scale from 0 to 100%. Training resulted in significant gains in script acquisition with maintenance of skills at three and six weeks posttreatment. Differences between cuing conditions were not significant. Three weeks of computer-based script training resulted in increased accuracy and rate of script production. The mean baseline performance was 50.0

(26.4)% for accuracy and 23.7 (20.6) for rate (words per minute, WPM). At the end of training, it had improved to 77.8 (19.6)% and 60.3 (30.5) WPM for accuracy and rate, respectively. Moreover, although there was a slight drop in performance noted at both three weeks and six weeks posttreatment, the decreases were small. At three weeks posttreatment, the mean scores for accuracy were 72.2 (22.4) and the mean scores for rate were 55.2 (34.0). By six weeks posttreatment, these scores had declined slightly to 68.6 (24.7) for accuracy and 51.4 (35.8) for rate [43].

The Web Oral Reading for Language in Aphasia (ORLA, Rehabilitation Institute of Chicago) [44] is a therapy program where patients repeatedly read aloud sentences, first in unison with a clinician and then independently. The program was developed to improve the patient's reading comprehension skills by providing practice in phonological and semantic reading routes. Following a no-treatment period, twenty-five individuals with chronic nonfluent aphasia were randomly assigned to receive twenty-four sessions of ORLA, 1–3 times per week, either by computer ($N = 11$) or by a speech language pathologist ($N = 14$) (SLP-ORLA). Results showed that the mean change in the Western Aphasia Battery-Aphasia Quotient scores (the primary outcome measure) from pre- to posttreatment was 3.29 (SD = 6.16) for the eleven participants receiving computer ORLA. In comparison, the mean change during the no-treatment phase from baseline to posttreatment was only −0.4. Student t-tests were used to compute the change from pretreatment to posttreatment between the computer ORLA and SLP-ORLA groups. No significant differences were found on any of the outcome measures (P values ranged from 0.2 to 0.6), suggesting good compatibility and feasibility of the VR version [45].

Sentactics (Sentactics Corporation, Concord, CA, USA) is a linguistic treatment which aims at improving sentence production and comprehension deficits through a virtual clinician. Patients are trained repeating and reading sentences and describing pictures presented on the screen. Thompson et al. [20] conducted a study to test the efficacy of Sentactics as an aphasia rehabilitation tool. Computer-delivered Sentactics was compared with a clinician-delivered therapy. Results showed that patients who received Sentactics training significantly improved in production and comprehension for both trained (0% to 90% production, 0% to 30% comprehension) and untrained sentences (0% to 30% production, 0% to 15% comprehension) [20].

More recently, a multiuser virtual world called EVA Park was designed for PWA. The authors wanted to investigate whether virtual environments would enable people with moderate aphasia to practice speech successfully with one or more conversational partners [32]. The results collected in twenty PWA, after five weeks of therapy intervention, revealed that the VR experience offered participants rich insights into aspects which go beyond the therapeutic outcomes. Indeed, PWAs experienced conversational initiative, positive emotional, and social outcomes and their therapeutic benefits were well-maintained on a measure of everyday communication (mean scores across the three time points: week 1: 6.5 vs. week 7: 7.2 vs. week 13: 7.4, Communication Activities of Daily Living (CADL-2) test). However, as also

observed by the authors [32], one limitation of their study was related to the lack of a control group inclusion which should have undergone a different treatment. This allows no conclusions to be drawn about the relative merits of the therapy delivered in VR compared to "conventional" face to face therapy.

Kurland et al. [46] investigated the effects of a tablet-based home practice program with telepractice on treatment outcomes in twenty-one individuals with chronic aphasia. The main outcome measure was percent accuracy on naming sets of treated and untreated objects and actions. Overall, results showed that home practice was effective for all participants with severity moderating treatment effects, such that individuals with the most severe aphasia made and maintained fewer gains (difference between post- and pretreatment in naming accuracy, severe: 0.067 vs. moderate: 0.057 vs. mild: 0.123 for treated items; severe: 0.099 vs. moderate: 0.157 vs. mild: 0.138 for untreated items).

Marshall et al. [47] reported two single case studies exploring the impact of daily language stimulation delivered through EVA Park platform [32] for treated and untreated word production, connected speech, and functional communication. After the therapy, outcomes varied across the different test measurements. The noun therapy significantly improved the naming of treated words in case study 1 but not in case study 2 (case 1, pre-posttreatment: 25 out of 50 items vs. 44 out of 50 items), with good maintenance after five weeks (case 1, 41 out of 50 items). There was no generalisation to untreated words (case 1, pre-posttreatment 27 out of 50 items vs. 25 out of 50 items), connected speech, or functional communication.

Within a case series ($N = 3$), Carragher et al. [48] explored the effect of storytelling intervention delivered in EVA Park [32]. The intervention dose was four sessions per week for a total of five weeks (twenty hours total). Following intervention, two participants ("Ange" and "Sally") showed substantial increases in the percentage of correct content words produced (Ange: 36.5%; Sally: 35.5%). The third participant demonstrated a more modest change with an increase of 12.1%.

Very recently, Palmer et al. [49] reported the first multicentre randomised controlled trial (BIG CACTUS) in patients with post stroke chronic aphasia (>6 months) to assess both the clinical and cost-effectiveness of self-managed computerised speech and language therapy (CSLT). Two hundred and seventy-five participants were randomly assigned to either six months of usual care (usual care group, $N = 101$), daily self-managed CSLT plus usual care (CSLT group, $N = 97$), or attention control plus usual care (attention control group, $N = 80$). Coprimary outcomes were changes, between baseline and 6 months after randomization, in lexical retrieval of personally relevant words in a picture naming test and in functional communication ability measured with the use of Therapy Outcome Measures (TOMs). The key secondary outcome was change in self-perception of communication and social participation measured through the Communication Outcomes After Stroke (COAST) questionnaire self-rated by the patient. Word finding improvement was 16. 2% higher in the CSLT group than in the usual care group and 14. 4% higher than in the attention control group. Improvement in word finding was maintained 6 months after the intervention period. However, CSLT did not have an effect on conversation, self-perceived improvements in everyday communication, social participation, and quality of life [49].

Maresca et al. [50] employed a VR tablet in order to evaluate the effectiveness of a rehabilitation training for aphasia. Thirty PWA were randomly assigned into either the control or the experimental group. The study lasted six months and included two phases. During the first phase, the experimental group was trained through the VR tablet, while the control group underwent traditional therapy. In the second phase, the experimental group was discharged but it was provided with the VR tablet, while the control group was assigned to community services. Results showed that the experimental group improved in all investigated tasks except in writing, while the control group improved only in comprehension, depression, and quality of life.

In summary, although in the field of aphasia rehabilitation, technical devices have begun to be employed, to date, digital versions of traditional language therapy exercises have been mostly used [17]. Very few studies have explored digital applications, including VR settings, for conversation in social interaction (but see [33, 51, 52]). More importantly, none of the cited studies has investigated the impact of VR technology on the patient's psychological well-being [but see 49].

Here, we report a video-based conversational training approach which makes use of semi-immersive VR environments to investigate their therapeutic benefits in enhancing language skills, communication efficacy, and psychosocial aspects (i.e., the self-esteem level; the patient's emotional, health, and humoral states) in a group of eighteen nonfluent chronic PWA. The efficacy of the VR approach was compared to the results of a matched control group of eighteen PWA who underwent the same conversational training without VR support.

1.1. Aims.
The study addressed the following research questions (RQs):

RQ1: does conversational therapy delivered via semi-immersive VR environments enhance language recovery in chronic post stroke aphasia?

RQ2: do therapy benefits generalize to measures of communication efficacy and psychological well-being?

RQ3: is VR therapy equivalent or more effective than conventional training?

1.2. Hypothesis.
In line with previous literature [8, 13, 14] which suggests that language treatment should enhance functional communication in ecological contexts, we hypothesize that conversational therapy combined with VR would be effective for aphasia. Since a central aspect of conversational approach is to set up communicative exchanges between the therapist and the patient in ecological contexts [15, 16], we further believe that treatment benefit would generalize to communication efficacy and, possibly, to psychological well-being.

2. Materials and Methods

2.1. Participants.
All patients were recruited from the neurological departments of different hospitals in Turin. Seventy-six have completed their speech therapy cycle and contacted the Experimental Laboratory of Aphasia of the Fondazione Carlo Molo Onlus in Turin in order to participate as volunteers in the research. A preliminary neuropsychological assessment was handled by an independent neuropsychologist who was blinded to the research. The inclusion criteria were fluent users of Italian, premorbidly right handed, a diagnosis of aphasia due to a single left hemisphere stroke occurring more than six months prior to the study; absence of cognitive impairment; ability to follow instructions; no hemispatial neglect; no articulatory disorder; no uncorrected visual impairment (self-report); and no hearing loss (screened via pure tone audiometry). Since our treatment was based on a conversational therapy approach aimed at enhancing verbal communication, we selected only nonfluent patients. Patients were not enrolled if they had a premorbid speech and language disorder caused by a neurological deficit other than stroke. Twenty patients were excluded because they did not meet the criteria. Fifteen people gave up for logistic reasons. Five had another stroke during the enrollment period. The thirty-six patients selected were randomly assigned to two different conditions by a researcher not involved in the research, using the Research Randomizer (https://www.randomizer.org/), a free web-based service that offers instant random sampling and random assignment. All have age between 32 and 77 years (59.75+/-11.21) with an educational level of 5 to 18 years (11.25+/-3.54). Eighteen patients were assigned to the experimental group and eighteen to the control group. In order to obtain more accurate results, the study included a sample size that would allow parametric statistics to be applied to the data.

Table 1 provides background details for the participants.

2.2. Ethical Approval.
The data analysed in the current study conformed with the Helsinki Declaration. Our named Institutional Review Board (Ethical Committee, University of Turin) specifically approved this study (protocol 100960) with the understanding and written consent of each subject.

2.3. Materials and Apparatus.
The semi-immersive VR scenarios were projected through a screen (50 inches). They were created with a NeuroVR 2.0 open source software (http://www.neurovr2.org) by the authors of the present study from the Afasia Experimental Laboratory of Carlo Molo Onlus Foundation in Turin. In order to favour the interaction between patients within the therapeutic setting, the authors opted for a semi-immersive virtual reality condition in which no patient wore a helmet. To limit the window effect typical of a nonimmersive virtual reality condition, a 50-inch curved screen was used to guarantee a sufficient level of image depth and sense of immersion for each patient [53]. The apparatus projects different virtual scenarios that can be explored by the patient. In order to elicit the ecological validity of the VR settings, each scenario represented everyday communication situations, such as different environments

TABLE 1: Demographic and clinical data of the thirty-six participants.

Participants	Age	Sex	Educational level	Time post onset	Etiology
S1	71	M	18	30	Frontotemporal hemorrhage
S2	50	F	8	28	Frontoparietal ischemia
S3	72	M	8	30	Frontotemporal ischemia
S4	68	M	13	40	Frontotemporal ischemia
S5	69	F	8	41	Frontal ischemia
S6	49	F	18	48	Temporoparietal hemorrhage
S7	53	M	13	36	Frontotemporal ischemia
S8	53	M	13	34	Frontoparietal ischemia
S9	71	M	13	54	Temporal ischemia
S10	32	M	15	40	Basal ganglia hemorrhage
S11	37	M	11	35	Temporoparietal hemorrhage
S12	51	M	13	30	Frontotemporal ischemia
S13	61	M	8	24	Temporoparietal ischemia
S14	48	M	8	24	Frontal hemorrhage
S15	72	F	5	30	Temporooccipital hemorrhage
S16	48	M	8	40	Frontal hemorrhage
S17	75	M	13	60	Temporoparietal ischemia
S18	70	M	8	30	Frontoparietal ischemia
S19	60	M	18	40	Frontotemporoparietal ischemia
S20	69	M	13	36	Frontotemporal ischemia
S21	56	F	13	35	Frontotemporal ischemia
S22	60	F	8	28	Temporal ischemia
S23	61	F	13	40	Frontotemporal ischemia
S24	53	M	13	42	Frontotemporal ischemia
S25	47	F	18	50	Frontotemporal ischemia
S26	61	M	13	54	Frontotemporal ischemia
S27	63	F	8	52	Frontotemporal hemorrhage
S28	70	F	8	60	Frontotemporal ischemia
S29	61	M	13	70	Frontotemporal ischemia
S30	38	M	13	54	Temporooccipital ischemia
S31	69	M	8	60	Frontotemporal ischemia
S32	70	M	8	58	Temporoparietal hemorrhage
S33	63	M	8	56	Frontotemporal ischemia
S34	60	M	9	52	Frontal ischemia
S35	77	F	13	50	Temporoparietal ischemia
S36	63	F	7	48	Temporoparietal ischemia

inside a city (i.e., a supermarket, a restaurant, an amusement park, the station, and the post office) (see Table 2). The apparatus was set up in order to integrate each scenario with different cognitive exercises, such as language (i.e., phonology, lexicon, semantics, and grammar), memory (i.e., working memory), attentional (i.e., sustained attention, selective attention), and executive function tasks. Cognitive exercises range from the simplest to the most complex ones. For example, the language tasks could require the patient to select the correct word among phonological (i.e., cappello (hat) and carrello (trolley)) or semantic (valigia (suitcase) and borsa (bag)) distractors, while the executive functions tasks involve the patient to manage unexpected events (see Table 2).

The interaction among patients was mediated by a speech therapist who operated in the VR scenario through the use of a personal computer. As the patient selects a virtual scenario (e.g., supermarket), the therapist presses the keyboard allowing the patient to explore it. Thus, the Neuro VR does not provide for the patient to explore the virtual environments without the help of the therapist. Within each scenario, different choices can be made by the patient (i.e., in the "Travel" scenario, patients could decide which sport to play (tennis or golf)). As the patient communicates to the therapist his/her choice, the therapist moves the mouse by clicking on the option chosen by the patient, thus opening a new screen in which the selected chooses appears. For example, if the

TABLE 2: Virtual scenarios.

Station
Patients explore the Porta Nuova railway station (Turin). They must proceed with the purchase of the railway ticket by providing their personal information, check the train track, and manage possible unexpected events (e.g., the train display board is not working, facing a stranger who is asking for help because he was robbed, and managing the seat occupied by another passenger).

Hotel
Patients are in the hotel, they have to check-in, decide how many days to stay, ask for breakfast time, and how to set the alarm clock. They must also decide which room they want and find their way around the hotel. In addition, they must manage possible unexpected events (e.g., a broken glass, a forgotten suitcase, and a mouse in the room).

Restaurant
Patients must initially make a phone reservation to reserve a table in the restaurant. At the restaurant, they have to choose what they want from the menu, order from the waiter, and pay the bill. In addition, they must handle possible unexpected events concerning the payment of the bill and the dishes ordered.

Supermarket
Patients must shop inside a supermarket with reference to a list of foods. They must, therefore, ask information to the clerks, choose the products, check that they have purchased everything, and go to the cash register. A possible unexpected event is represented by a thief who steals the wallet of an elderly lady. Patients must help the lady by contacting the police.

Amusement park
Patients are located inside an amusement park. They must go to the entrance desk, ask for tickets, decide on which rides to climb, and face possible unexpected events (e.g., they lose some objects while getting on the Ferris wheel).

Cinema
Patients are watching a movie: "Cinderella", and they are asked to tell the story and comment on the movie.

Travel
Patients must take a trip that will take them on a cruise to Egypt. During the cruise, they will be able to perform various sports (e.g., tennis). In Egypt, they will visit several archaeological sites.

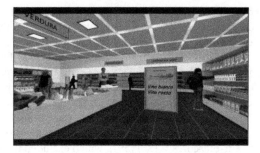

FIGURE 1: ScenePlayer NeuroVR: "Supermarket".

to select the food from the shelves and to perform a concomitant cognitive exercise, such as a semantic fluency task (i.e., "tell me all you need to get groceries" → money, wallet, bag, credit card, and so on). The different tasks are graded by difficulty. Thus, the item selection may result more or less difficult by the presence of phonological (i.e., cappello (hat) and carrello (trolley)) or semantic (valigia (suitcase) and borsa (bag)) distractors. If the patient is not able to retrieve the word, he/she can be facilitated through visual or verbal cues. The different cognitive exercises alternate with conversational phases in which the patient is asked to describe the scenario, to request information to the people which appear in the scenario (i.e., a policeman), to conversate with the speech therapist or the other patients available in the therapy room. The scenario can also sometimes present some contingencies that the patient has to face (i.e., a robbery to a lady → calling the policeman).

2.4. Procedure. The 36 participants were randomly assigned through a computer software program to one of two training: (1) conversational training combined with VR ($N = 18$) and (2) conversational training without VR (conventional therapy (CT)) ($N = 18$). Assessments were administered by an independent neuropsychologist who was blinded to the condition under which the patient was assigned. Within each condition, in order to facilitate their interaction, patients were organised into six groups of three people. Due to resource constraints, it was not feasible to run more than 3 participants simultaneously. For each training, participants completed twenty-four weeks of intensive language training (total=six months), each treatment lasted two hours, and it was performed twice a week.

2.5. Outcome Measures. A range of outcome measures was used to evaluate the effects of the two treatments (VR vs. CT). Language, communication skills, and psychosocial aspects were tested before and after the training via standardized test batteries. The primary outcome language measure was the Aachen Aphasia Test (A.A.T.) [54].

Secondary outcome measures included the Conversation Analysis Profile for People with Aphasia test (C.A.P.P.A. test, [55]) which evaluates the patient's communication skills both from the patient and of his/her caregiver perspective. The questionnaire investigates the frequency and the severity of the patient's communicative disorder with respect to four

patient chooses a tennis court, he/she can move the tennis ball by naming the objects placed on the side of the ball. Then, if the objects are correctly named, the therapist throws the ball to the other side. The response shift will thus be transferred to the patient who is playing together at that time and who, in turn, must name the objects placed on the other side of the field. Each virtual scenario includes the same number of cognitive exercises which train the different functions and the exercises vary in number and difficulty on the basis of the itinerary chosen. Thus, the apparatus automatically selects the exercises to be performed as the patient gets through the virtual environment and makes his/her choice (i.e., if the patient is at the greengrocer, he may be asked to indicate a fruit among semantic or phonological distractors or to perform a category fluency task).

For example, in the Supermarket scenario (see Figure 1), the first objective is to get groceries. Thus, the patient is asked different areas: language ability, self-correction, verbal initiative, and turn taking and topic management. Two different batteries for evaluating the psychosocial aspects of the patient's disability such as the Visual Analogue Self Esteem Scale [56] and the W.H.O.Q.O.L. Scale [57] were also included. Subjects were also administered memory tests (i.e., digit span, cut – off scores < 5), the Corsi test (cut – off scores < 4) and attentional tasks (attentional matrices, cut-off scores ≤ 30) [58], and the Trail Making test (B-A seconds, cut-off scores > 186) [59]), which excluded the presence of working memory and attention deficits that might have confounded the data. All subjects were classified nonfluent aphasics because of their reduced spontaneous speech with short sentences and frequent word-finding difficulties. They had no articulatory deficits that might have distorted their oral production.

2.6. Conversational Training with VR. The six-month training consisted of two-hour therapy sessions twice a week for twenty-four weeks (total = 48 hours of therapy). At the beginning of each session, the three patients jointly chose a virtual scenario (i.e., the restaurant) and the therapist moved the mouse by clicking on the chosen option and, thus, starting the sequence of events shown in the scenario. The participants were required to observe each VR environment and to come up with a dialogue with the help of the therapist. If no patient took the initiative to speak, the therapist described the situation and then asked each patient for some information about the scenario (e.g., which hotel location to select on a map displayed in the scenario). Then, each participant had to provide a feedback (e.g., repeat what he/she has understood) to the patient who has previously spoken. During the treatment, all patients had to perform both conversational therapy and cognitive exercises. For example, after completing the "Railway Station" block, which requires limited interaction among patients, the patients come to the "Travel" block which facilitates conversational exchanges and positive competition among participants (i.e., in the "Travel block," patients have to decide where they want to lodge (i.e., camping, hotel, camper) and each patient should convince the others about the best accommodation by trying to make his/her preference prevails; patients can also make a price estimation with respect to the different ways of travelling. Those who come closest to the correct price get the prevalence). In accordance with the principle of the Conversational Therapy approach [15, 16], no formal protocol is directed the therapist. The therapy adapted from time to time to the patient's needs, and the exercises went on based on the patient's responses. It was not possible to continue to the next block if all tasks of the previous one were not carried out. The main objective of the therapy was to set up a natural conversation on the virtual scenario in which all interlocutors participated using their available communicative resources. Both the patients and the therapist were left free to use verbal or nonverbal communication (e.g., orthographic or phonological cues, gestures, and drawings). This possibility of using any communication means was also supported by a whiteboard on which the patient could draw or write. The whiteboard was also used as a support for cognitive exercises

(e.g., in a naming task, the therapist could write on the whiteboard the first syllable of a word (orthographic cue) in order to facilitate lexical retrieval). The therapist had to accept all the information provided by the patient and try to relate it to the topic of conversation in order to improve its content and informativeness. The goal of the therapy was to enhance verbal communication, to make the patient more informative day-by-day with the context, and to enable him/her to talk about the video without the therapist's support. In order to facilitate communicative exchanges among patients, the three participants were half-moon seated. Thus, they were each watching the screen and at the same time interacting between each other in the room. Each patient, in turn, was required to take the floor.

2.7. Conversational Training without VR. The procedure and the training were the same as the one for the experimental group but without the VR scenarios. A total of six months of training and two-hour therapy sessions twice a week (total = 48 hours of therapy) were provided to each patient. During this treatment, patients were involved in cooperative conversations regarding different topics (i.e., hobbies, job, and holidays; what have you done during the week-end?) [14, 15]. As for the VR training, the conversation alternated with cognitive exercises but only with the support of the whiteboard.

2.8. Data Analysis. All statistical analyses were conducted with IBM SPSS Statistics 22 software. For the outcome measures, two ANOVA analyses were planned. The first was a mixed ANOVA with the within variable of time (two levels: pre vs. posttreatment), and the between variable of group (two levels: VR group vs. control group). This directly compared the results of the two groups at two time points (pre vs. posttreatment) on each test. The second analysis was a within-group ANOVA, with the within-variable TIME (two levels: pre vs. posttreatment) comparing, within each group separately, the mean scores at two time points on each test. If the ANOVA showed significant effects, respective post hoc Bonferroni tests were conducted. In order to investigate baseline differences between the two groups, one-way ANOVA comparisons for age, educational level, time post stroke, and screening measures were also applied. Since within each group, subjects were treated in groups of three, we had six comparisons, thus, the significance level was set at α 0.008 in all statistical analyses. To evaluate the extent of the effects for each variable, the values of the effect size were entered using partial η^2 index, which SPSS software automatically associates with ANOVA.

3. Results

One-way ANOVA comparisons for age, educational level, time post stroke, and screening measures found significant baseline differences between the groups only with respect to time post stroke ($F(1.34) = 14.186$, $P = 0.001$). Indeed, the time post stroke of the VR group (mean = 36.33, DS: 9.86) was significantly shorter than that of the control group (mean = 49.17, DS: 10.57).

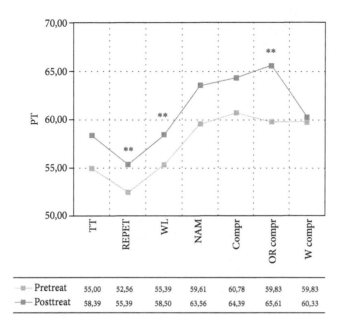

FIGURE 2: Normalized scores in the different subtests of the Aachen Aphasia Test (AAT) for the VR group. Legend: Pre-Treat: pretreatment; Post-Treat: posttreatment; TT: token test, REPET: repetition; WL = written Language; NAM: naming; Compr: comprehension; OR Compr: oral comprehension; W Compr: written comprehension; PT: normalized scores; Within-group ANOVA: $^*p \leq 0.008$.

TABLE 3: Summary of the results obtained in the different subtests of the AAT test in the two groups.

Tests	VR group	Partial η^2	Control group	Partial η^2
AAT—token test	0.018	0.385	0.094	0.216
AAT—repetition	0.002**	0.559	0.004**	0.505
AAT—written language	0.002**	0.552	0.045	0.296
AAT—naming	0.016	0.393	0.065	0.256
AAT—comprehension	0.027	0.347	0.019	0.382
AAT—oral comprehension	0.008**	0.462	0.428	0.053
AAT—written comprehension	0.699	0.013	0.102	0.208

Sig. within-group ANOVA: $^{**}p \leq 0.008$.

3.1. Outcome Measures

3.1.1. Aachen Aphasia Test. The mixed ANOVA revealed the main effect of time: token test ($F(1, 34) = 12.386$, $p = 0.001$, partial $\eta^2 = 0.267$); repetition ($F(1, 34) = 27.092$, $p < 0.001$, partial $\eta^2 = 0.443$); written language ($F(1, 34) = 18.417$, $p < 0.001$, partial $\eta^2 = 0.351$); naming ($F(1, 34) = 9.177$, $p = 0.005$, partial $\eta^2 = 0.213$); and comprehension ($F(1, 34) = 11.098$, $p = 0.002$, partial $\eta^2 = 0.246$).

No effect of GROUP and no interaction time*group for each AAT subtest were found.

So, participants improved between pre- and posttreatment on this measure, but both groups improved equally.

In the VR group, the within-group ANOVA showed a significant effect of time in repetition ($F(1, 12) = 15.211$, $p = 0.002$, partial $\eta^2 = 0.559$, mean = 52.56 (DS:8.09) pretreatment vs. 55.39 (DS: 10.07) posttreatment); written language ($F(1.12) = 14.792$, $p = 0.002$, partial $\eta^2 = 0.552$, mean = 55.39 (DS:10.98) pretreatment vs. 58.50 (DS:10.82) posttreatment; oral comprehension ($F(1, 12) = 10.291$, $p =$

0.008, partial $\eta^2 = 0.462$, mean = 59.83 (DS:9.33) pretreatment vs. 65.61 (DS: 10.72) posttreatment) (see Figure 2 and Table 3). According to the AAT cut-off score, before the treatment, for each subtest, patients were classified as moderate aphasics. After the treatment, they were still below the cut-off score but they were classified as mild aphasics (see Figure 2).

In the control group, the within-group ANOVA showed a significant effect of time only in repetition ($F(1, 12) = 12.255$, $p = 0.004$, partial $\eta^2 = 0.505$; mean = 54.28 (DS: 9.55) pretreatment vs. 57.06 (DS: 9.73) posttreatment (see Figure 3 and Table 3). According to the AAT cut-off score, before the treatment, for each subtest, patients were classified as moderate aphasics. After the treatment, they were still below the cut-off score but they were classified as mild aphasics (see Figure 3).

3.1.2. C.A.P.P.A. Test—Patient's Perspective. The mixed ANOVA revealed the main effect of time from the patient's perspective: language ability for frequency ($F(1, 34) = 21.564$,

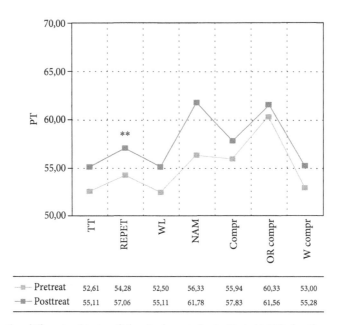

FIGURE 3: Normalized scores in the different subtests of the Aachen Aphasia Test (AAT) for the control group. Legend: Pre-Treat: pretreatment; Post-Treat: posttreatment; TT: token test, REPET: repetition; WL = written language; NAM: naming; Compr: comprehension; OR Compr: oral comprehension; W Compr: written comprehension; PT: normalized scores; within-group ANOVA: $^{**}p \le 0.008$.

$p < 0.001$, partial $\eta^2 = 0.388$) and severity ($F(1, 34) = 25.326$, $p < 0.001$, partial $\eta^2 = 0.427$), self-correction for severity ($F(1, 34) = 9.491$, $p = 0.004$, partial $\eta^2 = 0.218$), turn taking for frequency ($F(1, 34) = 13.209$, $p = 0.001$, partial $\eta^2 = 0.280$) and severity ($F(1, 34) = 18.570$, $p < 0.001$, partial $\eta^2 = 0.353$), and topic management for frequency ($F(1, 34) = 17.585$, $p < 0.001$, partial $\eta^2 = 0.341$) and severity ($F(1, 34) = 13.401$, $p = 0.001$, partial $\eta^2 = 0.283$).

No effect of group and no interaction time * group for each C.A.P.P.A. subtest were found.

So participants improved between pre- and posttreatment on this measure from the patient's perspective, but both groups improved equally.

In the VR group, the within-group ANOVA showed a significant effect of time: language ability ($F(1, 12) = 19.969$, $p = 0.001$, partial $\eta^2 = 0.625$; mean = 44.19 (DS: 21.54) pretreatment vs. 30.05 (DS: 16.95) posttreatment for frequency; $F(1, 12) = 27.844$, $p < 0.001$, partial $\eta^2 = 0.699$; mean = 42.17 (DS: 24.84) pretreatment vs. 27.27 (DS: 22.21) posttreatment for severity) and turn taking ($F(1, 12) = 13.394$, $p = 0.003$, partial $\eta^2 = 0.527$; mean = 27.78 (DS: 18.46) pretreatment vs. 18.25 (DS: 16.66) posttreatment for frequency; $F(1, 12) = 51.209$, $p < 0.001$, partial $\eta^2 = 0.810$; mean = 22.22 (DS: 20.04) pretreatment vs. 9.52 (DS: 12.49) posttreatment for severity) (see Figure 4 and Table 4).

In the control group, the within-group ANOVA revealed a significant effect of time only in the frequency of the topic management subtest ($F(1, 12) = 26.065$, $p < 0.001$, partial $\eta^2 = 0.685$, mean = 41.30 (DS: 26.13) pretreatment vs. 20.37 (DS: 17.83) posttreatment) (see Figure 5 and Table 4).

3.1.3. C.A.P.P.A. Test—Caregiver's Perspective. The mixed ANOVA revealed the main effect of time from the caregiver's

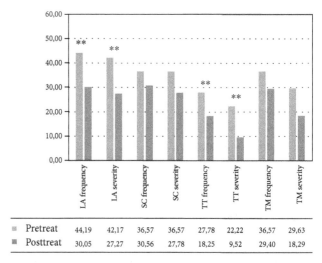

FIGURE 4: Mean percentage of scores in the different subtests of the C.A.P.P.A. test, for frequency and severity, in the VR Group from the patient's perspective. Legend: Pre-Treat: pretreatment. Post-Treat: posttreatment; LA: language ability; SC: ability to self-correct; TT: turn taking; TM: topic management; within-group ANOVA: $^{**}p \le 0.008$.

perspective: language ability, frequency ($F(1, 34) = 30.033$, $p < 0.001$, partial $\eta^2 = 0.476$) and severity ($F(1, 34) = 42.986$, $p < 0.001$, partial $\eta^2 = 0.566$); self-correction, frequency ($F(1, 34) = 31.314$, $p < 0.001$, partial $\eta^2 = 0.487$); and severity ($F(1, 34) = 18.257$, $p < 0.001$, partial $\eta^2 = 0.356$); and turn taking, frequency ($F(1, 34) = 14.082$, $p = 0.001$, partial $\eta^2 = 0.299$).

No effect of group and no interaction time * group for each C.A.P.P.A. subtest were found.

TABLE 4: Summary of the results obtained in the different subtests of the C.A.P.P.A. test, for frequency and severity, in the VR and control groups from the patient's perspective.

	VR group	Partial η^2	Control group	Partial η^2
Frequency				
(i) Language ability	0.001**	0.625	0.032	0.328
(ii) Self-correction	0.234	0.116	0.229	0.118
(iii) Turn taking	0.003**	0.527	0.102	0.207
(iv) Topic management	0.278	0.097	0.001**	0.685
Severity				
(i) Language ability	0.001**	0.669	0.021	0.372
(ii) Self-correction	0.092	0.218	0.021	0.370
(iii) Turn taking	0.001**	0.810	0.050	0.284
(iv) Topic management	0.046	0.291	0.034	0.322

Sig. within-group ANOVA: $^{**}p \le 0.008$.

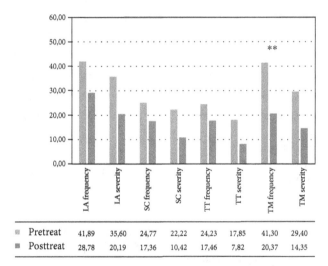

	LA frequency	LA severity	SC frequency	SC severity	TT frequency	TT severity	TM frequency	TM severity
Pretreat	41,89	35,60	24,77	22,22	24,23	17,85	41,30	29,40
Posttreat	28,78	20,19	17,36	10,42	17,46	7,82	20,37	14,35

FIGURE 5: Mean percentage of scores in the different subtests of the C.A.P.P.A. test, for frequency and severity, in the control group from the patient's perspective. Legend: Pre-Treat: pretreatment; Post-Treat: posttreatment; LA: language ability; SC: ability to self-correct; TT: turn taking; TM: topic management; within-group ANOVA: $^{**}p \le 0.008$.

So participants improved between pre- and posttreatment on this measure from the caregiver's perspective, but both groups improved equally.

In the VR group, the within-group ANOVA showed a significant effect of time: language ability ($F(1, 12) = 31.277$, $p < 0.001$, partial $\eta^2 = 0.740$; mean = 39.04 (DS: 15.83) pretreatment vs. 27.81 (DS: 16.85) posttreatment frequency; $F(1, 12) = 23.076$, $p = 0.001$, partial $\eta^2 = 0.677$; mean = 27.00 (DS: 23.37) pretreatment vs. 15.51 (DS: 17.61) posttreatment severity); self-correction ($F(1, 12) = 19.031$, $p = 0.001$, partial $\eta^2 = 0.634$; mean = 41.67 (DS: 24.52) pretreatment vs. 19.85 (DS: 17.15) posttreatment frequency; $F(1, 12) = 15.073$, $p = 0.003$, partial $\eta^2 = 0.578$; mean = 31.37 (DS: 33.56) pre-

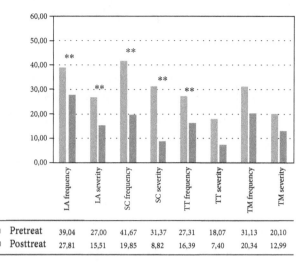

	LA frequency	LA severity	SC frequency	SC severity	TT frequency	TT severity	TM frequency	TM severity
Pretreat	39,04	27,00	41,67	31,37	27,31	18,07	31,13	20,10
Posttreat	27,81	15,51	19,85	8,82	16,39	7,40	20,34	12,99

FIGURE 6: Mean percentage of scores in the different subtests of the C.A.P.P.A. test, for frequency and severity, in the VR group from the caregiver's perspective. Legend: Pre-Treat: pretreatment; Post-Treat: posttreatment; LA: language ability; SC: ability to self-correct; TT: turn taking; TM: topic management; within-group ANOVA: $^{**}p \le 0.008$.

TABLE 5: Summary of the results obtained in the different subtests of the C.A.P.P.A. test, for frequency and severity, in the VR group and in the control group from the caregiver's perspective.

	VR group	Partial η^2	Control group	Partial η^2
Frequency				
(i) Language ability	0.001**	0.740	0.011	0.432
(ii) Self-correction	0.001**	0.634	0.001**	0.606
(iii) Turn taking	0.001**	0.662	0.085	0.227
(iv) Topic management	0.015	0.431	0.881	0.002
Severity				
(i) Language ability	0.001**	0.677	0.001**	0.614
(ii) Self-correction	0.003**	0.578	0.020	0.373
(iii) Turn taking	0.011	0.456	0.189	0.139
(iv) Topic management	0.062	0.281	0.230	0.118

Sig. within-group ANOVA: $^{**}p \le 0.008$.

treatment vs. 8.82 (DS: 14.50) posttreatment severity), and turn taking ($F(1, 12) = 21.576$, $p = 0.001$, partial $\eta^2 = 0.662$; mean = 27.31 (DS: 16.99) vs. 16.39 (DS: 13.07) posttreatment frequency) (see Figure 6 and Table 5).

In the control group, the within-group ANOVA showed a significant effect of time in language ability for severity ($F(1, 12) = 19.062$, $p = 0.001$, partial $\eta^2 = 0.614$; mean = 25.98 (DS: 16.60) pretreatment vs. 14.39 (DS: 12.59) posttreatment and in self-correction for frequency ($F(1, 12) = 18.432$, $p = 0.001$, partial $\eta^2 = 0.606$; mean = 36.80 (DS: 19.13) pretreatment vs. 22.69 (DS: 14.16) posttreatment (see Figure 7 and Table 5).

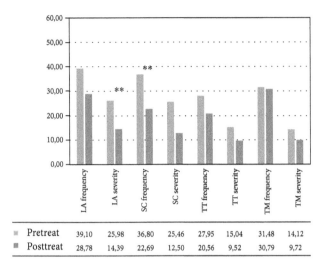

	LA frequency	LA severity	SC frequency	SC severity	TT frequency	TT severity	TM frequency	TM severity
Pretreat	39,10	25,98	36,80	25,46	27,95	15,04	31,48	14,12
Posttreat	28,78	14,39	22,69	12,50	20,56	9,52	30,79	9,72

FIGURE 7: Mean percentage of scores in the different subtests of the C.A.P.P.A. test, for frequency and severity, in the control group from the caregiver's perspective. Legend: Pre-Treat: pretreatment; Post-Treat: posttreatment; LA: language ability; SC: ability to self-correct; TT: turn taking; TM: topic management; within-group ANOVA: $**p \leq 0.008$.

3.1.4. Visual Analogue Self-Esteem Scale (VASES). The mixed ANOVA revealed the main effect of time ($F(1, 34) = 14.848$, $p < 0.001$, partial $\eta^2 = 0.304$) but no effect of group and no interaction time * group.

So participants improved between pre- and posttreatment on this measure, but both groups improved equally.

Only in the virtual group, the within-group comparison showed a significant effect of time ($F(1, 12) = 12.598$, $p = 0.004$, partial $\eta^2 = 0.512$; mean = 37.00 (DS: 5.46) pretreatment vs. 42.50 (DS: 6.31) posttreatment.

3.1.5. WHOQoL Questionnaire. The mixed ANOVA revealed the main effect of time: WHO physical area ($F(1, 34) = 12.622$, $p = 0.001$, partial $\eta^2 = 0.271$), WHO social area ($F(1, 34) = 12.027$, $p = 0.001$, partial $\eta^2 = 0.261$), and WHO environmental area ($F(1, 34) = 18.309$, $p < 0.001$, partial $\eta^2 = 0.350$).

No effect of group and no interaction time * group were found.

So participants improved between pre- and posttreatment on the different scales of the WHOQoL questionnaire, but both groups improved equally.

In the VR group, the within-group ANOVA revealed a significant effect of time in different areas: WHO physical area ($F(1, 12) = 15.030$, $p = 0.002$, partial $\eta^2 = 0.556$; mean = 66.87 (DS: 11.86) pretreatment vs. 77.38 (DS: 14.55) posttreatment), WHO psychological area ($F(1, 12) = 18.578$, $p = 0.001$, partial $\eta^2 = 0.608$; mean = 64.13 (DS: 15.34) pretreatment vs. 71.99 (DS: 14.85) posttreatment), and WHO environmental area ($F(1, 12) = 30.865$, $p < 0.001$, partial $\eta^2 = 0.720$; mean = 61.82 (DS: 13.50) pretreatment vs. 72.06 (DS: 13.32) posttreatment) (see Figure 8 and Table 6).

In the control group, the within-group ANOVA revealed a significant effect of time only in the social area ($F(1, 12) =$

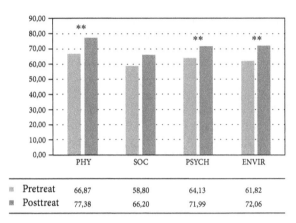

	PHY	SOC	PSYCH	ENVIR
Pretreat	66,87	58,80	64,13	61,82
Posttreat	77,38	66,20	71,99	72,06

FIGURE 8: Mean percentage of scores in the different subtests of the WHOQoL questionnaire (Word Health Organization Quality of Life—WHOQOL group, 1998) for the VR group. Legend: Pre-Treat: pretreatment; Post-Treat: posttreatment; PHY: physical; SOC: social; PSYCH: psychological; ENVIR: environmental; within-group ANOVA: $**p \leq 0.008$.

TABLE 6: Summary of the results obtained in the VASES and WHOQoL test for the VR group and the control group.

	VR group	Partial η^2	Without VR group	Partial η^2
VASES	0.004**	0.512	0.136	0.175
WHO physical	0.002**	0.556	0.629	0.228
WHO social	0.097	0.212	0.003**	0.525
WHO psychological	0.001**	0.608	0.737	0.010
WHO environmental	0.001**	0.720	0.114	0.194

Sig. within-group ANOVA $**p \leq 0.008$.

13.271, $p = 0.003$, partial $\eta^2 = 0.525$; mean = 55.09 (DS: 17.42) pretreatment vs. 70.37 (DS: 14.92) posttreatment) (see Figure 9 and Table 6).

4. Discussion

The present study investigated the usefulness of semi-immersive virtual environments combined with a conversational therapy approach for enhancing language recovery in a sample of post stroke chronic PWA. It employed a randomized controlled design which compared the results of eighteen PWA who received an intensive VR intervention combined with conversational therapy with the performance of eighteen matched controls who underwent the same conversational therapy but without VR. A broad range of outcome measures examined the impact of the two treatments (VR vs. without VR) not only on language-specific tasks (AAT test) but also on the patients' communication abilities (C.A.P.P.A. test) and on different psychosocial aspects measured through the VASES and WHOQoL. The study showed that substantial improvement can be achieved in the different domains for both groups. Indeed, after the treatment, no significant differences in the different measures were present

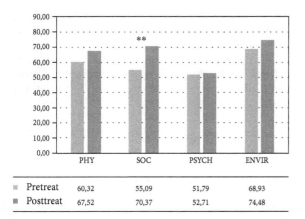

	PHY	SOC	PSYCH	ENVIR
▦ Pretreat	60,32	55,09	51,79	68,93
▪ Posttreat	67,52	70,37	52,71	74,48

FIGURE 9: Mean percentage of scores in the different subtests of the WHOQoL questionnaire (Word Health Organization Quality of Life–WHOQOL group, 1998) for the control group. Legend: Pre-Treat: pretreatment; Post-Treat: posttreatment; PHY: physical; SOC: social; PSYCH: psychological; ENVIR: environmental; within-group ANOVA: $**p \leq 0.008$.

between the two groups. Thus, these results replicate other findings indicating that even in chronic aphasia, language improvements can be achieved through intensive therapy [60, 61] which makes use of a pragmatic approach, such as conversational therapy [12–16]. Moreover, the fact that there was no difference between the VR group and the conventional therapy group suggests, in accordance with previous studies [see 44] good compatibility and feasibility of the VR version. Interestingly, the within-subject comparisons revealed that the amount of improvement found in the different areas was distributed over far more language, communicative, and psychological aspects in the VR group than in the control group. Indeed, the VR training had a positive impact on three out of six tasks of the AAT test (repetition, written language, and oral comprehension), while in the control group, only on the repetition task. With regard to the C.A.P.P.A. test, the conversational approach resulted efficacious on the PWA communicative abilities independent of the presence of a VR support but it impacted across the different areas (i.e., language ability, self-correction, and turn taking) only in the VR group. As reported in Introduction, in the past, several VR systems have been developed for cognitive rehabilitation; some of which have only gone through studies with a small number of participants [43, 47, 48] and/or without control groups [32]. Most of the existing studies with VR-based cognitive rehabilitation focused on specific language domains [25–28], such as word retrieval [18, 19, 43, 44, 46–48], sentence building [20, 21], and language comprehension [22]. So NeuroVR was developed to target rehabilitation of multiple cognitive domains (i.e., language, verbal communication, attention, concentration, memory, and executive functions) simultaneously requiring the execution of daily routines in progressive levels of cognitive complexity.

The impact of VR for language recovery is in line with recent proposals from the embodied theory which considers language as represented in a multimodal dimension in which word semantics are also made of sensorimotor properties

[62–68]. Thus, in order to facilitate language, it is efficacious to recreate a multimodal experience, such as the one that can be implemented through VR technology. Interestingly, self-reported data in the VASES and WHOQoL test revealed that, after the training, the VR group improved significantly in different psychological aspects such as their self-esteem, health, emotional, and humoral states and in their ability to maintain attention and concentration. These findings are especially relevant because our VR intervention targeted cognitive aspects but also improved the patients' emotional condition which is rarely taken into account when planning a language intervention. Indeed, the emotional and humoral states have consistently been associated with psychological well-being [69–74] and various authors have stressed that deficiencies in these psychological aspects are a crucial component in the development and course of depression in aphasia [75–78]. Given the high prevalence of depression following stroke (ranging from 25 to 79%, [77–79]) and the significant changes in physical, cognitive, and psychosocial functioning potentially experienced by the survivor [73, 74], it is easy to understand that stroke has a negative impact on psychological well-being. Indeed, the few available studies which have addressed this issue have suggested that a key personal resource contributing to psychosocial functioning after acquired brain injury is self-esteem [80–82]. Because the vast majority of instruments for mood evaluation are linguistically demanding, they have been of limited use in PWA. Consequently, right now, we know considerably less about how PWA feel than about how other stroke survivors feel. Most research on mood post stroke has either excluded PWA or relied on caregivers or health care staff to speak for them [80, 82]. In the present study, together with the WHOQoL, we used VASES [56] which is a reliable measure for identifying patients with a high risk for emotional dysfunction and in research on self-esteem after stroke due to the nonverbal nature of the test. Indeed, VASES [56] has been proven useful in identifying stroke survivors most at risk for emotional dysfunction and may be useful as a research tool in this population [56]. In our VR group, after the training, a significant increase in the level of self-esteem was found. Most probably, the possibility for the PWA to practice their communication skills within real situations and, above all, to interact among each other, has increased the patients' self-esteem helping them to overcome their language difficulties.

5. Conclusion

Overall, the results of this six-month study have revealed that language rehabilitation through an ecologically valid VR system can have a large impact in cognitive and psychological functioning. Thus, our results contribute with new evidence and provide further understanding on the use of VR in the rehabilitation of cognitive deficits. Despite the positive impact, some limitations of our study must be considered when interpreting the results. Concerning the sample, it can be observed that eighteen participants are still a small sample, though it is larger than previous studies. Moreover, the time post stroke comparison revealed that, although all patients were in the chronic phase (>36 months), the VR group was less chronic than the control group. Thus, there is still a need of further research considering other clinical populations, larger sample sizes, and more comparative studies. However, given the importance of a positive psychological state in PWA for motivating their participation in the therapy sessions, we believe that the use of VR, in the near future, should be pursued.

References

[1] M. Ali, P. Lyden, and M. Brady, "Aphasia and dysarthria in acute stroke: recovery and functional outcome," *International Journal of Stroke*, vol. 10, no. 3, pp. 400–406, 2015.

[2] K. Hilari, S. Byng, D. L. Lamping, and S. C. Smith, "Stroke and aphasia quality of life scale-39 (SAQOL-39), evaluation of acceptability, reliability, and validity," *Stroke*, vol. 34, no. 8, pp. 1944–1950, 2003.

[3] M. Cruice, R. Hill, L. Worrall, and L. Hickson, "Conceptualising quality of life for older people with aphasia," *Aphasiology*, vol. 24, no. 3, pp. 327–347, 2010.

[4] A. Basso, M. Forbes, and F. Boller, "Rehabilitation of aphasia," *Handbook of Clinical Neurology*, vol. 110, pp. 325–334, 2013.

[5] P. Marangolo and C. Caltagirone, "Options to enhance recovery from aphasia by means of non-invasive brain stimulation and action observation therapy," *Expert Review of Neurotherapeutics*, vol. 14, no. 1, pp. 75–91, 2014.

[6] A. Franzén-Dahlin, M. R. Karlsson, M. Mejhert, and A. C. Laska, "Quality of life in chronic disease: a comparison between patients with heart failure and patients with aphasia after stroke," *Journal of Clinical Nursing*, vol. 19, no. 13-14, pp. 1855–1860, 2010.

[7] M. C. Brady, H. Kelly, J. Godwin, P. Enderby, P. Campbell, and Cochrane Stroke Group, "Speech and language therapy for aphasia following stroke (review)," *Cochrane Database of Systematic Reviews*, vol. 1, pp. 1–45, 2016.

[8] R. M. Lazar, B. Minzer, D. Antoniello, J. R. Festa, J. W. Krakauer, and R. S. Marshall, "Improvement in aphasia scores after stroke is well predicted by initial severity," *Stroke*, vol. 41, no. 7, pp. 1485–1488, 2010.

[9] B. B. Johansson, "Current trends in stroke rehabilitation. A review with focus on brain plasticity," *Acta Neurologica Scandinavica*, vol. 123, no. 3, pp. 147–159, 2011.

[10] A. L. Holland, "Pragmatic aspects of intervention in aphasia," *Journal of Neurolinguistics*, vol. 6, no. 2, pp. 197–211, 1991.

[11] G. A. Davis, "Cognitive pragmatics of language disorders in adults," *Seminars in Speech and Language*, vol. 28, no. 2, pp. 111–121, 2007.

[12] T. Walker, J. Thomson, and I. Watt, "Displays and claims of understanding in conversation by people with aphasia," *Aphasiology*, vol. 30, no. 6, pp. 750–764, 2015.

[13] M. C. Savage and N. J. Donovan, "Comparing linguistic complexity and efficiency in conversations from stimulation and conversation therapy in aphasia," *International Journal of Language & Communication Disorders*, vol. 52, no. 1, pp. 21–29, 2017.

[14] P. Marangolo, V. Fiori, C. Caltagirone, and A. Marini, "How conversational therapy influences language recovery in chronic non-fluent aphasia," *Neuropsychological Rehabilitation*, vol. 23, no. 5, pp. 715–731, 2013.

[15] P. Marangolo and F. Pisano, "Conversational therapy in aphasia: from behavioral intervention to neuromodulation," *Seminars in Speech and Language*, vol. 41, no. 1, pp. 61–70, 2020.

[16] R. Wilkinson, "Intervening with conversation analysis in speech and language therapy: improving aphasic conversation," *Research on Language and Social Interaction*, vol. 47, no. 3, pp. 219–238, 2014.

[17] M. J. Choi, H. Kim, H. W. Nah, and D. W. Kang, "Digital therapeutics: emerging new therapy for neurologic deficits after stroke," *Journal of Stroke*, vol. 21, no. 3, pp. 242–258, 2019.

[18] S. Doesborgh, M. van de Sandt-Koenderman, D. Dippel, F. van Harskamp, P. Koudstaal, and E. Visch-Brink, "Cues on request: the efficacy of Multicue, a computer program for wordfinding therapy," *Aphasiology*, vol. 18, no. 3, pp. 213–222, 2010.

[19] R. Palmer, P. Enderby, C. Cooper et al., "Computer therapy compared with usual care for people with long-standing aphasia poststroke: a pilot randomized controlled trial," *Stroke*, vol. 43, no. 7, pp. 1904–1911, 2012.

[20] C. K. Thompson, J. W. J. Choy, A. Holland, and R. Cole, "Sentactics®: computer-automated treatment of underlying forms," *Aphasiology*, vol. 24, no. 10, pp. 1242–1266, 2010.

[21] M. Linebarger, D. McCall, T. Virata, and R. S. Berndt, "Widening the temporal window: processing support in the treatment of aphasic language production," *Brain and Language*, vol. 100, no. 1, pp. 53–68, 2007.

[22] L. M. D. Archibald, J. B. Orange, and D. J. Jamieson, "Implementation of computer-based language therapy in aphasia," *Therapeutic Advances in Neurological Disorders*, vol. 2, no. 5, pp. 299–311, 2009.

[23] M. Van Mourik and W. M. E. Van De Sandt-Koenderman, "Multicue," *Aphasiology*, vol. 6, no. 2, pp. 179–183, 1992.

[24] R. B. Fink, A. Brecher, M. F. Schwartz, and R. R. Robey, "A computer-implemented protocol for treatment of naming disorders: evaluation of clinician-guided and partially self-guided instruction," *Aphasiology*, vol. 16, no. 10-11, pp. 1061–1086, 2002.

[25] C. A. Des Roches, I. Balachandran, E. M. Ascenso, Y. Tripodis, and S. Kiran, "Effectiveness of an impairment-based individualized rehabilitation program using an iPad-based software platform," *Frontiers in Human Neuroscience*, vol. 8, p. 1015, 2015.

[26] R. D. Steele, A. Baird, D. McCall, and L. Haynes, "Combining teletherapy and on-line language exercises in the treatment of chronic aphasia: an outcome study," *International Journal of Telerehabilitation*, vol. 6, no. 2, pp. 3–20, 2015.

[27] B. C. Stark and E. A. Warburton, "Improved language in chronic aphasia after self-delivered iPad speech therapy," *Neuropsychological Rehabilitation*, vol. 28, no. 5, pp. 818–831, 2018.

[28] J. Kurland, A. R. Wilkins, and P. Stokes, "iPractice: piloting the effectiveness of a tablet-based home practice program in aphasia treatment," *Seminars in Speech and Language*, vol. 35, no. 1, pp. 51–63, 2014.

[29] S. Snell, N. Martin, and E. A. Keshner, "Engagement with a virtual clinician encourages gesture usage in speakers with aphasia," in *2017 International Conference on Virtual Rehabilitation (ICVR)*, vol. 6, pp. 20–25, 2017.

[30] Y. Zhang, P. Chen, X. Lin, G. Wan, C. Xie, and X. Yu, "Clinical research on therapeutic effect of virtual reality technology on Broca Aphasia patients," in *2017 2nd International Conference on Information Technology (INCIT)*, 2017.

[31] K. Grechuta, B. R. Ballester, R. E. Munne et al., "Augmented dyadic therapy boosts recovery of language function in patients with nonfluent aphasia," *stroke*, vol. 50, no. 5, pp. 1270–1274, 2019.

[32] J. Marshall, T. Booth, N. Devane et al., "Evaluating the benefits of aphasia intervention delivered in virtual reality: results of a quasi-randomised study," *PLoS One*, vol. 11, no. 8, article e0160381, 2016.

[33] V. Booth, T. Masud, L. Connell, and F. Bath-Hextall, "The effectiveness of virtual reality interventions in improving balance in adults with impaired balance compared with standard or no treatment: a systematic review and meta-analysis," *Clinical Rehabilitation*, vol. 28, no. 5, pp. 419–431, 2014.

[34] Y. Laufer and P. Weiss, "Virtual reality in the assessment and treatment of children with motor impairment: a systematic review," *Journal of Physical Therapy Education*, vol. 25, no. 1, pp. 59–71, 2011.

[35] T. E. Motraghi, R. W. Seim, E. C. Meyer, and S. B. Morissette, "Virtual reality exposure therapy for the treatment of posttraumatic stress disorder: a methodological review using CONSORT guidelines," *Journal of Clinical Psychology*, vol. 70, no. 3, pp. 197–208, 2014.

[36] P. Anderson, B. O. Rothbaum, and L. F. Hodges, "Virtual reality exposure in the treatment of social anxiety," *Cognitive and Behavioral Practice*, vol. 10, no. 3, pp. 240–247, 2003.

[37] E. Klinger, S. Bouchard, P. Légeron et al., "Virtual reality therapy versus cognitive behavior therapy for social phobia: a preliminary controlled study," *CyberPsychology & Behavior*, vol. 8, no. 1, pp. 76–88, 2005.

[38] P. L. Anderson, E. Zimand, L. F. Hodges, and B. O. Rothbaum, "Cognitive behavioural therapy for public-speaking anxiety using virtual reality for exposure," *Depression and Anxiety*, vol. 22, no. 3, pp. 156–158, 2005.

[39] S. B. Brundage and A. B. Hancock, "Real enough: using virtual public speaking environments to evoke feelings and behaviours targeted in stuttering assessment and treatment," *American Journal of Speech-Language Pathology*, vol. 24, no. 2, pp. 139–149, 2015.

[40] L. Millen, R. Edlin-White, and S. Cobb, "The development of educational collaborative virtual environments for children with autism," *UK.The 5th Cambridge workshop on universal access and assistive technology*, Cambridge, 2010.

[41] S. Parsons and S. Cobb, "State-of-the-art of virtual reality technologies for children on the autism spectrum," *European Journal of Special Needs Education*, vol. 26, no. 3, pp. 355–366, 2011.

[42] J. Stark, C. Pons, and D. Csaba, "Integrating face to face language therapy with virtual reality applications for persons with aphasia," in *Proceedings of the International Conference on Virtual Reality*, Philadelphia, 2013.

[43] L. R. Cherney, R. C. Kaye, and S. van Vuuren, "Acquisition and maintenance of scripts in aphasia: a comparison of two cuing conditions," *American Journal of Speech-Language Pathology*, vol. 23, no. 2, pp. S343–S360, 2014.

[44] L. Cherney and S. van Vuuren, "Telerehabilitation, virtual therapists, and acquired neurologic speech and language disorders," *Seminars in Speech and Language*, vol. 33, no. 3, pp. 243–257, 2012.

[45] L. R. Cherney, "Oral reading for language in aphasia (ORLA): evaluating the efficacy of computer-delivered therapy in chronic nonfluent aphasia," *Topics in Stroke Rehabilitation*, vol. 17, no. 6, pp. 423–431, 2015.

[46] J. Kurland, A. Liu, and P. Stokes, "Effects of a Tablet-Based Home Practice Program With Telepractice on Treatment Outcomes in Chronic Aphasia," *Journal of Speech, Language, and Hearing Research*, vol. 61, no. 5, pp. 1140–1156, 2018.

[47] J. Marshall, N. Devane, L. Edmonds et al., "Delivering word retrieval therapies for people with aphasia in a virtual communication environment," *Aphasiology*, vol. 32, no. 9, pp. 1054–1074, 2017.

[48] M. Carragher, R. Talbot, N. Devane, M. Rose, and J. Marshall, "Delivering storytelling intervention in the virtual world of EVA Park," *Aphasiology*, vol. 32, no. sup1, pp. 37–39, 2018.

[49] R. Palmer, M. Dimairo, C. Cooper et al., "Self-managed, computerised speech and language therapy for patients with chronic aphasia post-stroke compared with usual care or attention control (Big CACTUS): a multicentre, single-blinded, randomised controlled trial," *The Lancet Neurology*, vol. 18, no. 9, pp. 821–833, 2019.

[50] G. Maresca, M. G. Maggio, D. Latella et al., "Toward Improving Poststroke Aphasia: A Pilot Study on the Growing Use of Telerehabilitation for the Continuity of Care," *Journal of Stroke and Cerebrovascular Diseases*, vol. 28, no. 10, p. 104303, 2019.

[51] A. Al Mahmud and J. B. Martens, "Social networking through email: studying email usage patterns of persons with aphasia," *Aphasiology*, vol. 30, no. 2-3, pp. 186–210, 2016.

[52] M. Woudstra, A. Al Mahmud, and J. B. Martens, "A snapshot diary to support conversational storytelling for persons with aphasia," in *Proceedings of the 13th International Conference on Human Computer Interaction with Mobile Devices and Services*, Stockholm, 2011.

[53] F. Morganti and G. Riva, *Conoscenza, comunicazione e tecnologia: Aspetti cognitivi della realtà virtuale*, LED Lezioni Universitarie, 2006.

[54] C. Luzzatti, K. Poeck, D. Weniger, K. Willmes, R. De Bleser, and W. Huber, *AAT: Aachener aphasie test: manuale e dati normativi*, Organizzazioni Speciali, Florence, Italy, 1996.

[55] A. Whitworth, L. Perkins, and R. Lesser, *Conversation analysis profile for people with aphasia (CAPPA)*, Wiley-Blackwell Press, 1997.

[56] S. Brumfitt and P. Sheeran, *VASES: Visual Analogue Self-Esteem Scale*, Winslow Press Ltd, Bicester, England, 1999.

[57] The WHOQOL, "Group (1998b)Development of the World Health Organization WHOQOL-BREF Quality of Life Assessment," in *Psychological Medicine*, vol. 28, pp. 551–558, Cambridge Univerity Press, 1998.

[58] H. Spinnler and G. Tognoni, *Standardizzazione e taratura italiana di test neuropsicologici*, Masson Italia Periodici Press, 1987.

[59] S. Mondini, D. Mapelli, A. Vestri, and P. S. Bisiacchi, *Esame neuropsicologico breve*, Raffaello Cortina Editore, Una batteria di test per lo screening neuropsicologico, 2003.

[60] M. Meinzer, D. Djunda, G. Barthel, T. Elbert, and B. Rockstroh, *Intensive language training enhances brain plasticity in chronic aphasia*, BMC Biology, 2005.

[61] B. Stahl, B. Mohr, V. Büscher, F. R. Dreyer, G. Lucchese, and F. Pulvermüller, "Efficacy of intensive aphasia therapy in patients with chronic stroke: a randomised controlled trial,"

Journal of Neurology, Neurosurgery & Psychiatry, vol. 89, no. 6, pp. 586–592, 2018.

[62] L. W. Barsalou, W. K. Simmons, A. K. Barbey, and C. D. Wilson, "Grounding conceptual knowledge in modality-specific systems," *Trends in Cognitive Sciences*, vol. 7, no. 2, pp. 84–91, 2003.

[63] V. Boulenger, O. Hauk, and F. Pulvermüller, "Grasping ideas with the motor system: semantic somatotopy in idiom comprehension," *Cerebral Cortex*, vol. 19, no. 8, pp. 1905–1914, 2009.

[64] V. Gallese and G. Lakoff, "The brain's concepts: the role of the sensory-motor system in conceptual knowledge," *Cognitive Neuropsychology*, vol. 22, no. 3-4, pp. 455–479, 2005.

[65] G. Buccino, F. Lui, N. Canessa et al., "Neural circuits involved in the recognition of actions performed by nonconspecifics: an fMRI study," *Journal of Cognitive Neuroscience*, vol. 16, no. 1, pp. 114–126, 2004.

[66] G. Buccino, F. Binkofski, G. R. Fink et al., "Action observation activates premotor and parietal areas in a somatotopic manner: an fMRI study," *European Journal of Neuroscience*, vol. 13, no. 2, pp. 400–404, 2001.

[67] P. Marangolo, S. Cipollari, V. Fiori, C. Razzano, and C. Caltagirone, "Walking but not barking improves verb recovery: implications for action observation treatment in aphasia rehabilitation," *PLoS ONE*, vol. 7, no. 6, article e38610, 2012.

[68] P. Marangolo, S. Bonifazi, F. Tomaiuolo et al., "Improving language without words: first evidence from aphasia," *Neuropsychologia*, vol. 48, no. 13, pp. 3824–3833, 2010.

[69] G. Gainotti, "Emotional, psychological and psychosocial problems of aphasic patients: an introduction," *Aphasiology*, vol. 11, no. 7, pp. 635–650, 1997.

[70] C. Code, G. Hemsley, and M. Herrmann, "The emotional impact of aphasia," *Seminars in Speech and Language*, vol. 20, no. 1, pp. 19–31, 1999.

[71] A. Campbell, "Subjective measures of well-being," *American Psychologist*, vol. 31, no. 2, pp. 117–124, 1976.

[72] C. Code and M. Herrmann, "The relevance of emotional and psychosocial factors in aphasia to rehabilitation," *Neuropsychological Rehabilitation*, vol. 13, no. 1-2, pp. 109–132, 2003.

[73] M. T. Sarno, "Quality of life in aphasia in the first post-stroke year," *Aphasiology*, vol. 11, no. 7, pp. 665–679, 1997.

[74] G. V. Ostir, I. M. Berges, M. E. Ottenbacher, A. Clow, and K. J. Ottenbacher, "Associations between positive emotion and recovery of functional status following stroke," *Psychosomatic Medicine*, vol. 70, no. 4, pp. 404–409, 2008.

[75] W. A. Gordon and M. R. Hibbard, "Poststroke depression: an examination of the literature," *Archives of Physical Medicine and Rehabilitation*, vol. 78, no. 6, pp. 658–663, 1997.

[76] G. S. Seale, I.-M. Berges, K. J. Ottenbacher, and G. V. Ostir, "Change in positive emotion and recovery of functional status following stroke," *Rehabilitation Psychology*, vol. 55, no. 1, pp. 33–39, 2010.

[77] C. Benaim, B. Cailly, D. Perennou, and J. Pelissier, "Validation of the aphasic depression rating scale," *Stroke*, vol. 35, no. 7, pp. 1692–1696, 2004.

[78] H. E. Bennett, S. A. Thomas, R. Austen, A. M. S. Morris, and N. B. Lincoln, "Validation of screening measures for assessing mood in stroke patients," *British Journal of Clinical Psychology*, vol. 45, no. 3, pp. 367–376, 2006.

[79] L. M. Sutcliffe and N. B. Lincoln, "The assessment of depression in aphasic stroke patients: the development of the stroke aphasic depression questionnaire," *Clinical Rehabilitation*, vol. 12, no. 6, pp. 506–513, 2016.

[80] A. M. Bakheit, L. Barrett, and J. Wood, "SHORT REPORT The relationship between the severity of post-stroke aphasia and state self-esteem," *Aphasiology*, vol. 18, no. 8, pp. 759–764, 2010.

[81] J. D. Brown and M. A. Marshall, "The three faces of self-esteem," in *Self-esteem: Issues and Answers*, M. Kernis, Ed., pp. 4–9, Psychology Press, New York, NY, 2006.

[82] S. Cooper-Evans, N. Alderman, C. Knight, and M. Oddy, "Self-esteem as a predictor of psychological distress after severe acquired brain injury: an exploratory study," *Neuropsychological Rehabilitation*, vol. 18, no. 5-6, pp. 607–626, 2008.

3

Interhemispheric Plasticity following Intermittent Theta Burst Stimulation in Chronic Poststroke Aphasia

Joseph C. Griffis,[1] Rodolphe Nenert,[2] Jane B. Allendorfer,[2] and Jerzy P. Szaflarski[2,3]

[1]*Department of Psychology, University of Alabama at Birmingham, Birmingham, AL 35294-0021, USA*
[2]*Department of Neurology, University of Alabama at Birmingham, Birmingham, AL 35294-0021, USA*
[3]*Department of Neurology, University of Cincinnati Academic Health Center, Cincinnati, OH, USA*

Correspondence should be addressed to Joseph C. Griffis; joegriff@uab.edu

Academic Editor: Adriana Conforto

The effects of noninvasive neurostimulation on brain structure and function in chronic poststroke aphasia are poorly understood. We investigated the effects of intermittent theta burst stimulation (iTBS) applied to residual language-responsive cortex in chronic patients using functional and anatomical MRI data acquired before and after iTBS. Lateralization index (LI) analyses, along with comparisons of inferior frontal gyrus (IFG) activation and connectivity during covert verb generation, were used to assess changes in cortical language function. Voxel-based morphometry (VBM) was used to assess effects on regional grey matter (GM). LI analyses revealed a leftward shift in IFG activity after treatment. While left IFG activation increased, right IFG activation decreased. Changes in right to left IFG connectivity during covert verb generation also decreased after iTBS. Behavioral correlations revealed a negative relationship between changes in right IFG activation and improvements in fluency. While anatomical analyses did not reveal statistically significant changes in grey matter volume, the fMRI results provide evidence for changes in right and left IFG function after iTBS. The negative relationship between post-iTBS changes in right IFG activity during covert verb generation and improvements in fluency suggests that iTBS applied to residual left-hemispheric language areas may reduce contralateral responses related to language production and facilitate recruitment of residual language areas after stroke.

1. Introduction

Strokes of the left middle cerebral artery (LMCA) territory often lead to impairments in language function that are collectively referred to as aphasias [1]. Language recovery after LMCA stroke is highly variable, and many patients remain chronically aphasic despite optimal rehabilitative approaches [2, 3]. Aphasia following LMCA stroke typically results from lesions affecting frontal and/or temporal language regions in the left hemisphere and also often involves damage to white matter pathways connecting these regions [4–11].

Functional neuroimaging studies indicate that the recovery of language abilities after LMCA stroke involves the restoration of language-related processing in the remaining tissues near affected language areas as well as the compensatory recruitment of unaffected areas for language-related processing [12–14]. While downregulated responses in affected left-hemisphere language areas and upregulated responses in unaffected right-hemisphere homologues are commonly observed during language task performance in acute patients [12, 13, 15], the restoration of typical language-related responses in residual left-hemisphere language areas (which is thought to be marked by a restoration of left-hemisphere dominance for language-related processing) is likely critical for the successful long-term recovery of language functions [12, 15–20]. Thus, while the upregulation of right-hemisphere responses during language task performance might reflect a form of compensatory reorganization, it is likely less effective than the reinstatement of left-hemisphere processing for accomplishing language task performance [13, 16, 20–23].

Studies investigating how changes in cortical function relate to language recovery following stroke provide strong evidence indicating that the preservation and/or restoration of language-related processing in the residual left inferior frontal gyrus (IFG), a region that has been strongly implicated in various language processes such as word processing and word generation [24–26], is strongly related to the recovery of language functions in both the acute and chronic stages of recovery. For example, adult patients with acute injury who show preserved dominance of the residual left IFG for language task performance have less severe language impairments than patients who depend on the compensatory recruitment of the right IFG to accomplish the same task, indicating that the preservation of language-related processing in this region after LMCA stroke is an important factor in determining initial aphasia severity [21, 22]. In addition, adult patients that receive early poststroke aphasia rehabilitation show enhanced language-related responses in the residual left IFG compared to patients that do not receive early rehabilitation, and the magnitude of treatment-related increases in left IFG responses during language task performance is correlated with improvements in language function after treatment [23]. Similarly, increases in the left-lateralization of IFG activity related to language task performance from early to chronic recovery phases correlate with improvements in naming ability in adult patients with poststroke aphasia [17], and the level of language-related activity in left frontal areas correlates with improvements in naming ability subsequent to behavioral treatments in chronic patients [27]. The development of treatments that can facilitate the restoration of language-related processing in residual frontal language areas may, therefore, be an important step in improving both spontaneous and treatment-induced recovery in patients with poststroke aphasia.

Techniques such as transcranial magnetic stimulation (TMS) enable the noninvasive manipulation of cortical excitability in specific parts of cortex and may provide a means for facilitating beneficial cortical plasticity in patients with poststroke aphasia [28, 29]. Experimental interventions utilizing these techniques typically attempt to induce changes in cortical function that mirror those observed in successfully recovered patients by transiently enhancing the excitability of residual left-hemisphere language areas or suppressing responses in their right-hemisphere homologues [29–31]. High-frequency TMS stimulation protocols (e.g., >5 Hz) such as intermittent theta burst stimulation (iTBS) are delivered in short intervals to produce a rapid facilitation of synaptic transmission in the stimulated cortex that can persist for over an hour after the initial stimulation session [32]. In addition to facilitating changes in local synaptic transmission and evoked potential amplitude, iTBS may also alter the temporal characteristics of ongoing oscillatory activity, suggesting that it may lead to changes in ongoing neural dynamics at larger spatial scales that reflect changes in the functional organization of distributed functional networks [33].

Excitatory stimulation protocols are typically applied to the residual left IFG in order to facilitate language-related processing [34–36]. In contrast, low-frequency stimulation protocols (e.g., <1 Hz) that are delivered in continuous trains for longer periods of time have predominantly inhibitory effects on synaptic transmission and are typically applied to the right IFG in order to reduce contralateral compensation and/or interference during language-related processing [36–40]. Studies investigating the efficacy of these paradigms

for restoring language function after stroke have provided consistent evidence for improvements in language function subsequent to stimulation [34, 36–38]. Studies assessing the general effects of excitatory [34] and inhibitory [40] stimulation paradigms on neuroimaging measures of language-related responses in aphasic patients suggest that improvements in language function are accompanied by changes in the responses of both the residual left-hemisphere language network and homologous areas in the right hemisphere, although research in this area remains limited.

A previous behavioral and functional MRI (fMRI) study conducted by our laboratory found that after 10 sessions of iTBS applied to residual language-responsive left frontal cortex identified with a semantic decision/tone decision task, patients with chronic poststroke aphasia showed significant improvements in word generation as well as changes in fMRI responses during a semantic decision task that included a significant leftward shift in the lateralization of activity in the IFG [34]. In addition, a previous analysis of concurrently collected diffusion tensor imaging (DTI) data from the same patients found evidence for changes in white matter integrity in multiple regions including the left IFG following iTBS treatment [41]. However, a major limitation of our previous fMRI study is that it was restricted to changes in activation associated with the same task that was used to define language-responsive cortex for targeting with iTBS [34], and this limits inferences regarding whether or not similar effects might be observed for activation during other language tasks. Our previous fMRI analysis was also limited in that it only assessed changes in fMRI measures of activation, and it is increasingly recognized that the characterization of changes in measures of interregional connectivity is important for developing a full understanding of how changes in interregional interactions relate to the recovery of function after stroke [42, 43]. In addition, our previous structural analysis was restricted to investigating changes in white matter integrity after iTBS, although changes in cortical grey matter morphology might also be expected since excitatory TMS protocols have been found to result in measureable changes in cortical grey matter volume after as little as 5 days of treatment in individuals without stroke [44].

Here, we first analyzed the pre-/postintervention fMRI data to assess whether or not iTBS might have similar effects on fMRI responses elicited by a covert verb generation (VG) paradigm that was not used to define iTBS targets. Notably, while both the semantic decision paradigm used in our previous study and the VG paradigm used in the current study reliably evoke strong responses in the left IFG in healthy individuals [45] and in patients with poststroke aphasia [46], they target different functional domains (word comprehension versus word generation) and there is typically little overlap between the activations attained with these tasks beyond the left inferior frontal cortex [46]. We hypothesized that if iTBS has a general facilitatory effect on language-related processing in the residual left IFG (i.e., by modulating synaptic transmission to facilitate communication with other language-relevant areas or to suppress interference from language-irrelevant interactions with other areas), then patients should show increased responses in the left IFG during covert verb generation after treatment with iTBS and increased left-lateralization of IFG activity associated with covert verb generation. Because language lateralization in frontal cortex is associated with both higher levels of activity in the left hemisphere and lower levels of activity in the right hemisphere for language-related versus non-language-related tasks [47] and because our previous study also found evidence for decreased activity in the right IFG related to semantic decisions following iTBS [34], we expected that patients would also show reductions in right IFG activity during covert verb generation after iTBS. In addition, because studies of healthy individuals indicate that the presence of left-lateralized IFG activation during language tasks may be in part due to a task-dependent reduction in connectivity between left and right IFG [48] and because we are unaware of any studies that have investigated changes in functional MRI measures of connectivity in patients with poststroke aphasia subsequent to iTBS treatment, we also investigated whether or not interhemispheric connectivity between right and left IFG during covert verb generation was affected by iTBS. Finally, in order to fully characterize the structural effects of iTBS in these patients, we also tested whether or not patients showed changes in regional grey matter volume after iTBS treatment.

2. Materials and Methods

2.1. Patient Demographics and Language Testing. Eight prospectively identified patients (4 females; mean age = 54.4, SD = 12.7) with chronic aphasia resulting from LMCA stroke were recruited as described previously [34, 41]. The mean time since stroke for all patients included was 5.25 years (SD = 3.62). Aphasia types were determined by a linguistics expert following language testing. Four patients presented with anomic aphasias; of these subjects, two also presented with dysarthria and one also presented with conduction aphasia. The remaining four patients all presented with nonfluent Broca's type aphasias. Aphasia diagnoses and lesion characteristics are shown for each patient in Table 1. None of the patients had contraindications to MRI scanning, none had history of seizures, and all were right-handed prior to the stroke. The study was approved by the University of Cincinnati, Cincinnati Children's Hospital Medical Center, and University of Alabama at Birmingham Institutional Review Boards and adhered to the Declaration of Helsinki regarding human subject research. Each patient provided signed informed consent prior to inclusion in the study. Neuropsychological measures of language function were acquired before and after iTBS treatment as described in previous publications [34, 41]. Briefly, naming and word-finding abilities were evaluated using the Boston Naming Test (BNT) [49], receptive vocabulary was evaluated using the Peabody Picture Vocabulary Test (PPVT) [50], verbal fluency was evaluated using the Semantic Fluency Test (SFT) [51] and Controlled Oral Word Association Test (COWAT) [52], and comprehension was evaluated using the Complex Ideation Subtest of the Boston Diagnostic Aphasia Examination (BDAE CompId) [53]. Patients also completed the min-Communicative Abilities Log in order to provide subjective

TABLE 1: Patient characteristics.

Patient	Aphasia diagnosis	Total lesion volume (voxels)
P1	Anomia, mild dysarthria	29,243
P2	Nonfluent (Broca-type)	32,744
P3	Anomia, mild dysarthria	1,436
P4	Anomia	20,195
P5	Nonfluent (Broca-type)	52,452
P6	Anomia, conduction	13,208
P7	Anomia	36,479
P8	Nonfluent (Broca-type)	7,269

measurements of progress in verbal communication [54]. Pre- and posttreatment testing used different versions of the assessments in order to reduce the potential for learning-related effects.

2.2. Intermittent Theta Burst Stimulation Protocol. Detailed descriptions of all iTBS and neuronavigation protocols performed on these patients can be found in our previous publication [34]. Briefly, all patients received iTBS to residual language-responsive cortex in or near the left IFG as identified using an fMRI semantic decision/tone decision language localizer task described in our previous publication [34]. Stimulation intensities used for each patient were set at 80% of the active motor threshold obtained from stimulation of the right motor cortex. Stimulation sessions occurred each day for five consecutive weekdays over the course of two weeks, resulting in a total of 10 stimulation sessions. Each session consisted of 600 total pulses, with three pulses at 50 Hz given every 200 milliseconds in 2-second trains at 10-second intervals over a 200-second period. fMRI-guided neuronavigation using BrainSight2 (Rogue Research Inc., Montreal Canada) enabled the targeting of residual language-responsive cortex in the left frontal lobe near the IFG (frontal targets were used for 7 patients; language-responsive cortex in the left temporal lobe was targeted for one patient; see Figure 1 in [34]) that was identified using the fMRI localizer task, and allowed for reliable and precise localization of the same location at each session. A schematic illustrating the experimental timeline is shown in Figure 1.

2.3. MRI Data Acquisition. MRI data were acquired before and after the treatment sessions. The functional and anatomical MRI data presented in this study were acquired using a Varian 4 Tesla Unity INOVA whole body MRI/MRS scanner (Varian, Inc., Palo Alto, CA). For each patient, a high-resolution T1-weighted 3D-MDEFT (Modified Driven Equilibrium Fourier Transform) anatomical volume (scan parameters: repetition time/echo time = 13.1/6 ms, field of view = $25.6 \times 19.2 \times 19.2$ cm, flip angle = 22°, and voxel dimensions = $1 \times 1 \times 1$ mm) and T2*-weighted blood oxygen-level dependent (BOLD) volumes (scan parameters: repetition time/echo time = 3000/30 ms, FOV = 25.6×25.6 cm, matrix = 64×64 pixels, number of slices = 30, slice thickness = 4 mm, and flip angle = 75°) were obtained at both pretreatment and posttreatment sessions.

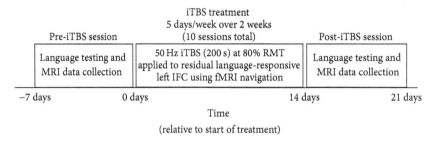

FIGURE 1: Experimental timeline. Patients underwent language testing and MRI scans during the week prior to treatment. Patients then received one session of iTBS each on weekday over a two-week period and underwent language testing and MRI scans again during the week following treatment.

FMRI data were collected while patients performed an alternating block-design covert verb generation (VG) task that consisted of alternating 30 s blocks of an active condition involving silent verb generation in response to binaurally presented nouns and a control condition involving bilateral sequential finger tapping (FT) in response to a frequency modulated tone centered on 400 Hz that was modulated by 25% every 5 s. This task was chosen because previous studies indicate that it reliably produces left-lateralized activation patterns [45] and because it has excellent test-retest (across time points) reliability for evoked activity patterns in patients with aphasia due to LMCA stroke [46]. The control condition served to control for the auditory stimulation during the noun presentation in the active condition and to distract patients from continuing to generate verbs outside of the active condition blocks while maintaining a task state. Each condition was performed 7 times. Each patient's understanding of and ability to perform the task were assessed prior to scanning by having the patients perform the task outside of the scanner. Patients had to be able to generate at least one verb in response to each noun prior to proceeding to scanning. Following each scan session, patients performed a forced-choice recognition test involving the nouns that were presented during the covert verb generation task, and the percentage of correctly remembered nouns was utilized as an indirect measurement of task performance.

2.4. MRI Data Preprocessing. All MRI data were preprocessed using MATLAB scripts implementing functions from the most recent release version of Statistical Parametric Mapping (SPM12, Wellcome Department of Cognitive Neurology, London, UK) running in MATLAB r2014B (The MathWorks Inc., Natick, MA). All statistical analyses were performed using statistical functions provided in MATLAB.

Functional MRI data from the baseline and follow-up scans were slice-time corrected, realigned and resliced, and coregistered to the structural image obtained during the same scan. Deformation fields containing the deformation differences between across-session average anatomical volume and the anatomical scan from each session were used to warp the coregistered functional volumes to the across-session average anatomical volume. The average anatomical scan was then normalized to Montreal Neurological Institute (MNI) template using unified normalization-segmentation

as implemented in the New Segment tool in SPM. The deformation parameters obtained from the warping of the anatomical volume were used to normalize the functional volumes to MNI template space. The functional volumes were resampled to $2 \times 2 \times 2$ millimeter isometric voxels and spatially smoothed with a 6-millimeter full-width half maximum (FWHM) Gaussian kernel. Functional volumes in which participants moved more than 0.5 mm in one frame (3 s) were replaced with a volume interpolated from adjacent time points. Volumes were to be rejected if they contained >3 mm of motion, but no volumes met criteria for rejection.

Individual patient lesion delineations were created from the pre-iTBS anatomical scans using an automated voxel-based Bayesian classification algorithm developed by our lab and implemented in the lesion_gnb toolbox for SPM12 [55]. The resulting lesion delineations were used to create a group-level lesion frequency map. The group-level lesion frequency map is provided in Figure 2 and illustrates the number of patients with lesioning at each voxel. The greatest across-patient lesion overlap was observed in the left insula, left putamen, and left precentral gyrus (Figure 2).

Anatomical data utilized in the voxel-based morphometry (VBM) analysis were preprocessed according to a recently described longitudinal preprocessing pipeline for VBM analyses [56]. First, probabilistic tissue segmentation implementing the New Segment + DARTEL (diffeomorphic automatic registration through exponentiated lie algebra) approach with an additional tissue prior (mean of white matter and CSF tissue probability maps) and medium bias regularization was used to obtain DARTEL-compatible tissue probabilistic maps (TPMs) encoding the grey matter (GM) and white matter (WM) probabilities for each voxel. The additional tissue prior and medium bias regularization were used since this has been shown to improve template-space normalization using the New Segment + DARTEL approach [57]. Next, patient-specific anatomical templates were created with DARTEL using the GM and WM tissue maps from the baseline and follow-up scans. For each patient, the baseline and follow-up TPMs were then warped to the subject-specific templates and modulated using the Jacobian determinant of the transformation to increase sensitivity to absolute differences in GM volume [58, 59]. The creation of the patient-specific templates was performed in order to enable more precise between-session spatial alignment of TPMs

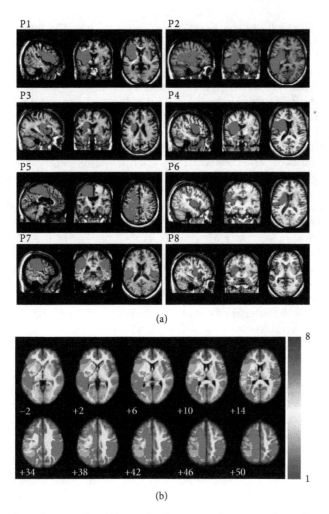

FIGURE 2: (a) Representative images from the normalized T1-weighted anatomical scans are shown for each patient; lesion delineations are shown in red. (b) A lesion frequency overlay for all 8 participants shown as a color-map overlaid on a template anatomical image. Colors represent the number of patients with a lesion at each voxel as indicated by the color bar.

[56]. A group template was then created by nonlinearly registering all of the patient-specific templates simultaneously using DARTEL. The modulated/warped GM and WM TPMs obtained from each patient were then nonlinearly normalized to the population template and modulated with the Jacobian determinant of the transformation. Finally, the population template was then registered to MNI space using an affine transformation, and each TPM was then coregistered to MNI space using an identical transformation and smoothed using an 8 mm FWHM Gaussian kernel.

2.5. *Functional MRI Data Analyses.* Functional MRI activity related to the covert verb generation task was quantified by contrasting the active condition blocks (VG) against the control condition blocks (FT). For each patient, the fMRI data were fit to a general linear model (GLM) [60] where each active block was modeled as a boxcar regressor convolved with a canonical hemodynamic response function. To account for temporal variability in the hemodynamic response, time and dispersion derivatives were modeled as basis functions in the first-level analyses [61]. Single-patient

statistical maps containing contrast estimates quantifying differences between the active and control conditions were computed for both pre- and post-iTBS scans. Statistical comparisons of the contrast estimate maps were used to evaluate changes in activation between the pre- and post-iTBS sessions.

FMRI data were first analyzed using a region of interest (ROI) approach in order to directly test our hypotheses regarding changes in IFG activity and connectivity between pre- and post-iTBS sessions. ROI masks were created using the marsbar toolbox for SPM (http://marsbar.sourceforge .net/), and ROIs in the left and right IFG were defined using peak activation coordinates obtained from an independent analysis of activation related to covert verb generation in healthy individuals [45]. 8 mm radius spherical ROIs were centered on voxels in the left IFG (MNI coordinates: $x = -50$, $y = 16$, and $z = 16$) and on mirrored coordinates in the right IFG (MNI coordinates: $x = 50$, $y = 16$, and $z = 16$). Only two patients (P1 and P4) had overlap between the left IFG ROI and their lesion delineation. P1's lesion encompassed nearly the entire left lateral prefrontal cortex and the left IFG ROI fell directly onto the perilesional rim, resulting in 100% lesion overlap with the left IFG ROI. P4's lesion was primarily localized to the left ventral IFG and the ROI overlapped by 60.2% with the perilesional rim. Nonetheless, for both patients, the 1st principal component of the signal extracted from the ROI showed phasic responses consistent with the design of the task. While anatomical overlap was noted, functional analyses indicated BOLD signal changes aligned with the box-car function of the fMRI task design indicating that the fMRI responses reflected the responses of perilesional cortex rather than CSF. Additionally, signal from the left IFG ROI was more strongly correlated with signal from the right IFG ROI than with the CSF signal, and this was only marginally influenced by partialling out variability accounted for by the CSF signal (Supplemental S1) (see Supplementary Material available online at http://dx.doi.org/10.1155/2016/4796906). Nonetheless, control analyses indicated that excluding these patients did not substantially change the statistical significance of results for any analysis involving the left IFG ROI, indicating that the presence of lesion-ROI overlaps for these patients did not strongly influence the outcome of the ROI analyses.

To test our hypothesis about whether patients showed changes in fMRI activity during covert verb generation in the left and right IFG ROIs after iTBS, we extracted the mean parameter estimates for the active versus control condition contrast and compared the estimates obtained for each ROI between the pre- and post-iTBS sessions. This analysis provided information about the mean level of activity in the IFG ROIs for each session, with positive values indicating stronger activation during the active condition and negative values indicating stronger activation during the control condition. To test our hypothesis that patients would show more strongly left-lateralized IFG activation following iTBS, laterality index (LI) analyses were performed to quantify the lateralization of activity related to covert verb generation. For each patient, changes in LI were evaluated using an adaptive threshold determination approach [62]. LI values range from −1 (complete right-lateralization) to 1 (complete left-lateralization), and LIs for each session were calculated according to the formula shown in

$$LI = \frac{(\sum activation_{left}/mwf) - \sum activation_{right}}{(\sum activation_{left}/mwf) + \sum activation_{right}}. \quad (1)$$

Using adaptive threshold determination, the term activation is defined as the values of voxels with intensities that are greater than the within-ROI average intensity for the contrast of interest. This method was chosen because it has been shown to provide reliable LI estimates that are more robust against interindividual variability in signal-to-noise ratio than approaches that employ arbitrary/fixed cut-off thresholds that are applied to all subjects (e.g., corrected P value thresholds); this method does not substantially increase susceptibility to false positives [62]. The mask weighting factor (mwf term in (1)) is used to adjust the LI estimates to account for differences in the volume of each ROI and is defined by the proportion of the volumes of the left- and right-hemisphere ROIs [62].

To test our hypothesis regarding the effects of iTBS on interhemispheric connectivity, we conducted a generalized psychophysiological interaction (gPPI) analysis using the gPPI toolbox for SPM [63]. gPPI enables the modeling of context-specific changes in the relationship of activity in one brain region, referred to as a seed region, to activity in other brain regions by including a term specifying an interaction effect between the seed region time series and the task time series in each first-level GLM [64]. gPPI effects are interpreted as changes in interregional connectivity which are driven by psychological states related to factors such as the task being performed [63, 65], making gPPI an appropriate tool for testing our hypothesis that iTBS would lead to changes in interhemispheric connectivity during covert verb generation. For each patient, the first principal component of the BOLD time series from each scan was extracted from the right IFG ROI and entered as a seed time series for the gPPI analysis. The right IFG ROI, rather than the left IFG ROI, was chosen in order to reduce potential confounds in the extracted time series related to lesion proximity since two patients showed substantial lesion overlap with the left IFG ROI. Cerebrospinal fluid (CSF) and WM signals were also included as nuisance variables in the gPPI model in order to reduce the influence of nonneural signals on estimates of task-dependent connectivity [66]. For each patient, gPPI estimates quantifying the level of condition-dependent connectivity from right to left IFG during each session were then extracted from the gPPI model using the marsbar tool for SPM and compared from pre- to post-iTBS sessions.

All between-session comparisons were tested for statistical significance using two-tailed dependent samples t-tests. Correlations between changes in fMRI measures of IFG function and behavioral measures were assessed using linear correlation analyses. Multiple-comparisons correction for all ROI-driven comparisons between pre-iTBS and post-iTBS scans was performed using the Benjamini-Hochberg procedure to control the false-discovery rate (FDR) at 0.05 [67, 68], and all associated P values presented are FDR-adjusted. Exploratory whole-brain GLM and gPPI analyses were also performed in order to provide a more thorough characterization of functional MRI measures of activity and right IFG connectivity related to the VG task at the pre-iTBS and post-iTBS sessions. Statistical tests for these analyses were performed using dependent samples t-contrasts. Exploratory and ad hoc partial correlational analyses were performed to further characterize the data and are presented with uncorrected P values.

2.6. Voxel-Based Morphometry Analyses. VBM is a technique that allows for the measurement of grey matter (GM) volume in T1-weighted MRI data [58, 69]. Here, we used VBM to address the question of whether or not patients showed changes in GM volume after iTBS treatment. The DARTEL-processed subject-level grey matter maps from baseline and follow-up scans were entered into a dependent samples t-contrast that also included each patient's lesion volume as a nuisance covariate. Changes in GM volume were assessed at the whole-brain level using dependent samples t-contrasts.

3. Results

3.1. Behavioral Results. Analyses evaluating performance on the out-of-scanner forced-choice noun recognition task revealed good performance for both pre-iTBS (mean % correct = 94.13; SEM = 1.63) and post-iTBS (mean % correct = 95.13; SEM = 2.05) sessions. Dependent samples t-test comparing pre-iTBS and post-iTBS evaluations did not reveal a significant change in noun recognition performance (t_7 = 0.415, P = 0.69). These results are consistent with previous studies that have reported good out-of-scanner noun recognition performance on this task in patients with poststroke aphasia [46, 70].

The effects of iTBS on neuropsychological measures of language function have been previously reported [34, 41] and will briefly be described here to provide details relevant to the current study. Our previous analysis revealed that patients showed a statistically significant (at $P < 0.05$) improvement on the Semantic Fluency Test, statistically nonsignificant (at $P < 0.05$) improvements in performance on the Boston Naming Test (Boston Diagnostic Aphasia Examination, Peabody Picture Vocabulary Test, and the Communicative Abilities Log), and a statistically nonsignificant (at $P < 0.05$) decrease in performance on the Controlled Oral Word Association Test (see Table 1 in [34]). Since statistically significant improvements were only observed for performance on the Semantic Fluency Test, exploratory analyses investigating the relationship between changes in functional MRI measures of IFG activation/connectivity and the behavioral effects of iTBS were restricted to this test. While ideally behavioral correlations would have been performed on the out-of-scanner noun recognition task, the miniscule change between sessions and globally good performance precluded this approach. Importantly, the Semantic Fluency Test, like the covert verb generation task, required patients to generate words in response to a prompt. For the Semantic Fluency Test, patients generated as many words as they could think of that were congruent with category prompt (e.g., animals) with a 1-minute time limit, and performance on the Semantic Fluency test was measured by the number of congruent words produced within the 1-minute time limit. Thus, whereas the covert verb generation task required patients to silently generate verbs in response to presented nouns, the Semantic Fluency Test required patients to generate words in response to a given category.

3.2. Functional MRI Results. To test our hypotheses regarding the effects of iTBS on the magnitudes of activity in left and right IFG during covert verb generation, we compared activation magnitudes at each ROI between pre- and post-iTBS sessions. It is worth noting that the ROIs used for these analyses were chosen *a priori* in order to avoid the introduction of bias by defining ROIs based on the GLM results. Our analyses revealed increased activation magnitudes in the left IFG (t_7 = 3.32; FDR P = 0.02; mean change = 0.54, SEM = 0.18) and decreased activation magnitudes in right IFG (t_7 = -2.3; FDR P = 0.05; mean change = -0.22, SEM = 0.09) related to covert verb generation after iTBS treatment. Left and right IFG activation magnitudes for each patient are

shown in Figures 3(b) and 3(c). On average, patients showed lower levels of activity in left IFG and higher levels of activity in right IFG during covert verb generation compared to finger tapping pre-iTBS. In contrast, patients showed higher levels of activity in left IFG and similar levels of activity in right IFG during covert verb generation compared to finger tapping post-iTBS. Accordingly, results from the LI analysis indicated that overall IFG responses during covert verb generation were more strongly left-lateralized after iTBS treatment (t_7 = 3.46, FDR P = 0.02; mean change = 0.48, SEM = 0.14). LI estimates for each patient at pre-iTBS and post-iTBS sessions are shown in Figure 3(d). On average, patients showed right-lateralized activation patterns in IFG pre-iTBS. In contrast, patients showed left-lateralized activation patterns in IFG post-iTBS.

To allow for a more thorough characterization of the data, whole-brain GLM analyses were also performed. Although no regions showed significant effects at a whole-brain FDR-corrected threshold of 0.05, the uncorrected statistical maps provide evidence for increased responses related to covert verb generation in left-hemisphere frontal, temporal, and parietal regions after iTBS (Figure 4(a)). While no regions showed changes that were significant after multiple-comparisons correction, the most reliable (voxelwise P < 0.001, uncorrected) increases in activity were observed in the left IFG pars opercularis (peak MNI coordinate: -40, 14, 10; 171 voxel clusters), the right thalamus (peak MNI coordinate: 10, -14, 20; 64 voxel clusters), and the right cerebellum VI (peak MNI coordinate: 30, -62, -30; 3 voxel clusters), and the most reliable (voxelwise P < 0.001, uncorrected) decreases in activity were observed in the right cerebellum crus 2 (peak MNI coordinate: 48, -52, -42; 12 voxel clusters), the right cerebellum VIII (peak MNI coordinate: 34, -44, -40; 6 voxel clusters), and the right inferior temporal gyrus (peak MNI coordinate: 54, -6, -30; 4 voxel clusters).

To test our hypothesis regarding the effects of iTBS on effective connectivity between the right and left IFG, we compared gPPI estimates between the right IFG seed region and the left IFG target region between pre- and post-iTBS sessions. It is important to note that gPPI estimates reflect the magnitude of condition-dependent changes in the relationship between activity in the seed region and activity in the target region [63]. Thus, the connectivity estimates for each session quantify how the relationship between responses in the right IFG and responses in the left IFG differed between conditions. These analyses revealed that compared to the pre-iTBS session, patients showed reductions in gPPI estimates between the right IFG seed region and the left IFG target region for the active condition contrast at the post-iTBS session (t_7 = -2.97; FDR P = 0.03; mean change = -0.24, SE = 0.09). The gPPI estimates for the active condition contrast for each patient are shown in Figure 3(e).

Since the gPPI measurement quantifies differences in the relationship between activity in the seed region (R IFG) and the target region (L IFG) that are moderated by task condition (VG-FT), a reduction in the gPPI estimate between right IFG and left IFG would indicate that the effect of right IFG activity on left IFG activity for covert verb generation relative to finger tapping was reduced after iTBS. Patients showed a small but positive mean effect of covert verb generation on connectivity

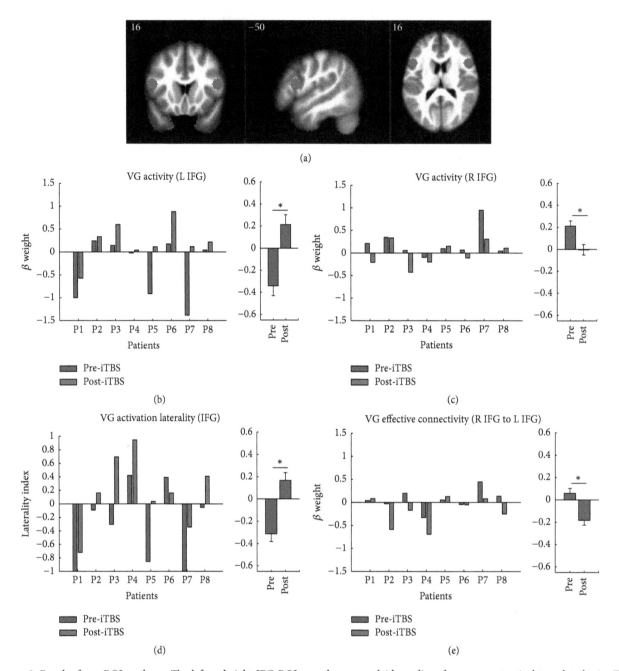

FIGURE 3: Results from ROI analyses. The left and right IFG ROIs are shown overlaid on slices from an anatomical template brain. The estimates of left (b) and right (c) IFG activation magnitudes, laterality indices (d), and effective connectivity from right to left IFG (e) are shown for the pre-iTBS (blue) and post-iTBS (red) sessions of each patient. For each plot in (b–e), bar graphs are shown on the right side that illustrate the mean and within-subjects standard error of the effect at pre-iTBS and post-iTBS sessions. *Significant at FDR $P = 0.05$.

between the right IFG and left IFG pre-iTBS, indicating that right IFG activity was more positively associated with left IFG activity during covert verb generation than during finger tapping. In contrast, patients showed a negative mean effect of covert verb generation on connectivity between the right IFG and left IFG post-iTBS, indicating that right IFG activity was more negatively associated with left IFG activity during covert verb generation than during finger tapping. Thus, the direction of the effect of task condition on the relationship between right IFG activity and left IFG activity changed

between pre-iTBS and post-iTBS sessions, with right IFG activity being more negatively associated with left IFG activity during covert verb generation than during finger tapping.

To allow for a more thorough characterization of the data, whole-brain gPPI analyses were also performed. Although no regions showed significant effects at a whole-brain FDR-corrected threshold of 0.05, the uncorrected statistical maps provide evidence for reduced connectivity between the right IFG and left-hemisphere frontal, temporal, and parietal regions after iTBS (Figure 4(b)). While no regions showed

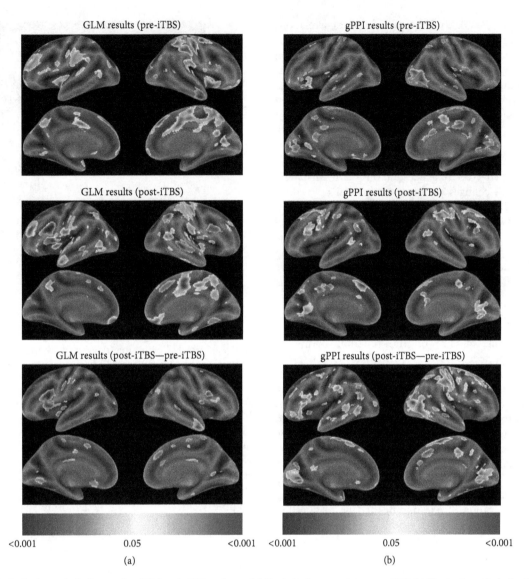

FIGURE 4: Whole-brain statistical maps for GLM and gPPI analyses. (a) Statistical parametric maps (SPMs) illustrating whole-brain activation for the VG > FT (red) and VG < FT (blue) contrasts from the pre-iTBS (top) and post-iTBS (middle) scan sessions are shown to illustrate overall activation patterns for each scan session (left, middle). An SPM illustrating changes in VG activation is also shown (bottom). (b) SPMs illustrating whole-brain gPPI results for the R IFG seed region for the VG > FT (red) and VG < FT (blue) contrasts from the pre-iTBS (top) and post-iTBS (bottom) scan sessions are shown to illustrate overall task-dependent connectivity patterns for each scan session. An SPM illustrating changes in task-dependent connectivity is also shown (bottom). Color bar values for all SPMs indicate uncorrected P values ranging from 0.05 to <0.001.

changes that were significant after multiple-comparisons correction, the most reliable (voxelwise $P < 0.001$, uncorrected) reductions in right IFG connectivity associated with the VG task were observed in the right middle temporal gyrus (peak MNI coordinate: 36, −74, 6; 65 voxel clusters), the right superior frontal gyrus (peak MNI coordinate: 16, −2, 60; 32 voxel clusters), the left IFG pars opercularis (peak MNI coordinate: −50, 8, 22; 8 voxel clusters), the right postcentral gyrus (peak MNI coordinate: 36, −32, 56; 7 voxel clusters), the left lingual gyrus (peak MNI coordinate: −14, −70, 0; 6 voxel clusters), the right cerebellum VI (peak MNI coordinate: 24, −60, −24; 4 voxel clusters), the left caudate (peak MNI coordinate: −12, −4, 10; 4 voxel clusters), and the left temporal

pole (peak MNI coordinate: −32, 10, −30; 1 voxel cluster). Interestingly, comparable (voxelwise $P < 0.001$, uncorrected) increases in right IFG connectivity associated with the VG task were not observed after iTBS.

3.3. Exploratory Behavioral Correlation Results. Prior to assessing behavioral correlations with fMRI measures of IFG function, correlations between total lesion volume and each measure were assessed. This revealed moderate but nonsignificant correlations between total lesion volume and changes in L IFG activity ($r = 0.5$, $P = 0.2$) and changes in connectivity ($r = 0.33$, $P = 0.43$) and weak but nonsignificant correlations between total lesion volume and right IFG activity ($r = 0.11$, $P = 0.79$). Thus, partial linear correlations were computed to investigate the relationship between the changes in functional MRI measurements of IFG function during covert verb generation and changes in performance on the Semantic Fluency Test following iTBS that were not attributable to total lesion volume. These analyses did not reveal significant correlations between overall changes in LI and changes in performance (partial $r = -0.03$, $P = 0.96$), changes in the magnitude of left IFG activity and changes in performance (partial $r = 0.16$, $P = 0.74$), or changes in the effects of covert verb generation on interhemispheric connectivity and changes performance (partial $r = 0.15$, $P = 0.76$). These analyses did reveal a strong negative correlation between changes in the magnitude of right IFG activity and changes in performance (partial $r = -0.82$, $P = 0.01$), indicating that decreases in right IFG activity during covert verb generation between pre/post-iTBS sessions were associated with concurrent improvements on the Semantic Fluency Test.

3.4. Ad Hoc Functional MRI Analysis Results. To further explore the effects of iTBS on IFG function, additional analyses were performed on the fMRI data. Our *a priori* analyses indicated that iTBS was associated with changes in the responses of both the left IFG and right IFG during covert verb generation and also indicated that iTBS was associated with reduced connectivity from right IFG to left IFG during covert verb generation. The exploratory behavioral correlation analyses also revealed the somewhat surprising result that post-iTBS improvements in performance on the Semantic Fluency Test were most strongly related to reductions in the responses of right IFG during covert verb generation. These findings led us to question whether the relationship between post-iTBS changes in the responses of left and right IFG during covert verb generation showed a consistent pattern across patients. They also led us to question whether the effects of iTBS on the responses of left and right IFG during covert verb generation might relate to the pretreatment levels of effective connectivity from right IFG to left IFG during covert verb generation. It might be expected, for example, that preexisting interhemispheric dynamics might influence the effects of high-frequency iTBS on the function of left and right IFG. These questions were addressed using additional exploratory partial correlation analyses that, while not related to our initial hypotheses, were included to more fully characterize the data.

First, we addressed the question of whether or not changes in left IFG activity after iTBS were correlated with changes in right IFG activity after iTBS while controlling for total lesion volume. This revealed a nonsignificant negative correlation between post-iTBS changes in left and right IFG activity (partial $r = -0.65$, $P = 0.12$). Second, we addressed the question of whether or not the effects of iTBS on left and right IFG activation magnitudes were correlated with the effects of covert verb generation on interhemispheric connectivity prior to iTBS treatment. This revealed a positive correlation between pre-iTBS effects of verb generation on interhemispheric connectivity and changes in left IFG activation magnitude after iTBS treatment (partial $r = 0.75$,

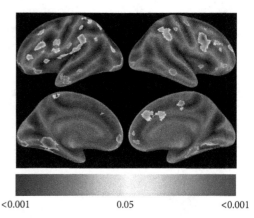

<0.001   0.05   <0.001

FIGURE 5: Whole-brain statistical maps VBM analyses. Statistical parametric maps (SPMs) illustrating increases (red) and decreases (blue) in GM volume following iTBS. Color bar values for all SPMs indicate uncorrected P values ranging from 0.05 to 0.001.

$P = 0.05$). A nonsignificant negative correlation was found between pre-iTBS connectivity and changes in right IFG activation magnitude after iTBS (partial $r = -0.60$, $P = 0.15$).

3.5. Voxel-Based Morphometry Analyses. VBM was used to test our hypothesis that patients would show changes in GM volume between pre- and post-iTBS sessions. An initial analysis using a voxelwise FDR threshold of 0.05 did not reveal any effects of iTBS on GM volume. An evaluation of the unthresholded statistical maps (Figure 5) revealed that the most reliable ($P < 0.001$, uncorrected) increases in GM volume occurred in the left medial orbital gyrus (peak MNI coordinates: −22, 52, −14; 123 voxel clusters) and in the left lingual gyrus (peak MNI coordinates: −20, −94, −14), and the most reliable ($P < 0.001$, uncorrected) decreases in GM volume occurred in the right superior frontal gyrus (peak MNI coordinates: 18, 66, 12; 8 voxel clusters) and in the right IFG pars opercularis (peak MNI coordinates: 36, 6, 30; 6 voxel clusters).

4. Discussion

Growing evidence supports the use of techniques that utilize the noninvasive modulation of cortical excitability to improve language functions in patients poststroke aphasia [28, 29, 34, 37, 40, 71–73]. However, the development and optimization of future treatment protocols that harness the full potential of these techniques are limited by a rudimentary understanding of the changes in neural function that enable their therapeutic effects [74]. The present study provides insights into this issue by characterizing changes in cortical function and structure following 10 sessions of iTBS applied to residual language-responsive cortex in a group of chronic poststroke aphasia patients. Our results show evidence for changes in language task-related responses in both the stimulated and unstimulated hemispheres following iTBS treatment that are characterized by a general shift from right-lateralized to left-lateralized responses. Moreover, we show evidence for changes in the language task-related connectivity of right-hemisphere homologues of residual left-hemisphere language areas subsequent to iTBS treatment. These findings both replicate our previously reported observations of post-iTBS changes in left- and right-hemisphere responses related to semantic decisions [34] and extend them by demonstrating that similar changes in activation as well as additional changes in interhemispheric connectivity are observed during a covert verb generation task. Importantly, the current study utilized a language task (covert verb generation) that targets different aspects of language function from our previous study, which focused on semantic decisions, and that is independent of the stimulation targeting paradigm [34]. In addition, behavioral partial correlation analyses revealed that post-iTBS changes in the function of contralesional cortex showed a strong relationship to improvements in neuropsychological measures of language function after treatment that could not be explained by interindividual differences in lesion extents. Although we only found preliminary evidence for changes in regional grey matter volume following treatment with iTBS, our results nonetheless provide evidence of structural and functional neuroplasticity subsequent to a short-duration iTBS treatment in patients with poststroke aphasia. While preliminary, these results provide important insights into the changes in cortical function that enable improvements in language abilities following iTBS treatment.

The rerecruitment of residual left-hemisphere cortex for language processes is likely an important factor for the optimal long-term recovery of language functions following LMCA stroke [12, 14–17, 19, 21, 23]. Noninvasive techniques such as iTBS may facilitate the reintegration of residual cortex into cortical language networks by promoting beneficial neuroplasticity [29, 40]. While the mechanisms underlying the neuroplastic effects of iTBS in stroke patients are not fully understood, they likely involve multiple factors including modulations of gene expression, growth factor production, neurotransmitter release, and the facilitation of synaptic plasticity [74]. Our findings provide support for the conclusion that iTBS can induce plastic changes in the function of both the stimulated and unstimulated hemispheres in patients with chronic poststroke aphasia. Indeed, our ROI results suggest that the application of iTBS to residual language-responsive cortex in the left hemisphere has the potential to reduce contralesional compensation, increase residual left-hemisphere recruitment for language task performance, and alter task-dependent interhemispheric connectivity (Figure 3). While exploratory in nature, the results from our whole-brain analyses support these conclusions. Our GLM analysis found evidence for distinct patterns of left versus right-hemisphere activity during pre-iTBS and post-iTBS sessions, with left-hemisphere frontotemporal areas showing increased activity related to covert verb generation post-iTBS (Figure 4(a)). Similarly, our gPPI analysis found evidence for large-scale changes in the connectivity of right IFG during covert verb generation between pre-iTBS and post-iTBS sessions, with widespread reductions in right IFG connectivity being observed after iTBS (Figure 4(b)).

A speculative explanation for the observed effects is that the changes in left versus right IFG activity and connectivity during covert verb generation reflect the reinstatement of balanced inhibitory interactions between left and right IFC [13, 75]. Disproportionate influences of right-hemisphere homologues on left-hemisphere language areas have been previously documented in patients with aphasia resulting from LMCA stroke [76], and it is possible that heightened right IFG activation during language tasks reflects the release of transcallosal inhibitory outputs from left to right IFG following left-hemisphere damage [14, 75]. While not reaching our threshold for statistical significance, the results of our post hoc analyses suggested that increases in left IFG activation were related to decreases in right IFG activation regardless of lesion extent. This suggests that changes in right IFG activation depended in part on changes in the function of the left IFG, although this result is preliminary and should be interpreted as such. More highly powered analyses of larger samples are therefore necessary before conclusions about this relationship can be definitively drawn.

Additionally, results from our post hoc analyses indicated that the effects of iTBS on left and right IFG function had opposite relationships with the pre-iTBS strength of right IFG to left IFG connectivity during covert verb generation. While exploratory and requiring additional validation, these results have important implications, as they suggest that preexisting interhemispheric dynamics contribute to the effects of iTBS on the function of both the stimulated and unstimulated hemispheres. This interpretation is consistent with results from a recent study that indicated that the preservation of frontal white matter tracts, specifically the left arcuate fasciculus, explains substantial interindividual variability in behavioral improvements following cathodal TDCS applied to right IFG in patients with left IFG lesions [77]. Our results indicate that patients that showed stronger right to left IFG connectivity during covert verb generation at the pre-iTBS session also showed the most pronounced effects of iTBS on both left and right IFG activation magnitudes at the post-iTBS session. While future studies comparing connectivity between stroke patients in healthy controls are necessary to fully understand the implications of these findings, the general implications are that iTBS treatment can lead to increased left IFG activity/reduced right IFG activity and reduced right IFG to left IFG connectivity during language task performance and that the effects of high-frequency iTBS on both left and right IFG activation likely depend on the preexisting interhemispheric state prior to treatment.

Nevertheless, it is pertinent to address the question of how such large-scale changes in cortical function might result from the passive stimulation of residual left-hemisphere areas. After stroke, the loss of large-scale neural populations is thought to result in an acute breakdown of function in large-scale cortical networks that enable complex cognitive functions such as language [78] and attention [79]. This abrupt disruption of neural communication and regulation might be conceptualized as a large-scale perturbation of the brain's functional state that alters the trajectory of ongoing neural signaling [42]. During recovery, adaptive changes in the residual neural populations are thought to allow for the restoration of interregional communication and regulation, and it has been proposed that successful recovery of function after stroke may reflect the restoration of a near-normal functional state, whereas poor recovery may reflect ineffective reorganization that results in an aberrant functional state that is maladapted to generating normal cognitive/behavioral outputs [42]. Thus, it might be speculated that by passively stimulating the residual left-hemisphere cortex iTBS might induce changes in the state of local neural populations that facilitate the restoration of a closer-to-normal functional brain state. An expected outcome in such a scenario would be that following iTBS patients would show task/stimulus-evoked responses that more closely resemble those observed in healthy individuals. While preliminary, the observed changes in language-related responses and interhemispheric connectivity resemble the patterns of language-related responses [24, 47] and task-dependent connectivity [48] that are observed in healthy individuals with typical language function.

While the combination of iTBS with active language therapy might also be expected to lead to an enhancement of beneficial neuroplasticity, the expectation that passive stimulation can lead to changes in task-driven responses and connectivity is not unfounded. Indeed, the cortical/subcortical networks that underlie cognitive and behavioral functions such as language and attention maintain ongoing interregional signaling even when tasks are not being performed [80–83]. Importantly, disruptions in resting state cortical networks are observed in stroke patients [43], and the structure of residual resting state networks is also altered by treatment [84]. Thus, it might be expected that passive high-frequency stimulation of a residual but dysfunctional language network node might lead to the strengthening of synaptic connections with other language network nodes and that this may facilitate the eventual reintegration of the stimulated node to the residual language network. Such an effect would be consistent with the capabilities of iTBS to induce LTP-like changes in synaptic transmission that persist beyond the stimulation period [32] and with reports that these effects are paralleled by changes in the temporal coordination of large-scale, low-frequency oscillatory activity [33].

4.1. Limitations. The present study has limitations that must be acknowledged and considered in interpreting the results and in designing future studies. Primarily, the lack of a sham-stimulation group precludes the ability to make definitive statements about whether the observed effects are specific to iTBS treatment. It is worth noting that activation patterns during the covert verb generation task have been found to be remarkably consistent across time in patients with chronic poststroke aphasia [46], and the presence of reliable effects across chronic stroke patients in the present study indicates that the observed effects are not likely due to spontaneous changes in IFG function. Nonetheless, future studies that employ a sham-stimulation control are necessary to make definitive statements regarding the neuroplastic effects of iTBS in patients with chronic poststroke aphasia.

While sham-controlled studies investigating the effects of neurostimulation on language function in patients with chronic poststroke aphasia have consistently reported behavioral improvements that are specific to real stimulation [36,

71, 73, 85], most of these have used stimulation protocols involving the application of low-frequency rTMS to the unaffected right IFG. This does make our finding that behavioral improvements subsequent to high-frequency stimulation of left IFG negatively correlated with changes in right IFG activation particularly noteworthy, as this finding supports the use of paradigms such as these that aim to suppress dysfunctional activity in right IFG. While it is possible that both approaches may be manipulating similar mechanisms to achieve improvements in behavior, it is important for future studies to characterize the similarities and differences in the neuroplastic effects induced by each approach and to identify the mechanisms by which beneficial behavioral effects are achieved. However, since iTBS increases local cortical excitability and potentiates cortical evoked responses [32, 33], it might potentiate language-related responses in residual IFG or lead to changes in LI estimates even in the absence of beneficial neuroplastic effects. For example, in the absence of some preserved interactions between left and right IFG, high-frequency stimulation of left IFG (or low-frequency stimulation of right IFG) might lead to unilateral changes in activation during language tasks that could present as a transient overall shift in LI estimates. This might provide an explanation for the absence of a relationship between overall changes in LI and improvements in SFT in the current study and for the absent [71] or weak [40] relationships between changes in LI and behavioral improvements reported by other studies that have applied low-frequency rTMS to right IFG. Indeed, while measurements such as LI provide useful summary statistics, they face intrinsic limitations that likely limit their utility in assessing the specific effects of iTBS [86]. Thus, future studies investigating the effects of iTBS in this population should consider independently the changes in left versus right-hemisphere function in addition to assessing changes in summary statistics such as LI.

A second limitation to this study is the relatively small sample size. Although some would argue that this property makes the observed significant effects more compelling since the likelihood of finding significant-but-trivial effects increases with sample size, our limited sample likely also led to the obscuration of real effects due to relatively low power [87]. Indeed, in the current study, the detrimental effects of having a small sample size would most likely manifest as insufficient power to detect real effects, especially for the whole-brain GLM, gPPI, and VBM analyses at multiple-comparisons corrected thresholds. As we did not find any significant effects at corrected P value thresholds for the whole-brain analyses, the results from these analyses should be interpreted with caution. As such, we have refrained from drawing strong conclusions about the effects of iTBS on GM volume or on activity/connectivity beyond those examined with our ROI analyses.

While the whole-brain results are exploratory and thus should not be used to draw strong conclusions about the effects of iTBS, they do merit discussion. Regarding the observed effects of iTBS on regional GM volume, it would not be surprising if iTBS did have an effect on GM morphology in these patients, as detectable changes following rTMS have been reported after in as little as five days by studies investigating the effects of rTMS on cortical morphology in healthy individuals [44]. It is also worth noting that the previously reported effects of iTBS on white matter integrity in these patients were obtained using similarly lenient thresholds [41], and given the large variability in lesion etiologies for the patients in this study, it is thus perhaps not surprising that stronger effects were not observed here. While the direction and locations of some of the most reliable VBM effects (increased GM in left prefrontal areas/decreased GM in right IFG) are in line with our expected results, the current results do not provide basis for strong conclusions but do provide support for future investigations into these effects. Similarly, as noted earlier in the discussion, the whole-brain GLM and gPPI results do show effects consistent with larger-scale changes in the responses and interactions of the residual language network during covert verb generation. Thus, future studies with larger sample sizes are necessary to provide a full characterization of the effects of iTBS in this population.

In conclusion, we investigated the effects of iTBS applied to residual language-responsive cortex in the left hemisphere on MRI measurements of cortical function and structure in eight patients with chronic poststroke aphasia. We found that iTBS was associated with increased left-lateralization of IFG activity during covert verb generation. Changes in lateralization were characterized by increases in left IFG activation magnitudes and decreases in right IFG activation magnitudes that presented as an overall shift in the lateralization of IFG activity during covert verb generation. iTBS also led to reduced right to left IFG connectivity during covert verb generation, consistent with our interpretation that the effects of iTBS are related in part to changes in context-dependent interhemispheric interactions. Interestingly, our post hoc analyses suggest that the effects of iTBS on left and right IFG function were negatively correlated across patients (increased left IFG activity was associated with decreased right IFG activity), and the changes in left versus right IFG responses had opposite relationships to pre-iTBS levels of right IFG to left IFG connectivity during covert verb generation. These data provide insights into the neuroplastic changes associated with iTBS applied to residual left-hemisphere language areas in the treatment of chronic poststroke aphasia and provide support for future research in this area. Randomized, blinded, and sham-controlled studies in a larger sample of patients are necessary and are currently in progress (e.g., NCT01512264) in order to better clarify the neuroplastic effects of iTBS in this population.

Acknowledgments

This study was supported in part by funds from the University Research Council at the University of Cincinnati (to Jerzy P. Szaflarski) and in part by R01 HD068488 (to Jerzy P. Szaflarski). The authors would like to thank anonymous reviewers for their helpful comments regarding this paper.

References

[1] P. Yarnell, P. Monroe, and L. Sobel, "Aphasia outcome in stroke: a clinical neuroradiological correlation," *Stroke*, vol. 7, no. 5, pp. 516–522, 1976.

[2] P. M. Pedersen, H. S. Jørgensen, H. Nakayama, H. O. Raaschou, and T. S. Olsen, "Aphasia in acute stroke: incidence, determinants, and recovery," *Annals of Neurology*, vol. 38, no. 4, pp. 659–666, 1995.

[3] A. Charidimou, D. Kasselimis, M. Varkanits, C. Selai, C. Potagas, and I. Evdokimidis, "Why is it difficult to predict language impairment and outcome in patients with aphasia after stroke?" *Journal of Clinical Neurology*, vol. 10, no. 2, pp. 75–83, 2014.

[4] H. C. Bastian, "On different kinds of aphasia, with special reference to their classification and ultimate pathology," *British Medical Journal*, vol. 2, no. 1401, pp. 985–990, 1887.

[5] J. P. Mohr, M. S. Pessin, S. Finkelstein, H. H. Funkenstein, G. W. Duncan, and K. R. Davis, "Broca aphasia: pathologic and clinical," *Neurology*, vol. 28, no. 4, pp. 311–324, 1978.

[6] E. A. Berker, A. H. Berker, and A. Smith, "Translation of Broca's 1865 report. Localization of speech in the third left frontal convolution," *Archives of Neurology*, vol. 43, no. 10, pp. 1065–1072, 1986.

[7] N. F. Dronkers, O. Plaisant, M. T. Iba-Zizen, and E. A. Cabanis, "Paul Broca's historic cases: high resolution MR imaging of the brains of Leborgne and Lelong," *Brain*, vol. 130, no. 5, pp. 1432–1441, 2007.

[8] H. Krestel, J.-M. Annoni, and C. Jagella, "White matter in aphasia: a historical review of the Dejerines' studies," *Brain and Language*, vol. 127, no. 3, pp. 526–532, 2013.

[9] D. Saur, B. W. Kreher, S. Schnell et al., "Ventral and dorsal pathways for language," *Proceedings of the National Academy of Sciences of the United States of America*, vol. 105, no. 46, pp. 18035–18040, 2008.

[10] D. Kümmerer, G. Hartwigsen, P. Kellmeyer et al., "Damage to ventral and dorsal language pathways in acute aphasia," *Brain*, vol. 136, no. 2, pp. 619–629, 2013.

[11] J. Fridriksson, P. Fillmore, D. Guo, and C. Rorden, "Chronic Broca's Aphasia is caused by damage to Broca's and Wernicke's areas," *Cerebral Cortex*, vol. 25, no. 12, pp. 4689–4696, 2015.

[12] D. Saur, R. Lange, A. Baumgaertner et al., "Dynamics of language reorganization after stroke," *Brain*, vol. 129, no. 6, pp. 1371–1384, 2006.

[13] W.-D. Heiss and A. Thiel, "A proposed regional hierarchy in recovery of post-stroke aphasia," *Brain and Language*, vol. 98, no. 1, pp. 118–123, 2006.

[14] P. E. Turkeltaub, S. Messing, C. Norise, and R. H. Hamilton, "Are networks for residual language function and recovery consistent across aphasic patients?" *Neurology*, vol. 76, no. 20, pp. 1726–1734, 2011.

[15] H. Karbe, A. Thiel, G. Weber-Luxenburger, K. Herholz, J. Kessler, and W.-D. Heiss, "Brain plasticity in poststroke aphasia: what is the contribution of the right hemisphere?" *Brain and Language*, vol. 64, no. 2, pp. 215–230, 1998.

[16] H. J. Rosen, S. E. Petersen, M. R. Linenweber et al., "Neural correlates of recovery from aphasia after damage to left inferior frontal cortex," *Neurology*, vol. 55, no. 12, pp. 1883–1894, 2000.

[17] C. A. M. M. van Oers, M. Vink, M. J. E. van Zandvoort et al., "Contribution of the left and right inferior frontal gyrus in recovery from aphasia. A functional MRI study in stroke patients with preserved hemodynamic responsiveness," *NeuroImage*, vol. 49, no. 1, pp. 885–893, 2010.

[18] J. Fridriksson, "Preservation and modulation of specific left hemisphere regions is vital for treated recovery from anomia in stroke," *The Journal of Neuroscience*, vol. 30, no. 35, pp. 11558–11564, 2010.

[19] J. Fridriksson, L. Bonilha, J. M. Baker, D. Moser, and C. Rorden, "Activity in preserved left hemisphere regions predicts anomia severity in aphasia," *Cerebral Cortex*, vol. 20, no. 5, pp. 1013–1019, 2010.

[20] J. P. Szaflarski, J. B. Allendorfer, C. Banks, J. Vannest, and S. K. Holland, "Recovered vs. not-recovered from post-stroke aphasia: the contributions from the dominant and non-dominant hemispheres," *Restorative Neurology and Neuroscience*, vol. 31, no. 4, pp. 347–360, 2013.

[21] L. Winhuisen, A. Thiel, B. Schumacher et al., "Role of the contralateral inferior frontal gyrus in recovery of language function in poststroke aphasia: a combined repetitive transcranial magnetic stimulation and positron emission tomography study," *Stroke*, vol. 36, no. 8, pp. 1759–1763, 2005.

[22] L. Winhuisen, A. Thiel, B. Schumacher et al., "The right inferior frontal gyrus and poststroke aphasia: a follow-up investigation," *Stroke*, vol. 38, no. 4, pp. 1286–1292, 2007.

[23] F. Mattioli, C. Ambrosi, L. Mascaro et al., "Early aphasia rehabilitation is associated with functional reactivation of the left inferior frontal gyrus: a pilot study," *Stroke*, vol. 45, no. 2, pp. 545–552, 2014.

[24] J. R. Binder, J. A. Frost, T. A. Hammeke, R. W. Cox, S. M. Rao, and T. Prieto, "Human brain language areas identified by functional magnetic resonance imaging," *The Journal of Neuroscience*, vol. 17, no. 1, pp. 353–362, 1997.

[25] R. A. Poldrack, A. D. Wagner, M. W. Prull, J. E. Desmond, G. H. Glover, and J. D. E. Gabrieli, "Functional specialization for semantic and phonological processing in the left inferior prefrontal cortex," *NeuroImage*, vol. 10, no. 1, pp. 15–35, 1999.

[26] S. G. Costafreda, C. H. Y. Fu, L. Lee, B. Everitt, M. J. Brammer, and A. S. David, "A systematic review and quantitative appraisal of fMRI studies of verbal fluency: role of the left inferior frontal gyrus," *Human Brain Mapping*, vol. 27, no. 10, pp. 799–810, 2006.

[27] J. Fridriksson, J. D. Richardson, P. Fillmore, and B. Cai, "Left hemisphere plasticity and aphasia recovery," *NeuroImage*, vol. 60, no. 2, pp. 854–863, 2012.

[28] M. A. Naeser, P. I. Martin, M. Ho et al., "Transcranial magnetic stimulation and aphasia rehabilitation," *Archives of Physical Medicine and Rehabilitation*, vol. 93, no. 1, supplement, pp. S26–S34, 2012.

[29] P. P. Shah, J. P. Szaflarski, J. Allendorfer, and R. H. Hamilton, "Induction of neuroplasticity and recovery in post-stroke aphasia by non-invasive brain stimulation," *Frontiers in Human Neuroscience*, vol. 7, article 888, 2013.

[30] E. Raffin and H. R. Siebner, "Transcranial brain stimulation to promote functional recovery after stroke," *Current Opinion in Neurology*, vol. 27, no. 1, pp. 54–60, 2014.

[31] G. Di Pino, G. Pellegrino, G. Assenza et al., "Modulation of brain plasticity in stroke: a novel model for neurorehabilitation," *Nature Reviews Neurology*, vol. 10, pp. 597–608, 2014.

[32] Y.-Z. Huang, M. J. Edwards, E. Rounis, K. P. Bhatia, and J. C. Rothwell, "Theta burst stimulation of the human motor cortex," *Neuron*, vol. 45, no. 2, pp. 201–206, 2005.

[33] O. Papazachariadis, V. Dante, P. F. M. J. Verschure, P. Del Giudice, and S. Ferraina, "iTBS-induced LTP-like plasticity parallels oscillatory activity changes in the primary sensory and motor areas of macaque monkeys," *PLoS ONE*, vol. 9, no. 11, Article ID e112504, 2014.

[34] J. P. Szaflarski, J. Vannest, S. W. Wu, M. W. DiFrancesco, C. Banks, and D. L. Gilbert, "Excitatory repetitive transcranial magnetic stimulation induces improvements in chronic post-

stroke aphasia," *Medical Science Monitor*, vol. 17, no. 3, pp. CR132–CR139, 2011.

[35] R. Holland, A. P. Leff, O. Josephs et al., "Speech facilitation by left inferior frontal cortex stimulation," *Current Biology*, vol. 21, no. 16, pp. 1403–1407, 2011.

[36] E. M. Khedr, N. Abo El-Fetoh, A. M. Ali et al., "Dual-hemisphere repetitive transcranial magnetic stimulation for rehabilitation of poststroke aphasia: a randomized, double-blind clinical trial," *Neurorehabilitation and Neural Repair*, vol. 28, no. 8, pp. 740–750, 2014.

[37] M. A. Naeser, P. I. Martin, M. Nicholas et al., "Improved picture naming in chronic aphasia after TMS to part of right Broca's area: an open-protocol study," *Brain and Language*, vol. 93, no. 1, pp. 95–105, 2005.

[38] C. H. S. Barwood, B. E. Murdoch, B.-M. Whelan et al., "Improved language performance subsequent to low-frequency rTMS in patients with chronic non-fluent aphasia post-stroke," *European Journal of Neurology*, vol. 18, no. 7, pp. 935–943, 2011.

[39] J. Kindler, R. Schumacher, D. Cazzoli et al., "Theta burst stimulation over the right Broca's homologue induces improvement of naming in aphasic patients," *Stroke*, vol. 43, no. 8, pp. 2175–2179, 2012.

[40] A. Thiel, A. Hartmann, I. Rubi-Fessen et al., "Effects of noninvasive brain stimulation on language networks and recovery in early poststroke aphasia," *Stroke*, vol. 44, no. 8, pp. 2240–2246, 2013.

[41] J. B. Allendorfer, J. M. Storrs, and J. P. Szaflarski, "Changes in white matter integrity follow excitatory rTMS treatment of post-stroke aphasia," *Restorative Neurology and Neuroscience*, vol. 30, no. 2, pp. 103–113, 2012.

[42] A. R. Carter, G. L. Shulman, and M. Corbetta, "Why use a connectivity-based approach to study stroke and recovery of function?" *NeuroImage*, vol. 62, no. 4, pp. 2271–2280, 2012.

[43] A. K. Rehme and C. Grefkes, "Cerebral network disorders after stroke: evidence from imaging-based connectivity analyses of active and resting brain states in humans," *The Journal of Physiology*, vol. 591, no. 1, pp. 17–31, 2013.

[44] A. May, G. Hajak, S. Gänßbauer et al., "Structural brain alterations following 5 days of intervention: dynamic aspects of neuroplasticity," *Cerebral Cortex*, vol. 17, no. 1, pp. 205–210, 2007.

[45] J. P. Szaflarski, S. K. Holland, L. M. Jacola, C. Lindsell, M. D. Privitera, and M. Szaflarski, "Comprehensive presurgical functional MRI language evaluation in adult patients with epilepsy," *Epilepsy and Behavior*, vol. 12, no. 1, pp. 74–83, 2008.

[46] K. P. Eaton, J. P. Szaflarski, M. Altaye et al., "Reliability of fMRI for studies of language in post-stroke aphasia subjects," *NeuroImage*, vol. 41, no. 2, pp. 311–322, 2008.

[47] M. L. Seghier, F. Kherif, G. Josse, and C. J. Price, "Regional and hemispheric determinants of language laterality: implications for preoperative fMRI," *Human Brain Mapping*, vol. 32, no. 10, pp. 1602–1614, 2011.

[48] M. L. Seghier, G. Josse, A. P. Leff, and C. J. Price, "Lateralization is predicted by reduced coupling from the left to right prefrontal cortex during semantic decisions on written words," *Cerebral Cortex*, vol. 21, no. 7, pp. 1519–1531, 2011.

[49] E. Kaplan, H. Goodglass, S. Weintraub, O. Segal, and A. van Loon-Vervoorn, *Boston Naming Test*, 2001.

[50] D. M. Dunn and L. M. Dunn, *Peabody Picture Vocabulary Test*, Manual. Pearson, 2007.

[51] E. Kozora and C. M. Cullum, "Generative naming in normal aging: total output and qualitative changes using phonemic and

semantic constraints," *Clinical Neuropsychologist*, vol. 9, no. 4, pp. 313–320, 1995.

[52] M. D. Lezak, D. B. Howieson, D. W. Loring, J. H. Hannay, and J. S. Fischer, *Neuropsychological Assessment (3)*, Oxford University Press, New York, NY, USA, 1995.

[53] H. Goodglass, E. Kaplan, and B. Barresi, *The Assessment of Aphasia and Related Disorders*, Lea & Febiger, Philadelphia, Pa, USA, 1972.

[54] F. Pulvermüller, B. Neininger, T. Elbert et al., "Constraint-induced therapy of chronic aphasia after stroke," *Stroke*, vol. 32, no. 7, pp. 1621–1626, 2001.

[55] J. C. Griffis, J. B. Allendorfer, and J. P. Szaflarski, "Voxel-based Gaussian naïve Bayes classification of ischemic stroke lesions in individual T1-weighted MRI scans," *Journal of Neuroscience Methods*, vol. 257, pp. 97–108, 2016.

[56] T. Asami, S. Bouix, T. J. Whitford, M. E. Shenton, D. F. Salisbury, and R. W. Mccarley, "Longitudinal loss of gray matter volume in patients with first-episode schizophrenia: DARTEL automated analysis and ROI validation," *NeuroImage*, vol. 59, no. 2, pp. 986–996, 2012.

[57] P. Ripollés, J. Marco-Pallarés, R. de Diego-Balaguer et al., "Analysis of automated methods for spatial normalization of lesioned brains," *NeuroImage*, vol. 60, no. 2, pp. 1296–1306, 2012.

[58] J. Ashburner and K. J. Friston, "Voxel-based morphometry—the methods," *NeuroImage*, vol. 11, no. 6, pp. 805–821, 2000.

[59] D. R. Gitelman, J. Ashburner, K. J. Friston, L. K. Tyler, and C. J. Price, "Voxel-based morphometry of herpes simplex encephalitis," *NeuroImage*, vol. 13, no. 4, pp. 623–631, 2001.

[60] K. J. Friston, A. P. Holmes, K. J. Worsley, J.-P. Poline, C. D. Frith, and R. S. J. Frackowiak, "Statistical parametric maps in functional imaging: a general linear approach," *Human Brain Mapping*, vol. 2, no. 4, pp. 189–210, 1994.

[61] M. Meinzer, P. M. Beeson, S. Cappa et al., "Neuroimaging in aphasia treatment research: consensus and practical guidelines for data analysis," *NeuroImage*, vol. 73, pp. 215–224, 2013.

[62] M. Wilke and K. Lidzba, "LI-tool: a new toolbox to assess lateralization in functional MR-data," *Journal of Neuroscience Methods*, vol. 163, no. 1, pp. 128–136, 2007.

[63] D. G. McLaren, M. L. Ries, G. Xu, and S. C. Johnson, "A generalized form of context-dependent psychophysiological interactions (gPPI): a comparison to standard approaches," *NeuroImage*, vol. 61, no. 4, pp. 1277–1286, 2012.

[64] K. J. Friston, C. Buechel, G. R. Fink, J. Morris, E. Rolls, and R. J. Dolan, "Psychophysiological and modulatory interactions in neuroimaging," *NeuroImage*, vol. 6, no. 3, pp. 218–229, 1997.

[65] J. X. O'Reilly, M. W. Woolrich, T. E. J. Behrens, S. M. Smith, and H. Johansen-Berg, "Tools of the trade: psychophysiological interactions and functional connectivity," *Social Cognitive and Affective Neuroscience*, vol. 7, no. 5, Article ID nss055, pp. 604–609, 2012.

[66] A. Bartels and S. Zeki, "The chronoarchitecture of the cerebral cortex," *Philosophical Transactions of the Royal Society B: Biological Sciences*, vol. 360, no. 1456, pp. 733–750, 2005.

[67] Y. Benjamini and Y. Hochberg, "Controlling the false discovery rate: a practical and powerful approach to multiple testing," *Journal of the Royal Statistical Society: Series B*, vol. 57, pp. 289–300, 1995.

[68] C. R. Genovese, N. A. Lazar, and T. Nichols, "Thresholding of statistical maps in functional neuroimaging using the false discovery rate," *NeuroImage*, vol. 15, no. 4, pp. 870–878, 2002.

[69] A. Mechelli, C. J. Price, K. J. Friston, and J. Ashburner, "Voxel-based morphometry of the human brain: methods and applica-tions," *Current Medical Imaging Reviews*, vol. 1, no. 2, pp. 105–113, 2005.

[70] J. B. Allendorfer, B. M. Kissela, S. K. Holland, and J. P. Szaflarski, "Different patterns of language activation in post-stroke aphasia are detected by overt and covert versions of the verb generation fMRI task," *Medical Science Monitor*, vol. 18, no. 3, pp. CR135–CR147, 2012.

[71] N. Weiduschat, A. Thiel, I. Rubi-Fessen et al., "Effects of repetitive transcranial magnetic stimulation in aphasic stroke: a randomized controlled pilot study," *Stroke*, vol. 42, no. 2, pp. 409–415, 2011.

[72] P. Marangolo, V. Fiori, M. A. Calpagnano et al., "tDCS over the left inferior frontal cortex improves speech production in aphasia," *Frontiers in Human Neuroscience*, vol. 7, article 539, 2013.

[73] C.-L. Ren, G.-F. Zhang, N. Xia et al., "Effect of low-frequency rTMS on aphasia in stroke patients: a meta-analysis of randomized controlled trials," *PLoS ONE*, vol. 9, no. 7, Article ID e102557, 2014.

[74] K. A. Bates and J. Rodger, "Repetitive transcranial magnetic stimulation for stroke rehabilitation-potential therapy or misplaced hope?" *Restorative Neurology and Neuroscience*, vol. 33, no. 4, pp. 557–569, 2015.

[75] A. Thiel, B. Schumacher, K. Wienhard et al., "Direct demonstration of transcallosal disinhibition in language networks," *Journal of Cerebral Blood Flow and Metabolism*, vol. 26, no. 9, pp. 1122–1127, 2006.

[76] G. Uruma, W. Kakuda, and M. Abo, "Changes in regional cerebral blood flow in the right cortex homologous to left language areas are directly affected by left hemispheric damage in aphasic stroke patients: evaluation by Tc-ECD SPECT and novel analytic software," *European Journal of Neurology*, vol. 17, no. 3, pp. 461–469, 2010.

[77] C. Rosso, V. Perlbarg, R. Valabregue et al., "Broca's area damage is necessary but not sufficient to induce after-effects of cathodal tDCS on the unaffected hemisphere in post-stroke aphasia," *Brain Stimulation*, vol. 7, no. 5, pp. 627–635, 2014.

[78] D. Saur and G. Hartwigsen, "Neurobiology of language recovery after stroke: lessons from neuroimaging studies," *Archives of Physical Medicine and Rehabilitation*, vol. 93, no. 1, pp. S15–S25, 2012.

[79] B. J. He, A. Z. Snyder, J. L. Vincent, A. Epstein, G. L. Shulman, and M. Corbetta, "Breakdown of functional connectivity in frontoparietal networks underlies behavioral deficits in spatial neglect," *Neuron*, vol. 53, no. 6, pp. 905–918, 2007.

[80] M. D. Fox, A. Z. Snyder, J. L. Vincent, M. Corbetta, D. C. Van Essen, and M. E. Raichle, "The human brain is intrinsically organized into dynamic, anticorrelated functional networks," *Proceedings of the National Academy of Sciences of the United States of America*, vol. 102, no. 27, pp. 9673–9678, 2005.

[81] M. D. Fox, M. Corbetta, A. Z. Snyder, J. L. Vincent, and M. E. Raichle, "Spontaneous neuronal activity distinguishes human dorsal and ventral attention systems," *Proceedings of the National Academy of Sciences of the United States of America*, vol. 103, no. 26, pp. 10046–10051, 2006.

[82] J. D. Power, A. L. Cohen, S. M. Nelson et al., "Functional network organization of the human brain," *Neuron*, vol. 72, no. 4, pp. 665–678, 2011.

[83] A. U. Turken and N. F. Dronkers, "The neural architecture of the language comprehension network: converging evidence from lesion and connectivity analyses," *Frontiers in Systems Neuroscience*, vol. 5, article 1, 2011.

[84] S. van Hees, K. McMahon, A. Angwin, G. de Zubicaray, S. Read, and D. A. Copland, "A functional MRI study of the relationship between naming treatment outcomes and resting state functional connectivity in post-stroke aphasia," *Human Brain Mapping*, vol. 35, no. 8, pp. 3919–3931, 2014.

[85] P.-Y. Tsai, C.-P. Wang, J. S. Ko, Y.-M. Chung, Y.-W. Chang, and J.-X. Wang, "The persistent and broadly modulating effect of inhibitory rTMS in nonfluent aphasic patients: a sham-controlled, double-blind study," *Neurorehabilitation and Neural Repair*, vol. 28, no. 8, pp. 779–787, 2014.

[86] M. L. Seghier, "Laterality index in functional MRI: methodological issues," *Magnetic Resonance Imaging*, vol. 26, no. 5, pp. 594–601, 2008.

[87] K. Friston, "Ten ironic rules for non-statistical reviewers," *NeuroImage*, vol. 61, no. 4, pp. 1300–1310, 2012.

4

Verbal Comprehension Ability in Aphasia: Demographic and Lexical Knowledge Effects

Panagiotis G. Simos,[1] **Dimitrios Kasselimis,**[1]
Constantin Potagas,[2] **and Ioannis Evdokimidis**[2]

[1] *School of Medicine, University of Crete, Voutes Campus, 71003 Heraklion, Greece*
[2] *Department of Neurology, University of Athens Medical School, Greece*

Correspondence should be addressed to Panagiotis G. Simos; akis.simos@gmail.com

Academic Editor: Argye E. Hillis

Background. Assessment of sentence-level auditory comprehension can be performed with a variety of tests varying in response requirements. A brief and easy to administer measure, not requiring an overt verbal or a complex motor response, is essential in any test battery for aphasia. *Objective.* The present study examines the clinical utility of receptive language indices for individuals with aphasia based on the Comprehension of Instructions in Greek (CIG), a variant of the Token Test, and the Greek version of PPVT-R. *Methods.* Normative data from a large community sample of Greek adults aged 46–80 years was available on both measures. A word-level-independent measure of auditory comprehension was computed as the standard score difference between the two tests and used to compare patients with and without comprehension deficits as indicated by their Boston Diagnostic Aphasia Examination profile. *Results and Conclusions.* Indices of internal consistency and test-retest reliability were very good. Education and age effects on performance were significant, with the former being stronger. The potential clinical utility of differential ability indices (contrasting sentence- and word-level auditory comprehension tests) is discussed.

1. Introduction

Auditory comprehension is one of the major components of general linguistic ability and many individuals with aphasia demonstrate comprehension deficits. These deficits are commonly associated with lesions in various left hemisphere regions, including the posterior middle temporal gyrus, the anterior superior temporal gyrus, the superior temporal sulcus, the angular gyrus, and frontal areas BA 46 and BA 47 [1]. In general, auditory comprehension is assessed at two levels: at the word level (word level auditory comprehension, henceforth WLAC) and at the sentence level (sentence level auditory comprehension, henceforth SLAC). In clinical settings, comprehension of spoken sentences is considered more critical and predictive of overall linguistic and social functioning and requires a set of intact cognitive functions, including lexical/semantic access (primarily tapped by WLAC tasks), syntactic processing, and working memory [2–4].

The ability to extract meaning from spoken sentences can be assessed with a variety of task formats. Some tests were specifically designed to assess processing of particular syntactic sentence frames, such as the Sentence Comprehension Test of the Northwestern Assessment of Verbs and Sentences [5, 6], the Subject-relative, Object-relative, Active, Passive syntactic battery [7], and the Syntactic Comprehension test included in the Bilingual Aphasia Battery ([8] also available in Greek: [9, 10]). The majority of tests employed in routine clinical practice, however, were designed to provide a global measure of comprehension of spoken language. Such tests include the Complex Ideational Material and Commands subtests of the Boston Diagnostic Aphasia Examination (BDAE; [11] also available in Greek: [12] Papathanasiou, Kasselimis, and Simos, in preparation). Similar tasks are included in the Western Aphasia Battery [13]. Stand-alone tests of SLAC assessing the ability to understand and respond to simple verbal commands, such as the Token Test [14], are also available. Although these tests were not designed to identify deficits in the appreciation of particular syntactic structures, they correlate highly with auditory comprehension and language production scores [2], are rather sensitive to even mild aphasic impairments [2, 15], and, given that they do not require a verbal response, are considered very useful in the evaluation of persons with severe nonfluent aphasia, particularly in the presence of significant time constraints on the assessment procedure.

One key issue involved in the interpretation of deficits documented on single SLAC tests concerns the specificity of results, which may be limited by the concurrent presence of word-level comprehension deficits in some patients. In principle, combining performance on separate scales to assess WLAC and SLAC separately may help improve sensitivity for a more global assessment of auditory comprehension, as well as specificity for detecting sentence-level comprehension difficulties. Such an approach requires normative data on both WLAC and SLAC tests, preferably in the same representative population sample. Given the wealth of evidence demonstrating age and education level effects on both types of tests [12, 16–20], the use of age- and education-adjusted norms is also important in this endeavor. Few studies thus far have contrasted the ability to comprehend verbal instructions with lexical knowledge in order to provide a more informative measure of sentence comprehension, controlling for individual variability in word-level comprehension [21–24].

In the present study, we assessed the psychometric properties (including demographic effects) of a stand-alone SLAC test, consisting of a modified version of the Token Test (originally developed in [14], henceforth referred to as Comprehension of Instructions in Greek-CIG). Further, the psychometric properties and clinical application of a differential measure of SLAC (controlling for WLAC ability) were examined. The Peabody Picture Vocabulary Test-R (PPVT-R, [25]), adapted in Greek by Simos et al. [20], was chosen as measure of WLAC, as it features identical response requirements (manual pointing to target) with CIG. The PPVT-R was designed as a receptive vocabulary test and performance on this test loads primarily on verbal comprehension-related factors [26]. Further, the two tasks pose similar demands for decision making (given that the participant is asked to choose between several alternative stimuli). While acknowledging the obvious limitations of assessing such a complex function, as auditory comprehension, through a single task, we argue that such a test could be a useful neuropsychological tool for assessing SLAC, since it engages most, if not all, of the fundamental processes involved in this function. The clinical sample consisted of 22 individuals with aphasia secondary to stroke who were classified as comprehension-impaired or comprehension-unimpaired based on their BDAE profiles. Data from a large (N = 480) community sample of Greek adults were used to compute standard scores on both tests, making it possible to assess group effects on performance differences between CIG and PPVT-R. It was hypothesized that use of a word-level-independent measure of auditory comprehension could improve detection of global comprehension deficits in persons with aphasia and be better equipped to discriminate such difficulties from deficits restricted to sentence comprehension with preserved word

comprehension. It was predicted that a sizable percentage of aphasia patients who displayed global comprehension deficits (as assessed by BDAE) would score in the impaired range on CIG despite normal-range performance on word comprehension. Conversely, encountering patients who show the reverse performance profile would be much less likely.

2. Methods

2.1. Participants

2.1.1. Community Cohort. Participants were 480 individuals aged 46–83 years recruited from 8 broad geographic areas of mainland Greece. All participants reportedly had normal or corrected to normal vision and hearing and were native Greek speakers. To further ensure that sensory deficits did not affect performance, examiners were trained to observe signs of hearing loss during the preliminary clinical interview. Individuals who appeared to have trouble understanding the examiners' queries at normal, conversational voice level were not included in the data set. Additional exclusion criteria included history of neurological or psychiatric disease or head injury resulting in loss of consciousness >10 min. Test-retest data were obtained from 20 participants within a period of 1-2 weeks. Data collection was performed between 9-2007 and 2-2009. Detailed demographic information on the normative sample has been reported previously by our group [20].

Individuals with aphasia included 22 men aged 33–80 years (mean: 57.82, SD: 10.88 years) with 6–17 years of formal education (mean: 10.45, SD: 4.18 years). All patients reported normal or corrected to normal vision and hearing and were native Greek speakers. All individuals with aphasia were evaluated by a trained neuropsychologist at the Eginition University Hospital. Testing was performed between 4 and 12 months after stroke and included the Greek adaptation of the Boston Diagnostic Aphasia Examination [12]. With the exception of two, all participants were evaluated >6 months after stroke. On the basis of their BDAE scores, standard BDAE profiles were generated, according to which patients were classified into five taxonomic categories: Broca's (n = 9), Wernicke's (n = 2), global (n = 8), transcortical motor (n = 2), and transcortical sensory (n = 1) aphasia. Patients were then divided into two groups: comprehension unimpaired (CU group consisting of patients with Broca's and transcortical motor aphasia; n = 11) and comprehension impaired (CI group consisting of patients with Wernicke's, global, and transcortical sensory aphasia; n = 11). The two groups did not differ in age (P > .07) or years of formal education (P > .85; see Table 1).

2.2. Materials. Several versions of the Token test are available [28–34] featuring sets of plastic tokens of various sizes, shapes, and colors. For the purposes of the present study, we adopted the pictorial format of the Token Test introduced by Korkman et al. [35] and included in the NEPSY battery. Initially, 14 verbal instructions were devised to represent

TABLE 1: Demographic characteristics of the community and patient samples.

	Community sample	Comprehension rating[3]	
		Impaired[4] (N = 11)	Nonimpaired (N = 11)
Age (years)[1]	62.88 (9.18)	61.45 (12.08)	54.17 (8.57)
	46–83	33–80	38–67
Education (years)	11.22 (4.62)	10.54 (4.63)	10.36 (3.90)
	0–20	6–17	6–16
Gender			
Men	195	11	11
Women	285	0	0
Occupation[2]			
Manual labor	122	3	2
Clerical	176	7	7
Homemaker	64	0	0
Scientific[3]	118	1	2
Geographic area			
Urban	168	9	10
Rural/small town	112	2	1

[1]Mean (SD) and range. [2]Current occupation or main occupation prior to retirement. [3]Professional occupation requiring a university degree, such as doctor, architect, pharmacist, and teacher. [4]Based on BDAE comprehension domain.

increasing levels of difficulty (in verbal complexity and short-term/working memory load). The stimulus consisted of a plate depicting five crosses and four circles varying in color (blue, yellow, red, black, and white) and arranged in a 3 × 3 grid. The participant was asked to point to one or two shapes in a particular sequence specified by the examiner. In pilot testing, all items were administered to 70 men and women aged 50–70 years without history of neurological or psychiatric disorder. Pilot data (item difficulty estimates based on proportion of individuals responding correctly and item-total correlations) did not indicate the need to eliminate any items or change the order of item presentation. All CIG items were administered.

The Greek adaptation of the PPVT-R was used to assess WLAC [20] consisting of 173 stimulus plates. Changes in the target stimulus were deemed necessary on several plates following pilot testing as well as changes in the order of presentation of several items. Cronbach's alpha was .98 and test-retest reliability was estimated at $r = .88$. PPVT-R administration to adult participants started with item 50. The administration was discontinued after 8 errors on 10 consecutive responses. In case of an incorrect response within the first 6 items (items 50–55), reverse administration was implemented until a baseline of 6 consecutive correct responses was reached.

Test administration was conducted individually by trained examiners. Short breaks were taken as required. Participation in the testing was voluntary and participants were informed that they could discontinue at any time.

2.3. Analyses. Item-level exploratory analyses on CIG were first performed on the data from the community sample (N = 480). The stability index for the total score was satisfactory (test-retest $r = .70$). Chronbach's alpha was .76 (all item-total correlation coefficients were >.3 with the exception of item no. 1 which was associated with near perfect performance and close to zero variance in this sample). Zero-order and partial correlation coefficients were used to estimate the effects of demographic variables and divide the sample into age- and education-level subgroups. Further, linear multiple regression analyses were implemented in order to ensure that age and education did not, independently, exert significant influence on CIG scores within each subgroup. Next, the effect of gender as well as the interaction between age and education on CIG raw scores was assessed through an ANOVA with gender age group, and education level group as the between-subjects variables. Finally, demographically adjusted standard scores were computed for PPVT-R and CIG, as well as difference scores reflecting differential ability on SLAC and WLAC. Two sets of difference scores were computed: simple algebraic difference and using Payne and Jones' [27] method which takes into account the intercorrelation between the original test scores in the normative population using the formula $Z_D = Z_{CIG} - Z_{PPVT}/\sqrt{2 - 2r_{xy}}$.

Finally, the utility of each set of standard scores for identifying subtle SLAC deficits in the absence of word-level comprehension difficulties was examined in the patient data. This aim was pursued at both the group level and for individual patients. At the group level, we assessed the magnitude of aphasia subgroup differences on the three metrics (CIG, PPVT, and CIG-PPVT difference scores). We also cross-tabulated aphasia subgroup against the proportions of patients demonstrating impaired performance on PPVT alone, CIG alone, and on both tests (as indicated by scores falling below the 5th percentile in the respective normative distributions).

3. Results

3.1. Normative Data. Correlations of raw CIG scores were moderate with both age ($r = -.36$, $P < .0001$, partial correlation controlling for years of education: $r = -.29$) and years of formal education ($r = .43$, $P < .0001$, controlling for age: $r = .37$). Accordingly, correction for education was deemed necessary in order to obtain standard scores, which were especially important for evaluating performance differences between CIG and PPVT-R. Demographic correction was achieved by dividing the community sample into 9 age (46–56, 57–67, and 68–83 years) by education subgroups (0–6, 7–12, and 13+ years). With group size >45 in all cases, this breakdown ensured that the independent effect of each of the two demographic variables (controlling for the other variable) was nonsignificant ($|\beta| < .3$, $P > .05$).

Descriptive information on CIG performance as a function of age and education level is presented in Table 2. The gender (2) by age (3) by education level (3) ANOVA on CIG raw scores revealed significant main effects of the latter two factors ($P < .001$) which were superseded by a significant

TABLE 2: Means (SD) and interquartile range of CIG total score as a function of age and education in the community sample.

	Age (years)		
	46–56	57–67	68–83
Education (years)			
0–6	10.20 (2.39)	9.06 (2.28)	8.01 (2.70)
	9.0–12.0	7.0–11.0	6.0–10.0
7–12	11.43 (2.09)	11.32 (2.37)	9.71 (2.56)
	9.1–13.0	9.0–14.0	8.0–11.5
13+	11.74 (1.89)	11.64 (1.99)	11.60 (1.83)
	11.0–13.0	11.0–13.0	10.0–13.0

age by education level interaction, $F(4,471) = 5.31$, $P = .0001$. Follow up tests revealed that the simple main effect of age (indicating decreasing performance with advancing age) was significant for persons with elementary, $F(2,158) = 8.58$, $P = .0001$, $\eta^2 = .10$, or high-school education, $F(2,142) = 7.98$, $P = .001$, $\eta^2 = .10$, and not for participants with tertiary education, $F(2,173) = 2.68$, $P = .06$, $\eta^2 = .04$. In the two former education level groups significant performance differences (Bonferroni-corrected at $a = .05$) were restricted between the youngest and oldest groups. The effect of gender was negligible ($P > .9$).

However, CIG raw score distributions were positively skewed (skewness = −.50, kurtosis = .48, and Kolmogorov-Smirnov index significantly different from 0, $P < .001$). In order to correct this problem, raw scores were first converted to percentiles, separately for each subgroup. These age and education level-adjusted percentile scores were subsequently normalized using Blom's [36] formula. The resulting distributions of scores displayed the features of the normal distribution (skewness and kurtosis ranging between −.3 and +.3 and Kolmogorov-Smirnov indices not significantly different from 0 at the .05 level). For the entire community sample, the mean of the resulting z score distribution was −.01 (SD = .94).

Importantly, the association between CIG and PPVT-R scores in the community sample was in the moderate range (zero order $r = .56$; controlling for age and education $r = .39$). Having confirmed that performance on a measure of receptive vocabulary, that does not require an overt verbal response (PPVT-R), contributed significantly to scores on our measure of auditory comprehension at the sentence level, we explored the distribution and potential clinical utility of difference scores between the two tests in the patient sample. Age- and education-level-corrected z scores were used in these analyses. PPVT-R scores were normalized separately for the 9 subgroups, according to the results of the corresponding normative study [20]. Difference scores (CIG minus PPVT-R z score) were subsequently computed for each participant. These scores were distributed normally (skewness = −.02, kurtosis = .30, and Kolmogorov-Smyrnov = .63, $P = .8$) with a mean of −.03 and a standard deviation of 1.03 and were therefore suitable for estimating critical values indicating extremely poor SLAC in the presence of adequate WLAC. Correlations between each single test and the difference score

were in the moderate range ($r = .56$ for CIG and −.58 for PPVT-R).

3.2. Patient Data. Table 3 summarizes raw and demographically adjusted scores (PPVT-R, CIG, and CIG-PPVT-R difference scores) for controls, patients with comprehension deficits, and patients without comprehension deficits. Correlations between each single test and the difference score were in the moderate range ($r = .42$ for CIG and −.59 for PPVT-R). Nonparametric Mann-Whitney tests for two independent samples were used to compare the two patient groups, given that the normality assumption was not met (Shapiro-Wilk statistic >.73, $P < .002$). As shown in Table 3, patients with clinically evident comprehension deficits showed lower PPVT-R (raw scores: M-W $U = 11.0$, $z = −3.10$, $P = .001$; demographically adjusted scores: M-W $U = 20.0$, $z = −2.47$, $P = .014$) and CIG-PPVT difference scores (M-W $U = 22.0$, $z = −2.32$, $P = .02$) than patients without such deficits. However, the group difference failed to reach significance for CIG scores (raw or adjusted, $P > .1$). As expected, the two approaches for computing difference scores provided virtually identical results.

Inspection of Table 4 reveals that, among CU patients, only 3/11 showed deficits on CIG and PPVT-R as compared to 8/11 CI patients. Among the remaining CU patients, four scored above the 5th percentile on both tests and four showed significantly reduced performance on CIG in the presence of relatively spared word-level auditory comprehension ability. Conversely, all CI patients scored below the 5th percentile on CIG with three showing relatively unimpaired word-level auditory comprehension ability.

4. Discussion

Two key issues which could be addressed through the current data set are discussed in turn below: (a) the dependence of test performance upon demographic factors and (b) the clinical utility of CIG and CIG-PPVT difference scores.

4.1. Effects of Demographic Variables. Age effects on SLAC tests (decreasing performance with increasing age) have been reported as minimal (and nonsignificant) for middle- and older-aged individuals [17, 18, 29, 37, 38]. To our knowledge, only one study found significant age effects [39]. However, age effects have been reported for differently designed SLAC tests. For example, Beaumont et al. [16] did find that performance on the Putney Auditory Comprehension Screening Test (PACST) decreased with age. But PACST, although a SLAC test, does not require execution of complex commands but simple yes/no answers. Like age, gender effects are reported as minimal and nonsignificant by many authors [18, 37]. There are also conflicting reports on the effects of years of formal education on SLAC test performance. For instance, Strauss et al. [40] detected minimal educational-level effects on the Token Test with a sample of adults with at least 8 years of education. Other studies, however, have found education-level effects on SLAC test performance [17, 18]. Mansur et al. [19] analyzed the performance of 162 normal subjects

TABLE 3: Performance of patients presenting with and without comprehension deficits and controls on the demographically adjusted CIG, PPVT-R, and CIG-PPVT-R difference scores.

	Controls (N = 480)	Individuals with aphasia: comprehension rating	
		Impaired (N = 11)	Nonimpaired (N = 11)
CIG			
Raw (mean, SD)	10.29 (2.70)	0.63 (0.92)	3.81 (4.11)
z (mean, SD)	0.07 (0.95)	−1.79 (0.03)	−1.57 (0.34)
Range	−1.83 to 1.43	−1.86 to −1.75	−1.80 to −0.84
PPVT-R			
Raw (mean, SD)	151.03 (21.08)	87.18 (35.53)**	136.36 (18.85)
z (mean, SD)	0.06 (0.96)	−1.61 (0.18)	−0.99 (1.00)
Range	−1.75 to 1.63	−1.75 to −1.11	−1.68 to 1.47
Simple algebraic difference			
CIG-PPVT difference score			
z (mean, SD)	0.01 (1.10)	−0.17 (0.19)*	−0.57 (0.72)
Range	−3.34 to 2.95	−0.73 to −0.05	−2.31 to 2.07
Payne and Jones' [27] method			
CIG-PPVT difference score			
z (mean, SD)	0.013 (1.22)	−0.19 (0.22)	−0.36 (1.17)
Range	−3.70 to 3.26	−0.81 to −0.05	−2.56 to 2.29

Patient group differences: *P = .02, **P = .01.

TABLE 4: Cross-tabulation of the number of patients scoring in the deficient range on CIG and PPVT-R against comprehension-deficit subgroup.

	Comprehension rating			
	Impaired (n = 11)		Nonimpaired (n = 11)	
	PPVT			
	High	Low	High	Low
CIG				
High	0	0	4	0
Low	3	8	4	3

on BDAE and found that years of formal education had an effect on WLAC (comprehension of forms, colors, and numbers), while both age and education had an effect on SLAC (Complex Ideational Material).

In the present data set, age effects were relatively small, yet statistically significant, suggesting that SLAC is not resistant to aging in contrast with a number of previous studies [17, 18, 29, 37, 38]. Changes in the functional capacity of the brain with normal aging have been widely reported, and include neuronal loss and generalized atrophy, myelin changes, and the appearance of sporadic neurofibrillary tangles [41–43]. Further, ageing is associated with increased frequency and severity of a host of medical problems, the impact of which on test performance was explored in more detail in a recent report [44]. Additionally, a reduction in everyday level of mental and/or physical activity among older participants (all individuals aged 68–83 years in the current cohort were retirees) should also be considered as a potential contributing factor to age-related decline in test performance [45–47]. It should be noted, however, that age effects were notably weaker for participants with more than 10 years of education. This finding is in accordance with the notion that life-span cognitive changes are moderated by education [48].

Our results agree with previous studies concerning the existence of a substantial effect of formal education on test scores [17, 18]. Indeed, the effects of level of education, indexed by years of formal schooling, outweighed those of age. This result confirms previous studies [17, 18], reporting significant effects of educational level on SLAC test performance. Thus, our data challenge the claim of Strauss et al. [40], who suggested that, for testing subjects who have received at least 8 years of education with the Token Test, a score correction is not needed. Strong effects of education level (and age) have been reported in previous studies on Greek community cohorts on naming [20, 49]. Educational level may affect performance on verbal tests, and especially those measuring lexical knowledge, indirectly as a proxy for higher professional attainment, further formal linguistic experience, cognitive reserve, and, even, as an indicator of higher experience with formal testing situations [50]. In addition, years of education may be considered as a reflection of intrinsic intellectual abilities fostering educational advancement. Some researchers, however, regard educational level with skepticism, suggesting instead the use of performance-based measures of intellectual capacity to adjust test scores [51].

4.2. Clinical Utility of CIG and CIG-PPVT Difference Scores. Estimates of internal consistency and test-retest reliability for the entire standardization sample on both tests (i.e., PPVT-R, CIG: [20], and present study) were adequate for clinical use [52]. In this context, both tests could be very useful in clinical practice. First, they are rather brief (administration time does not exceed 7 minutes for CIG and PPVT-R short form) and do not require a verbal or a complex motor response. Therefore, they are suitable for assessing severely nonfluent individuals with aphasia or stroke patients with hemiplegia. Moreover, the partial correlation between PPVT-R and CIG, controlling for age and education, was in the moderate range, suggesting that a significant proportion of individual variance in an SLAC measure can be accounted for by word-level (lexical) knowledge.

Having met minimum psychometric requirements, we then sought to explore the potential clinical utility of differential ability indices across the two tests. Very few studies have thus far directly compared measures of auditory comprehension at the word and sentence level, which do not require an overt verbal response. A common problem when testing individuals with aphasia is that their premorbid verbal IQ is difficult to estimate reliably. Thus, the clinician cannot measure the effect of lexical knowledge on sentence comprehension. By administering two tests (one SLAC test and one WLAC test), both not requiring a verbal response, and by computing the difference between the z-scores of these two tests one could, in principle, obtain a more "pure" index of sentence-level comprehension. In the present data set, 11/22 patients were classified as impaired on PPVT-R and 18/22 on CIG, using age- and education-adjusted normative scores. However, only 11/22 patients scored in the impaired range on both tests. This finding is in agreement with the notion that auditory comprehension is not unidimensional, but rather a complex function served by several component processes [1, 53–55]. This notion is consistent with the observation that some patients encounter severe difficulty in appreciating complex syntactic structures (even in tasks that pose minimal demands on single-word lexical/semantic knowledge), while their comprehension of single words is relatively spared. The opposite trend is less common, however.

While the comprehension-impaired group was expected to have low scores on both tests, nonimpaired patients' auditory comprehension abilities are ipso facto considered to be intact. However, this was not the case. Overall, 7/11 patients scored lower than expected on CIG, with 3/11 demonstrating impaired performance also on PPVT-R. This is in accordance with the notion that a clinical, screening battery such as BDAE may not possess adequate sensitivity to reveal the full extent of a given patient's language deficits (see also [49, 56]). It may also be the case, however, that results of a single test, such as CIG, are not sufficient to draw firm conclusions on the integrity of a highly complex language function.

In this context, the present paper argues that the combined use of WLAC and SLAC test scores may provide a comprehensive description of auditory language comprehension disturbance after stroke. At first glance, the results in Table 4 may appear inconclusive. The two groups could not be easily differentiated in terms of CIG performance. This was confirmed by the lack of a significant difference between the two groups on CIG scores (see Table 3). But when performance on PPVT-R was taken into account, the two groups became evidently distinct on the basis of differential performance patterns (see Table 4). It should also be noted that a criterion of low performance on both tasks—thus indicating a "global"

auditory comprehension deficit encompassing both lexical/semantic knowledge and syntactic processing—may be of further use to differentiate between the two groups. While the majority of comprehension-impaired patients (8/11) scored in the deficient range on both tasks, this was not the case for the nonimpaired group, where only 3 patients demonstrated comparably low performance. Interestingly, deficient performance on PPVT-R was not observed among patients in the comprehension-nonimpaired group. The three patients in this group who scored below the 5th percentile on CIG may thus be considered as presenting with a pure syntactic deficit, where lexical/semantic knowledge was preserved, but syntactic processing was affected. The fact that the CIG score difference between the two groups failed to reach significance may be explained in terms of syntactic processing difficulties of the nonimpaired group, considering that 9 out of 11 patients were classified as Broca's aphasics (such deficits have been well described in Broca's aphasia; see, for example, [57]). This argument is further supported by the fact that the two groups differed significantly regarding CIG-PPVT difference score (with the nonimpaired group showing greater discrepancy between CIG and PPVT scores). However, no significant difference was found for the corrected difference score.

One final remark should be made with regard to the use of difference scores in this study and neuropsychological research in general. Difference scores derived from simple subtraction may be unreliable. In the present analyses, the use of the correction formulas suggested by Payne and Jones [27] eliminates many psychometric shortcomings, by adjusting for the intercorrelation between the two measures. However, there are still limitations of the formula, because it presumes that the two scores are normally distributed. This latter assumption may lead to overestimation of the abnormality of an individual's difference score. Crawford et al. [58] have created another formula to overcome this issue which, for samples with $N > 10$, as in the present study, is expected to produce comparable results. In any case, the validity of difference scores is an empirical question that should be assessed in practice (for a detailed discussion on the use of difference scores in neuropsychological research, see [59]).

5. Conclusion

In conclusion, the present data confirm previous studies reporting significant educational effects on SLAC. Moreover, results contradict previous findings by demonstrating deterioration in SLAC with advancing age. It should also be pointed out that, as with the majority of similar field studies, the present study was based on a sample of convenience composed of volunteers recruited from a variety of sources, a procedure that carries all the potential limitations of nonrandom sampling. However, care was taken to represent major elderly population groups as indicated by geographical distribution, educational level, and current/past occupation.

Finally, preliminary patient data support the potential clinical utility of the combined use of CIG and PPVT-R, for identifying patients with pure sentence-level comprehension deficits.

Acknowledgments

This research has been cofunded by the European Union (European Social Fund (ESF)) and Greek national funds through the Operational Program "Education and Lifelong Learning" of the National Strategic Reference Framework (NSRF)—Research Funding Program: Heracleitus II. investing in knowledge society through the European Social Fund.

References

[1] N. F. Dronkers, D. P. Wilkins, R. D. Van Valin Jr., B. B. Redfern, and J. J. Jaeger, "Lesion analysis of the brain areas involved in language comprehension," *Cognition*, vol. 92, no. 1-2, pp. 145–177, 2004.

[2] M. D. Lezak, D. B. Howieson, and D. W. Loring, *Neuropsychological Assessment*, Oxford University Press, New York, NY, USA, 2004.

[3] J. D. Noll and S. R. Randolph, "Auditory semantic, syntactic, and retention errors made by aphasic subjects on the token test," *Journal of Communication Disorders*, vol. 11, no. 6, pp. 543–553, 1978.

[4] R. Lesser, "Verbal and non verbal memory components in the token test," *Neuropsychologia*, vol. 14, no. 1, pp. 79–85, 1976.

[5] S. Cho-Reyes and C. K. Thompson, "Verb and sentence production and comprehension in aphasia: Northwestern Assessment of Verbs and Sentences (NAVS)," *Aphasiology*, vol. 26, pp. 1250–1277, 2012.

[6] C. K. Thompson, A. Meltzer-Asscher, S. Cho et al., "Syntactic and morphosyntactic processing in stroke-induced and primary progressive aphasia," *Behavioural Neurology*, vol. 26, pp. 35–54, 2013.

[7] T. Love and E. Oster, "On the categorization of aphasie typologies: the SOAP (a test of syntactic complexity)," *Journal of Psycholinguistic Research*, vol. 31, no. 5, pp. 503–529, 2002.

[8] M. Paradis, "Principles underlying the bilingual aphasia test (BAT) and its uses," *Clinical Linguistics and Phonetics*, vol. 25, no. 6-7, pp. 427–443, 2011.

[9] M. Kambanaros and K. K. Grohmann, "BATting multilingual primary progressive aphasia for Greek, English, and Czech," *Journal of Neurolinguistics*, vol. 25, pp. 520–537, 2012.

[10] K. Tsapkini, G. Jarema, and E. Kehayia, "A morphological processing deficit in verbs but not in nouns: a case study in a highly inflected language," *Journal of Neurolinguistics*, vol. 15, no. 3–5, pp. 265–288, 2002.

[11] H. Goodglass and E. Kaplan, *Boston Diagnostic Aphasia Examination*, Lea & Febiger, Philadelphia, Pa, USA, 1983.

[12] K. Tsapkini, C. H. Vlahou, and C. Potagas, "Adaptation and validation of standardized aphasia tests in different languages: lessons from the Boston diagnostic aphasia examination—short form in Greek," *Behavioural Neurology*, vol. 22, no. 3-4, pp. 111–119, 2009.

[13] A. Kertesz, *Western Aphasia Battery*, The Psychological Corporation, San Antonio, Tex, USA, 1982.

[14] E. de Renzi and L. A. Vignolo, "The token test: a sensitive test to detect receptive disturbances in aphasics," *Brain*, vol. 85, no. 4, pp. 665–678, 1962.

[15] O. Spreen and E. Strauss, *A Compendium of Neuropsychological Tests: administration, Norms, and Commentary*, Oxford University Press, New York, NY, USA, 1998.

[16] J. G. Beaumont, J. Marjoribanks, S. Flury, and T. Lintern, "Assessing auditory comprehension in the context of severe physical disability: the PACST," *Brain Injury*, vol. 13, no. 2, pp. 99–112, 1999.

[17] R. J. Ivnik, "Neuropsychological tests' norms above age 55: COWAT, BNT, MAE Token, WRAT-R Reading, AMNART, STROOP, TMT, and JLO," *Clinical Neuropsychologist*, vol. 10, no. 3, pp. 262–278, 1996.

[18] B. Orgass and K. Poeck, "Clinical validation of a new test for aphasia: an experimental study on the Token Test," *Cortex*, vol. 2, pp. 222–243, 1966.

[19] L. L. Mansur, M. Radanovic, L. Taquemori, L. Greco, and G. C. Araújo, "A study of the abilities in oral language comprehension of the Boston Diagnostic Aphasia Examination—Portuguese version: a reference guide for the Brazilian population," *Brazilian Journal of Medical and Biological Research*, vol. 38, no. 2, pp. 277–292, 2005.

[20] P. G. Simos, D. Kasselimis, and A. Mouzaki, "Age, gender, and education effects on vocabulary measures in Greek," *Aphasiology*, vol. 25, no. 4, pp. 475–491, 2011.

[21] H. Gardner, M. L. Albert, and S. Weintraub, "Comprehending a word: the influence of speed and redundancy on auditory comprehension in aphasia," *Cortex*, vol. 11, no. 2, pp. 155–162, 1975.

[22] K. M. Heilman and R. J. Scholes, "The nature of comprehension errors in Broca's conduction and Wernicke's aphasics," *Cortex*, vol. 12, no. 3, pp. 258–265, 1976.

[23] D. B. Hier, S. I. Mogil, N. P. Rubin, and G. R. Komros, "Semantic aphasia: a neglected entity," *Brain and Language*, vol. 10, no. 1, pp. 120–131, 1980.

[24] G. L. Wallace and J. H. Stapleton, "Analysis of auditory comprehension performance in individuals with severe aphasia," *Archives of Physical Medicine and Rehabilitation*, vol. 72, no. 9, pp. 674–678, 1991.

[25] L. M. Dunn and E. S. Dunn, *Peabody Picture Vocabulary Test—Revised*, American Guidance Service, Circle Pines, Minn, USA, 1981.

[26] J. P. Culbert, R. Hamer, and V. Klinge, "Factor structure of the Wechsler Intelligence scale for Children-Revised, Peabody Picture Vocabulary Test, and the Peabody Individual Assessment Test in a psychiatric sample," *Psychology in the Schools*, vol. 26, pp. 331–336, 1989.

[27] R. W. Payne and G. Jones, "Statistics for the investigation of individual cases," *Journal of Clinical Psychology*, vol. 13, no. 2, pp. 115–121, 1957.

[28] J. C. Arvedson, M. R. McNeil, and T. L. West, "Prediction of revised Token Test overall, subtest, and linguistic unit scores by two shortened versions," in *Clinical Aphasiology Conference*, pp. 57–63, BRK Publishers, Rockville, Md, USA, 1985.

[29] E. de Renzi and P. Faglioni, "Normative data and screening power of a shortened version of the token test," *Cortex*, vol. 14, no. 1, pp. 41–49, 1978.

[30] B. Hallowell, R. T. Wertz, and H. Kruse, "Using eye movement responses to index auditory comprehension: an adaptation of the Revised Token Test," *Aphasiology*, vol. 16, no. 4–6, pp. 587–594, 2002.

[31] M. M. McNeil and T. E. Prescott, *Revised Token Test*, Pro-Ed, Austin, Tex, USA, 1978.

[32] B. Orgass, "Eine Revision des Token Tests II. Validitätsnachweis, Normierung und Standardisierung," *Diagnostica*, vol. 22, pp. 141–156, 1976.

[33] O. Spreen and A. L. Benton, The Neurosensory Center Comprehensive Examination for Aphasia. Neuropsychology Laboratory, University of Victoria, 1969, 1977.

[34] A. L. Benton, Hamsher, K. de S, and A. B. Sivan, *Multilingual Aphasia Examination*, AJA Associates, Iowa City, Iowa, USA, 3rd edition, 1994.

[35] M. Korkman, U. Kirk, and S. Kemp, *NEPSY*, The Psychological Corporation, San Antonio, Tex, USA, 1998.

[36] G. Blom, *Statistical Estimates and Transformed Beta Variables*, John Wiley and Sons, New York, NY, USA, 1958.

[37] J. A. Lucas, R. J. Ivnik, G. E. Smith et al., "Mayo's older African Americans normative studies: Norms for Boston naming test, controlled oral word association, category fluency, animal naming, token test, WRAT-3 reading, trail making test, stroop test, and judgment of line orientation," *Clinical Neuropsychologist*, vol. 19, no. 2, pp. 243–269, 2005.

[38] J. B. Rich, *Pictorial and verbal implicit and recognition memory in aging and Alzheimer's disease: a transfer-appropriate processing account [Doctoral dissertation]*, University of Victoria, 1993.

[39] O. B. Emery, "Linguistic decrement in normal aging," *Language and Communication*, vol. 6, no. 1-2, pp. 47–64, 1986.

[40] E. Strauss, E. M. S. Sherman, and O. Spreen, *A Compendium of Neuropsychological Tests: Administration, Norms, and Commentary*, Oxford University Press, New York, NY, USA, 3rd edition, 2006.

[41] H. Braak and E. Braak, "Frequency of stages of Alzheimer-related lesions in different age categories," *Neurobiology of Aging*, vol. 18, no. 4, pp. 351–357, 1997.

[42] R. L. Buckner, "Memory and executive function in aging and ad: multiple factors that cause decline and reserve factors that compensate," *Neuron*, vol. 44, no. 1, pp. 195–208, 2004.

[43] F. A. Schmitt, D. G. Davis, D. R. Wekstein, C. D. Smith, J. W. Ashford, and W. R. Markesbery, "'Preclinical' AD revisited: neuropathology of cognitively normal older adults," *Neurology*, vol. 55, no. 3, pp. 370–376, 2000.

[44] P. G. Simos, D. Kasselimis, and A. Mouzaki, "Effects of demographic variables and health status on brief vocabulary measures in Greek," *Aphasiology*, vol. 25, no. 4, pp. 492–504, 2011.

[45] K. W. Schaie, "The development of intelligence in adulthood," *Zeitschrift für Gerontologie*, vol. 13, no. 4, pp. 373–384, 1980.

[46] C. Schooler, "Psychosocial factors and effective cognitive functioning in adulthood," in *Handbook of the Psychology of Aging*, J. E. Birren and K. W. Schaie, Eds., pp. 347–358, Academic Press, San Diego, Calif, USA, 3rd edition, 1990.

[47] R. F. Zec, "The neuropsychology of aging," *Experimental Gerontology*, vol. 30, no. 3-4, pp. 431–442, 1995.

[48] A. Ardila, F. Ostrosky-Solis, M. Rosselli, and C. Gómez, "Age-related cognitive decline during normal aging: the complex effect of education," *Archives of Clinical Neuropsychology*, vol. 15, no. 6, pp. 495–513, 2000.

[49] A. Patricacou, E. Psallida, T. Pring, and L. Dipper, "The Boston naming test in Greek: normative data and the effects of age and education on naming," *Aphasiology*, vol. 21, no. 12, pp. 1157–1170, 2007.

[50] F. Ostrosky-Solis, A. Ardila, M. Rosselli, G. Lopez-Arango, and V. Uriel-Mendoza, "Neuropsychological test performance in illiterate subjects," *Archives of Clinical Neuropsychology*, vol. 13, no. 7, pp. 645–660, 1998.

[51] B. A. Steinberg, L. A. Bieliauskas, G. E. Smith, C. Langellotti, and R. J. Ivnik, "Mayo's Older Americans Normative Studies: age- and IQ-adjusted norms for the Boston Naming Test, the MAE Token Test, and the Judgment of Line Orientation Test," *Clinical Neuropsychologist*, vol. 19, no. 3-4, pp. 280–328, 2005.

[52] D. V. Cicchetti, "Multiple comparison methods: establishing guidelines for their valid application in neuropsychological research," *Journal of Clinical and Experimental Neuropsychology*, vol. 16, no. 1, pp. 155–161, 1994.

[53] S. Gao and K. Sun, "The special-category semantic disturbance of auditory comprehension of aphasics," *Chinese Journal of Neurology*, vol. 35, no. 6, pp. 330–332, 2002.

[54] C. Humphries, J. R. Binder, D. A. Medler, and E. Liebenthal, "Syntactic and semantic modulation of neural activity during auditory sentence comprehension," *Journal of Cognitive Neuroscience*, vol. 18, no. 4, pp. 665–679, 2006.

[55] K. Jodzio, D. Biechowska, and B. Leszniewska-Jodzio, "Selectivity of lexical-semantic disorders in Polish-speaking patients with aphasia: evidence from single-word comprehension," *Archives of Clinical Neuropsychology*, vol. 23, no. 5, pp. 543–551, 2008.

[56] E. Peristeri and K. Tsapkini, "A comparison of the BAT and BDAE-SF batteries in determining the linguistic ability in Greek-speaking patients with Broca's aphasia," *Clinical Linguistics and Phonetics*, vol. 25, no. 6-7, pp. 464–479, 2011.

[57] D. Caplan, "Aphasic deficits in syntactic processing," *Cortex*, vol. 42, no. 6, pp. 797–804, 2006.

[58] J. R. Crawford, D. C. Howell, and P. H. Garthwaite, "Payne and Jones revisited: estimating the abnormality of test score differences using a modified paired samples t test," *Journal of Clinical and Experimental Neuropsychology*, vol. 20, no. 6, pp. 898–905, 1998.

[59] A. M. Poreh, *The Quantified Process Approach to Neuropsychological Assessment*, Taylor and Francis, New York, NY, USA, 2006.

5

Bilingual Language Control and General Purpose Cognitive Control among Individuals with Bilingual Aphasia: Evidence Based on Negative Priming and Flanker Tasks

Tanya Dash and Bhoomika R. Kar

Centre of Behavioural and Cognitive Sciences, Senate Hall Campus, University of Allahabad, Allahabad-211002, India

Correspondence should be addressed to Bhoomika R. Kar; bhoomika@cbcs.ac.in

Academic Editor: Jubin Abutalebi

Background. Bilingualism results in an added advantage with respect to cognitive control. The interaction between bilingual language control and general purpose cognitive control systems can also be understood by studying executive control among individuals with bilingual aphasia. *Objectives.* The current study examined the subcomponents of cognitive control in bilingual aphasia. A case study approach was used to investigate whether cognitive control and language control are two separate systems and how factors related to bilingualism interact with control processes. *Methods.* Four individuals with bilingual aphasia performed a language background questionnaire, picture description task, and two experimental tasks (nonlinguistic negative priming task and linguistic and nonlinguistic versions of flanker task). *Results.* A descriptive approach was used to analyse the data using reaction time and accuracy measures. The cumulative distribution function plots were used to visualize the variations in performance across conditions. The results highlight the distinction between general purpose cognitive control and bilingual language control mechanisms. *Conclusion.* All participants showed predominant use of the reactive control mechanism to compensate for the limited resources system. Independent yet interactive systems for bilingual language control and general purpose cognitive control were postulated based on the experimental data derived from individuals with bilingual aphasia.

1. Introduction

Bilingualism and cognitive control are two widely studied phenomena. Numerous studies have examined the interaction between bilingualism and cognitive control using different methodologies and paradigms [1–11]. Juggling two or more languages makes our brain more flexible [10]. The bilingual advantage has been well established not only with respect to studies comparing monolingual and bilingual individuals [6, 12–14] but also among different bilingual groups [6–9]. Interestingly, a review by Adesope et al. [15] suggested that different aspects of bilingualism influence distinct levels of cognitive control mechanisms. Moreover, several cognitive outcomes may be attributed to bilingualism, including increased attentional control, working memory, metalinguistic awareness, and abstract and symbolic representational skills. Researchers have differentiated between bilingual language control and domain general cognitive control [2, 16]. Miller and Cohen [17] proposed that to provide top-down support to language control, processes such as attention, working memory, response selection, and inhibition function as different manifestations of domain general cognitive control. Moreover, bilingual language control (bLC) may not be a subsidiary to domain general cognitive control [16]; however, bLC may still show some overlap with domain general control mechanisms [2, 18].

Different frameworks have been suggested to study the interaction between bilingualism and cognitive control. A few studies have examined the interaction between bilingualism and cognitive control in the context of bilingual aphasia [18–20]. Aphasia is a language impairment caused by brain damage. Language-related deficits are well explained in the literature targeting auditory comprehension, naming skills, spontaneous speech, and repetition as well as reading and writing skills. There are lines of evidence supporting the presence of cognitive impairment in individuals with aphasia [19, 21]; however, most of these studies refer to the independence of deficits in language skills and other cognitive processes. In one such study, Helm-Estrabrooks [22] argued that clinicians cannot predict the relative integrity of other domains of cognition on the basis of language deficits observed in aphasic patients. Another group of researchers [23] discussed the implications of different aspects of cognition in language-related treatment approaches. They employed a global aphasic neuropsychological battery (nonlinguistic tests) and a test of auditory comprehension. The battery of tests assessed attention, memory, intelligence, visual recognition, and non-verbal auditory recognition. The authors concluded that the score on this battery was independent of spoken language comprehension.

Communicative success among individuals with aphasia may be dependent on the integrity of the executive functions that allow us to plan, sequence, organise, and monitor goal-directed activities in a flexible manner. While emphasising the role of executive functions in communicative processes, Helm-Estrabrooks and Ratner [24] suggested that deficits in executive functions may result in a failure in the generalisation of skills, which are similar to those learned in therapy sessions to those learned in everyday life situations. Similarly, Purdy [19] conducted a study investigating the efficiency, speed, and accuracy of individuals with aphasia while performing executive function tasks (i.e., Porteus Maze Test, Wisconsin Card Sorting Test, and Tower of London). Their deficits were predominantly related to cognitive flexibility and, to a lesser extent, planning.

Until recently, cognitive impairments in aphasia were studied in isolation; however, this can be well explored through empirical research by examining the underlying mechanisms that manifest as cognitive impairments. A study by Penn et al. [25] supports this notion of bilingual advantage, in which they compared monolingual and bilingual individuals with aphasia. If bilingualism is a cognitive advantage, then bilingual aphasics may demonstrate a faster rate of language recovery compared to monolingual aphasics. However, bilingual aphasics exhibited pathological code switching and code mixing behaviours. In one of their studies, Abutalebi and Green [2] highlighted the need to investigate the performance of bilingual aphasics on a range of control tasks. They suggested that individuals with parallel recovery may demonstrate problems with control without having problems related to language interference.

In addition to the language processing deficits evident among individuals with aphasia, there are subtle cognitive-communicative deficits, which are not due to the faulty language processing system but may be due to general problems in resolving conflict. Green et al. [26] reported that there are two distinct control-related impairments, one for naming and another for control. Green and colleagues compared two bilingual aphasics who demonstrated a parallel form of recovery to a similar extent. However, their performance on three explicit control tasks indicated that different control mechanisms were involved in recovery. One of the patients showed an impaired verbal, but spared nonverbal control,

whereas the other patient demonstrated deficits in the selection of the manual response. Thus, two separate circuits may exist for naming and control, and the recovery patterns may be dependent on damage to these control circuits [2].

According to Abutalebi et al. [18], language control and cognitive control mechanisms may act as the primary determinants of cognitive-linguistic recovery in aphasia. This is because the effect of treatment is dependent on the integrity of the naming and control pathways as previously described by Abutalebi and Green [2]. To understand this distinction between naming and control networks, Abutalebi et al. [18] studied the neural correlates of selective language therapy in a Spanish-Italian bilingual aphasic in a longitudinal study consisting of three time points. An improvement in naming performance was evident in the naming network only. Another study [20] emphasised the role of the dorsal anterior cingulate in both language control and while resolving nonverbal conflict. Using a combined functional and structural neuroimaging method, a structural overlap between the two networks (i.e., naming and control) was demonstrated. These studies demonstrated that there was a dissociation as well as an overlap between the mechanisms that were involved while resolving verbal and nonverbal conflict.

Conflict resolution tasks involve two modes of control mechanisms, namely, proactive and reactive controls. The proactive mode of control is prospective or future-oriented, helping to prepare the cognitive system for upcoming events via the predictive use of context. Reactive control is retrospective, responding to the presence of salient events by engaging control only when it is needed, via the reactivation of previously stored information [27]. In the context of bilingualism, these two modes of control might be operating in cases of conflict and during increasing demand on the inhibitory control system while using activation-suppression mechanisms. Thus, this study aimed to address the relationship between language control and general purpose cognitive control with respect to the recruitment of proactive and reactive control mechanisms among bilingual aphasics.

The current study was designed to test patients on a range of executive function tasks that bear on the circuits implicated in language control and general purpose cognitive control. The specific objective was to examine differences in performance across executive control tasks with linguistic and nonlinguistic stimuli. Flanker and negative priming paradigms were employed to show the distinction in performances with different cognitive outcomes between the two paradigms. One way to understand how control mechanisms are recruited by bilingual aphasics is to examine the slow and fast trials, which indicate the use of reactive and proactive control mechanisms, respectively. Special emphasis was placed on accuracy, efficiency, and speed-related measures, unlike previous studies, which focused on one of the three aspects of performance. Predominant involvement of reactive control compared to proactive control mechanisms in the context of both linguistic and nonlinguistic stimuli was expected. Differences in performance were expected with respect to negative priming and flanker effects in the two paradigms, indicating variability in different control processes. Thus, the present study helps to understand the interactive yet independent control mechanisms in the clinical population, particularly in language disorders, such as aphasia, which provide the appropriate context to examine the relationship between bilingualism and cognitive control. In addition, such an investigation also helps to understand the broad cognitive-linguistic mechanisms that underlie a disease process and its recovery patterns.

2. Method

2.1. Screening Measures

2.1.1. Language Background Questionnaire [28]. This questionnaire was employed to collect information on the languages in use, frequency of use, self-reported proficiency, and the linguistic environment at home, work, and so forth. Domains assessed in the questionnaire included acquisition history (age of acquisition and at what age the subject became fluent), contexts of acquisition (modality: oral/written/both; environment of acquisition: informal/formal/both), language use (%), language preference (1–3 rating scale; where 1 = never, 2 = sometimes, 3 = most of the time), and the proficiency rating on different tasks (a 0–10 rating scale was provided for each descriptive task, for example, asking for directions, counting up to 100 in both languages, and so forth, which resulted in a composite score for proficiency). Apart from these questions, a contribution of various other factors, such as the use of language with family, friends, extended family, and neighbours was assessed by asking the participants to name the language predominantly used in different contexts. The participants also indicated the medium of instruction and self-reported proficiency level in the domains of speaking, understanding, reading, and writing (1–5 point rating) (see Table 1 for language background information for all the participants).

2.1.2. Picture Description Task. This test is a subtest of the language proficiency test [29]. In this task, the participants were instructed to carefully describe a picture by focusing on the overall theme of the picture along with the individual items in that particular picture. A grand rubric score was calculated by summing the scores on the following aspects: overall impact and achievement of purpose (whether the participant establishes the main idea), organisation and techniques (coherence and cohesion, method of organisation), and mechanics (focusing on grammar, pronunciation, presence of pause). Pictures were selected from the Western Aphasia Battery [30] and Boston Diagnostic Aphasia Examination [31] for L1 and L2, respectively. A total score of 18 could be achieved by each participant (Table 5 presents the scoring method).

2.1.3. Western Aphasia Battery [30]. WAB is a tool used to assess language functions in adults and discerns the presence and type of aphasia. Four major components of the aphasia quotient are spontaneous speech, auditory verbal comprehension, repetition, and naming. Table 3 presents the scores obtained on each of the subtasks in WAB for the four participants.

2.1.4. Aphasia Severity Rating Scale [31]. This is a severity rating scale that is often used in clinical routine as well as in scientific studies. Administration of this scale takes 5–15 minutes and is very simple to perform. It is a 5-point rating scale where the communication profile is described and based on the clinical observation that one can make a judgment about severity. Table 2 presents the ratings indicating the severity of aphasia for each of the four participants.

2.2. Participants. We report data from four male bilingual right-handed individuals with aphasia. English was the second language for all the participants. L1 was Telugu for two participants and Hindi for the other two participants. All four participants were considered for the current study based on the following inclusion criteria: (a) diagnosis of aphasia based on the Western Aphasia Battery [30], (b) above chance level performance on the experimental tasks, (c) average level of intellectual functions on Raven's Coloured Progressive Matrices test (as a subtask in WAB), (d) being able to perform the picture description task from the test of language proficiency, which provides a composite rubric score [29], (e) similar degree of impairment in L1 and L2, and (f) postmorbid daily usage of both languages in the speaking/understanding domain as well as in the reading/writing domain. These criteria were met using the subjective and objective measures mentioned above as well as the clinician's report.

All participants showed parallel recovery based on their performance on the language skills tasks as well as the self-reported information on the language background questionnaire [28]. All four participants were highly educated and were able to perform the activities of daily living. The experimental and language proficiency tasks were performed on the same day with many rest pauses (see Table 2 for a summary of the demographic information of all the participants).

2.2.1. Participant 1. CR was a 33-year-old, right-handed Telugu-English bilingual male, who was a banker prior to his illness. He had resumed his work on a part-time basis a few days from the time of his current evaluation. CR reported a complaint of a loss of speech due to a postmeningitis squeal. It had resulted in diffuse damage to the left frontal and parietal regions as per the clinician's report. CR was initially diagnosed with Broca's aphasia and is currently diagnosed with anomic aphasia. CR had been undergoing speech and language therapy for 15 months prior to the time of his current evaluation on a regular basis. On the WAB subtests, his language skills were affected in all four WAB subtasks; namely, spontaneous speech, auditory verbal comprehension, repetition, and naming. His repetition subtask score was below the 50th percentile, and his naming subtask score was at the 50th percentile level. His auditory verbal comprehension skills were better than the rest of his skills. Performance on the picture description task in both languages showed an impairment at the discourse level with rubric scores of 11 and 9 for L1 and L2, respectively (maximum score of 18). His spontaneous speech showed the presence of both circumlocutions and paraphasic errors (semantic). Language switching or mixing was neither observed nor reported.

TABLE 1: Language background information based on current state (poststroke aphasia data).

Participants	CR	MMH	SC	MU
Languages exposed at home	Telugu (sometimes Kannada)	Urdu/Hindi	Telugu (sometimes Tamil with extended family)	Hindi/Urdu
Languages exposed at office/workplace/college	English, Kannada, Hindi	English, Hindi, Kannada	English, Telugu, Hindi	English, Hindi
Age of acquisition:	L1 (Telugu): since birth L2 (English): 10th standard L3 (Kannada): after arriving at Kannada speaking state due to occupational needs in 2008	L1 (Hindi/Urdu): since birth L2 (English): 3.5 years L3 (Kannada): after arriving at Kannada speaking state (10 years)	L1 (Telugu): since birth L2 (Tamil): exposed since birth L3 (English): since school that is 1st standard	L1 (Hindi/Urdu): since birth L2 (English): since school that is 1st standard
Order of dominance (premorbid):				
L1	Telugu (60%)	Hindi/Urdu (70%)	Telugu (50%)	Hindi (50%)
L2	English (40%)	English (30%)	English (50%)	English (50%)
Order of dominance (postmorbid):				
L1	Telugu (30%)	Hindi/Urdu (85%)	Telugu (60%)	Hindi (90%)
L2	English (70%)	English (15%)	English (40%)	English (10%)
	Sporadic usage of Kannada and Hindi	Sporadic usage of Kannada	Sporadic usage of Tamil and Hindi	
Modality of language acquisition:				
L1	both (oral/written and formal/informal)	both (oral/written and formal/informal)	both (oral/written and formal/informal)	both (oral/written and formal/informal)
L2	both (oral/written and formal/informal)	both (oral/written and formal/informal)	both (oral/written and formal/informal)	both (oral/written and formal/informal)
Family members uses following languages:				
Grandparents, parents, siblings-	Telugu	Hindi/Urdu	Telugu/Tamil	Hindi
Neighbours/children-	Kannada	Kannada	Hindi/Telugu	Hindi
Language use choice: 3 point rating (composite scores)	(can perform 3/10 tasks)	(can perform 6/10 tasks)	(can perform 6/10 tasks)	(can perform 5/10 tasks)
L1	3	1	1	2.7
L2	2	2.7	3	2
Language proficiency 5 point rating (composite scores)	(can perform 5/15 tasks)	(can perform 7/15 tasks)	(can perform 6/15 tasks)	(can perform 10/15 tasks)
L1	2.25	2.53	3.1	4.25
L2	4.25	3.25	2.83	2.25
Self-reported proficiency (5-point rating)				
Reading (L1 L2)	4 4	4 4	2 2	2 3
Writing (L1 L2)	3 4	3 4	1 2	2 2
Speaking (L1 L2)	3 4	3 4	2 2	3 2
Understanding (L1 L2)	4 4	4 4	4 3	4 4

TABLE 2: Demographic information.

Participants	CR	MMH	SC	MU
Age	33 years	34 years	35 years	59 years
Etiology	Bacterial meningitis	CVA	Trauma	CVA
Time post stroke	17 months	26 months	15 months	20 months
Native language	Telugu	Hindi/Urdu	Telugu	Hindi
Educational and work background	MBA and currently employed as a banker	Postgraduate and currently unemployed	B. Tech and own a construction business	Retired as assistant controller of examination for an university
Languages known (in order of dominance)	Telugu, English, Hindi	Hindi, English, Urdu	Telugu, English, Tamil, Hindi	Hindi, English, Urdu
Aphasia type	Anomic aphasia	Anomic aphasia	Broca's aphasia	Anomic aphasia
Rehabilitation period	15 months	20 months	3 months	17 months
Aphasia severity	2	3	1	3
Language for therapy	L2	Both L1 and L2	Both L1 and L2, more emphasis L1.	L1

TABLE 3: Scores on the Western Aphasia battery.

Participants WAB task (maximum scores)	CR	MMH	SC	MU
Spontaneous speech				
Information content (10)	7	9	4	8
Fluency (10)	4	9	5	9
Auditory verbal comprehension				
Yes/no question (60)	48	60	20	58
Auditory word recognition (60)	60	58	53	48
Sequential commands (80)	40	72	21	74
Repetition (100)	45	81	26	79
Naming				
Object naming (60)	40	59	4	45
Word fluency (20)	3	12	2	15
Sentence completion (10)	4	7	2	8
Responsive speech (10)	3	10	5	9

2.2.2. Participant 2. MMH was a 34-year-old right-handed male and presented with a history of cerebrovascular disease. He was diagnosed with aphasia and was undergoing therapy. He was initially diagnosed with global aphasia and is currently diagnosed with anomic aphasia. He had a lesion in the left cerebral hemisphere involving the insular cortex, frontal, and frontoparietal region, which was suggestive of an infarct in the left middle cerebral artery territory. MMH had been undergoing speech and language therapy for 17 months prior to the time of his current evaluation. He was unemployed at the time of his current evaluation and had been undergoing speech and language therapy as well as physiotherapy and occupational therapy due to right hemiparesis. On the WAB, his spontaneous speech was greatly affected, with a score in the 70th percentile, whereas his scores were greater than the 80th percentile on rest of the tasks, namely, the auditory verbal comprehension, repetition, and naming subtasks. His spontaneous speech showed problems in fluency as well as in speech initiation. Performance on the picture description task in both languages resulted in a composite rubric score

of 14 and 12 in Hindi and English, respectively. No significant problems were observed in language selection.

2.2.3. Participant 3. SC was a 35-year-old right-handed male who presented with a history of head trauma, which resulted in a subdural hematoma in the left hemisphere involving the frontal regions. At the time of the current evaluation, SC was actively participating in the family business. His initial diagnosis was global aphasia, and his current diagnosis was Broca's aphasia. He had been regularly attending speech and language therapy sessions for three months since the injury. He demonstrated difficulties in the naming (26%) and repetition (13%) subtasks on the WAB, similar to Participant 1. Circumlocution and paraphasia were also observed more in English than Telugu. His auditory comprehension skills were better than the rest of the subtasks on the WAB with 94% accuracy. There was a difference in his performance between L1 and L2 on the picture description task. He showed a greater impairment in L2 compared to L1 with composite rubric scores of 11 and 6 for L1 and L2, respectively.

TABLE 4: Mean reaction time and standard deviations on control tasks.

Participants	CR	MMH	SC	MU
Flanker task (nonlinguistic)				
Congruent	964.42	608.85	737.2	911.98
	(556.89)	(153.17)	(181.92)	(140.86)
Incongruent	1183	580.62	877.63	915.65
	(767.47)	(158.50)	(269.85)	(183.13)
Neutral	1221.61	672.70	708.56	941.3
	(597.01)	(186.53)	(153.81)	(217.62)
Flanker task (linguistic)				
L1 congruent	1488.6	1003.08	1269.2	1467
	(450.91)	(178.79)	(270.48)	(381.61)
L1 incongruent within	1319.52	999.71	1136.62	1406.38
	(476.38)	(231.41)	(229.28)	(342.35)
L1 incongruent across	1318.94	1023.84	1303.63	1639.66
	(423.27)	(154.55)	(296.71)	(387.03)
L2 congruent	1439.38	896.9	1218.21	1336.71
	(503.12)	(143.40)	(283.56)	(380.55)
L2 incongruent within	1578.68	910.13	1171.92	1130.87
	(569.45)	(149.55)	(256.05)	(252.92)
L2 incongruent across	1476.91	903.64	1208.93	1312.33
	(526.39)	(173.09)	(292.72)	(340.48)
Negative priming task				
Attended repetition	1651.69	607.45	648.08	832.27
	(769.31)	(117.23)	(301.44)	(284.72)
Control	1939.81	933.05	791.27	1626.32
	(681.08)	(131.70)	(334.3)	(269.32)
Ignored repetition	1751.57	807.33	1091.83	1232.01
	(732.14)	(201.76)	(554.43)	(434.35)

TABLE 5: Rubric for picture description: for spoken discourse analysis.

Strong: 3 points	Average: 2 points	Weak: 1 point
Overall impact and achievement of purpose		
3 Presents a vivid, memorable picture of a person, place or things	**2** Presents a clear picture of a person, place, or thing	**1** Presents an unclear or confusing picture of a person, place and thing
3 Establishes a dominant, or main, impression of the picture	**2** Focuses on important characteristic(s) of the picture	**1** Presents an unfocused array of characteristics of the picture
3 Conveys a clear sense of purpose	**2** Suggests the speakers purpose	**1** Unclear or inadequate indication of speakers' purpose
Organization and techniques		
3 Uses a clear, consistent method of organization of event	**2** Method of organization is usually clear and consistent	**1** Method of organization is difficult to identify or follow
3 Coherence and cohesion demonstrated through some appropriate use of devices (transitions, pronouns, causal linkage, etc.)	**2** Coherence and cohesion (sentence to sentence) evident; may depend on holistic structure, most transitions are appropriate	**1** Evidence of coherence may depend on sequence. If present, transitions may be simplistic or even redundant
Mechanics		
3 Very few, if any errors in grammar and pronunciation and presence of few pauses (filled and unfilled)	**2** Small number of errors in grammar and pronunciation and presence of indefinable pauses (filled and unfilled)	**1** Numerous errors in grammar and pronunciation and presence of pauses (filled and unfilled)

Note: a composite score on the picture description task is the sum of ratings across the three aspects of discourse analysis.

2.2.4. Participant 4. MU, a 59-year-old right-handed male was working at a higher administrative position at an academic institution prior to his stroke. He had experienced an ischemic stroke involving the MCA territory, which caused a typical lesion in the left frontal areas as well as white matter lesions. He presented with hemiparesis and an inability to speak. His initial diagnosis was global aphasia, and his current diagnosis was anomic aphasia. He had undergone therapy for a period of 20 months. On the auditory verbal comprehension subtask, his score was more than 90% similar to the scores of Participants 2 and 3. However, his WAB profile matched more with Participant 2. He showed a similar performance in L1 and L2 on the picture description task with scores of 14 and 12, respectively (see Table 3 for scores on the WAB for all participants).

2.3. Control Tasks

2.3.1. Nonlinguistic Negative Priming Task. Negative priming describes the phenomenon of a prolonged reaction time (RT) and/or a greater number of errors when the participants have to respond to a target that was ignored in the preceding trial [32, 33]. In this task, the participants were required to process pairs of trials that were structured according to a prime-probe schema. Two picture stimuli (line drawings of animate or inanimate objects) were displayed in the form of overlapping pictures in shades of grey on both trials: one picture was the target in which the participants must respond and the other was the distracter, which must be ignored. In the present experiment, the participants were required to respond to one of the shades of grey (dark grey with the RGB coordinates 60, 60, 60, or light grey with the RGB coordinates 157, 157, 157) by suggesting the identity of the picture as being animate or inanimate.

The stimuli were presented on a $17''$ monitor in a quiet dimly lit room. The stimuli appeared at the centre of the screen, which measured within the frame of 106 pixels * 52 pixels. The horizontal and vertical resolutions were fixed at 71 dpi. The participants were seated comfortably at a distance of 60 cm from the computer monitor. The experiment was programmed using E prime version 2.0 to record the reaction time and accuracy of each trial. Each trial began with a fixation point for a duration of 400 milliseconds (ms) followed by a prime-probe stimuli, which was presented on a white background for a duration of 500 ms. These stimuli were each separated by a 300 ms blank screen. During the probe trial, the blank screen remained until the response or 3000 ms, whichever came first, and then the next trial began with a fixation point. The participants were required to press the right arrow key for animate and left arrow key for inanimate targets using the first and second fingers of their dominant hand. They were instructed to respond as quickly and as accurately as possible.

The experiment consisted of a total of 180 trials with 60 trials for the attended repetition condition, 60 trials for the ignored repetition condition, and 60 trials for the control condition. The attended repetition measured the facilitation effect in performance. In such a condition, the picture being attended in the prime trial was attended again on the probe trial, resulting in faster reaction times compared to the control and ignored repetition conditions. The ignored repetition measured the inhibitory effect on performance. In such a condition, the picture being ignored in the previous trial was attended in the probe/current trial, resulting in an increase in reaction time (slowing of the response) compared to the other two conditions.The control condition acts as a baseline measure for the experiment in which the pictures (two overlapping pictures) in the prime trial were different from the probe trial. Thus, there was no effect of priming, whether positive or negative priming. The accuracy and reaction times were recorded for each condition for all four participants. The analysis was performed based on these three conditions. A linguistic counterpart of the negative priming task with a similar design could not be performed because it involved perceptually complex stimuli with overlapping words, and these stimuli appeared to be difficult for individuals with aphasia during the pilot phase of the study.

2.3.2. Flanker Task with Linguistic and Nonlinguistic Stimuli. The flanker task is a response inhibition task that is used to assess the ability to suppress responses that are inappropriate in a particular context. The flanker paradigm was originally introduced as a way to study the cognitive processes involved in the detection and recognition of targets in the presence of distracting information or noise [34]. In the present study, Eriksen's Flanker task [34] was employed to measure executive control to examine conflict resolution with two comparable tasks using linguistic and nonlinguistic stimuli. To introduce a conflict resolution component, the central arrow is "flanked" by congruent or incongruent stimuli. The target is flanked on either side by two arrows in the same direction (congruent condition) or in the opposite direction (incongruent condition). On some trials, the target is flanked by neutral flankers (neutral condition), which were neither similar to the target nor to the flankers in the incongruent condition. The same conditions were used in the current study. Both the target and flankers appeared simultaneously. The participants were required to respond to the direction of the central target arrow, which could be facing in the same direction as the flankers (congruent condition) or in the opposite direction compared to the flankers (incongruent condition). There was also a neutral condition, which consisted of a central target arrow that faced either left or right with dashes as the flankers on either side of the target, thus resulting in a no conflict condition. Each trial began with a fixation cross for 400 ms followed by the stimuli (target and flankers), which were presented for 500 ms followed by a blank screen that stayed until the response or 3000 ms, whichever came first. The participants were required to respond by pressing the right arrow key on the keyboard if the target was facing towards the right, and the left arrowkeyif the target was facing towards the left. There were 180 trials in total, with 60 trials in each condition. There were approximately 30 practice trials in the beginning of the session prior to starting with the main experimental trials.

The linguistic version of the flanker task in different language pairs was designed with letters from the two languages (L1 and L2) known to each participant (Hindi-English and Telugu-English). This task was based on the standard flanker task, but with two flanker compatibility conditions (congruent and incongruent). It did not include the neutral condition because it would have resulted in an unequal number of incongruent trials for both the languages (because the incongruent condition also had two levels). The number of flankers was the same as the nonlinguistic version. The only addition was the presence of two types of incongruent trials: those with within-language incongruence (HHSHH) and those with across language incongruence (HHतHH).

We determined the appropriateness of the stimuli (letters) in the pilot study using normal healthy participants. Each trial began with a fixation cross for 400 ms followed by the target letter flanked by congruent (flanking letters were the same as the target letter) or incongruent flankers (flanking letters were different from the target letter). The stimuli were presented against a white background for 500 ms followed by a blank screen. The blank screen remained until the response or 3000 ms, whichever came first, and then the next trial began with a fixation cross. The participants were required to press the right arrow key for "H," left arrow key for "S," up arrow key for "म," and down arrow key for "त" for the flanker task with stimuli in Hindi and English languages. A similar design was used for the Telugu-English version of this task. A total of 360 trials were presented, with 120 trials in each condition, which were congruent, incongruent within a language, and incongruent across language. These conditions were equally divided for both the languages. The response level inhibition resulted in slowing of the responses on the incongruent trials and varied as a function of language. Eriksen's flanker task has also been reported for linguistic stimuli, but only with one language [34].

In both versions of the flanker task (linguistic and nonlinguistic), the stimuli were presented on a 17″ monitor with a refresh rate of 85 Hz in a quiet and dimly lit room. The participants were comfortably seated at a distance of 60 cm from the computer monitor. In the linguistic version of the task, the array of letters appeared on the centre of the screen within the frame of 140 pixels ∗ 45 pixels, whereas in the nonlinguistic version arrows appeared within the frame of 135 pixels ∗ 25 pixels. The experiment was programmed using E prime version 2.0 to record the reaction time and accuracy for each trial.

3. Results

The current study focused on the performance patterns of each participant on the cognitive control tasks, and the subjective and objective measures of language proficiency. The data obtained with the language background questionnaire and the composite rubric scores on the picture description task are provided in Table 1. Data based on the performance of each participant on the respective cognitive control tasks are shown in Table 4. We discussed the results based on the variations in the performance of each participant on the cognitive control tasks as well as their language background information. Statistical inference was generated via visual analysis of the data (mean RT scores as well as CDF plots of different conditions) for each participant for each specific

experiment. Correlation analysis was performed to test the relationship between objective and subjective task performance. The variability in a single case study method was controlled using experimental tasks and tools for language proficiency, which have been well adapted for Indian conditions. Negative priming and the flanker paradigm are well established paradigms employed across populations; thus there is a limited chance of variability because of the measurement instrument. This language history questionnaire has been employed in an Indian population [29, 35] in both qualitative and quantitative bilingual studies.

The cumulative frequency distribution was employed as an important tool for the interpretation of individual data to examine the performance patterns of each task across the four participants. To analyse the reaction time data, the cumulative frequency data were used to gain insight into how often a specific phenomenon was either below or above a specific value. The RT distributions were computed using the cumulative distribution function (CDF) in MATLAB. We examined the RT-based differences at the 5th percentile (fast trials) and 95th percentile (slow trials) across conditions for each participant. In a few instances, a different range of percentiles was used to indicate patterns in the performance of specific experimental conditions. Slow and fast reaction times were used as measures of the proactive and reactive modes of control. Slow trials are known to reflect the involvement of the reactive control mechanisms and fast trials are known to reflect the involvement of proactive control mechanisms [27].

The results are discussed with respect to the patterns in the performance on each experimental task across the four participants. In this study, the primary objective was not to compare the performance of the four participants but to illustrate the variations in each participant's performance across tasks and across conditions (experimental manipulations) within a task.

3.1. Negative Priming Task with Nonlinguistic Stimuli. All four participants performed the negative priming task with a good overall accuracy except for SC who showed a below chance level performance on one of the tasks. However, variations in performance across participants were observed with respect to the engagement of proactive and reactive control mechanisms as revealed by the RT distributions on the 5th and 95th percentiles.

CR's performance on the negative priming task with superimposed line drawings of objects (with reaction times as a measure of performance) suggests the presence of a facilitation effect in the absence of a negative priming effect (see Figure 1(a)). However, error analysis showed a greater number of errors for the ignored repetition trials compared to the control condition, suggesting the presence of a negative priming effect (see Figure 1(b)). In addition, CDF plots further supported these results. CDF curves showed facilitation or a positive priming effect more prominently in the fast trials (i.e., 5th percentile) (see Figure 1(c)). This effect was persistent throughout the distribution except at the 95th percentile level (i.e., slow trials) where the distribution appeared to be very similar across conditions. These results indicated that

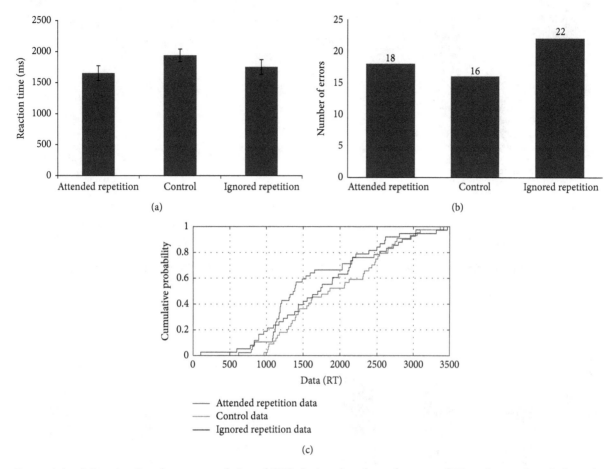

FIGURE 1: (a–c): Reaction time data, error analysis, and CDF plot based on the performance of CR on the negative priming task.

when the time to respond to a target is less, then the facilitation effect is greater compared to when the time available is more. These results indicated the presence of proactive control in a minimal conflict condition (i.e., attended repetition condition). Similarly, ignored repetition reaction times were faster compared to the control condition throughout the distribution except for the 95th percentile level.

Taken together, these results indicated that although the overall mean RTs showed an absence of a negative priming effect, the negative priming or persistent inhibitory effect surfaced only on the slow trials, when the time available was more, indicating a dependence on the reactive control mechanism. The proactive control mechanisms appeared to be compromised. However, because the error analysis showed a negative priming effect with a greater number of errors on the ignored repetition trials compared to the control trials, this in itself may be the reason why fast trials did not show a negative priming effect. Thus, when the participant takes less time during a more demanding condition (i.e., ignored repetition), it may result in a greater number of errors.

MMH's performance on the negative priming task showed facilitation or a positive priming effect, and a negative priming effect was not observed (see Figure 2(a)). CDF analysis only showed the presence of a facilitation effect and the absence of a negative priming effect based on the observation that there was no difference between the RT distributions for the ignored repetition condition and control condition (see Figure 2(b)). Furthermore, the facilitation effect was greater on the slow trials compared to the fast trials. An absence of an inhibitory effect was observed in both the fast and slow trials. The results based on MMH's performance indicated a potential dependence on reactive control mechanisms and showed a partial correspondence with the RT distributions observed on the nonlinguistic flanker task, as discussed later in this section.

The third participant, SC, performed at a below chance level on the negative priming task. However, interestingly, his performance (RTs) indicated both facilitation and inhibitory effects (see Figure 3(a)). Error analysis suggested the presence of an inhibitory effect with a greater number of errors on the ignored repetition condition compared to the control and attended repetition conditions, and an absence of the facilitation effect (no difference in errors between the attended repetition condition and control condition) (see Figure 3(b)). CDF plots also showed a uniform distribution for all three conditions (attended repetition < control < ignored repetition) showing no variations in performance with respect to the fast and slow trials across conditions (see Figure 3(c)). However, visual inspection of the CDF plots suggested a greater inhibition on the slow trials compared to the fast trials.

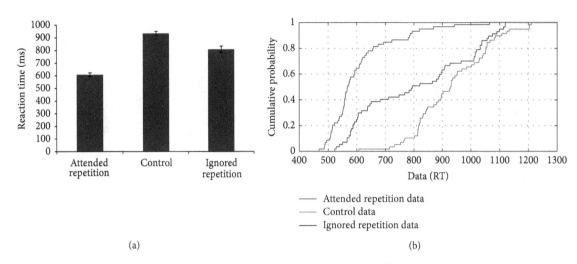

(a)   (b)

FIGURE 2: (a-b): Reaction time data and CDF plot based on the performance of MMH on the negative priming task.

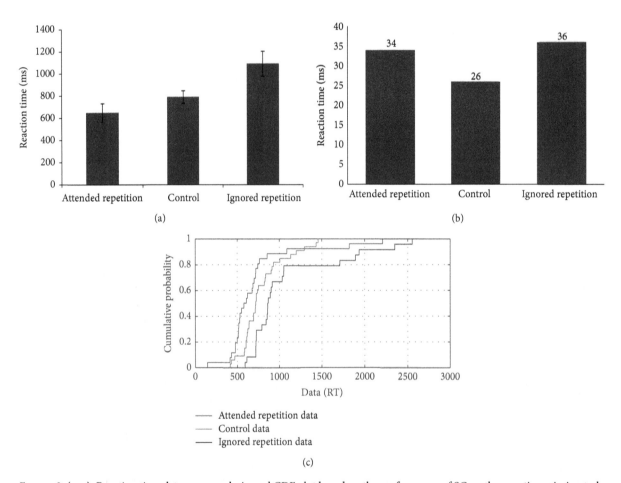

(a)   (b)

(c)

FIGURE 3: (a–c): Reaction time data, error analysis, and CDF plot based on the performance of SC on the negative priming task.

MU's performance on the negative priming task with nonlinguistic stimuli, similar to CR and MMH, showed the presence of a facilitation effect and the absence of a persisting inhibitory effect (see Figure 4(a)), which was translated in the same manner in the CDF analysis. However, for the ignored repetition condition, there were variations in performance throughout the distribution compared to the control condition. CDF plots indicated that the inhibitory or negative priming effect only appeared on the slow trials, indicating the involvement of reactive control mechanisms (see Figure 4(b)).

Thus, the performance of all the participants on the negative priming task primarily reflected the involvement of reactive control mechanisms. Proactive control mechanisms

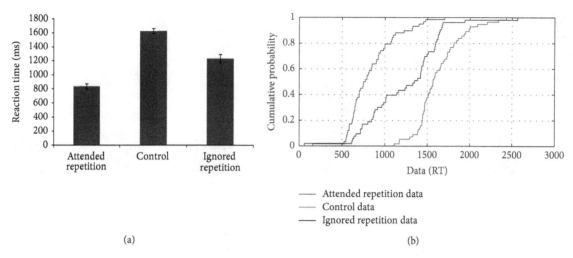

(a)   (b)

FIGURE 4: (a-b): Reaction time data and CDF plot based on the performance of MU on the negative priming task.

appear to be affected with respect to the persistent inhibitory effects as indicated by the subjects' performance on the negative priming task.

3.2. Flanker Task with Nonlinguistic Stimuli. All of the participants performed the flanker task with nonlinguistic stimuli with good accuracy except for SC, who showed less accuracy but at an above chance level.

CR's performance on the nonlinguistic flanker task showed a congruency effect (i.e., mean reaction times on the congruent trials were faster than incongruent trials) (see Figure 5(a)). Unlike the usual effects observed on flanker tasks, neutral trials were slower compared to the incongruent trials. Error analysis showed a greater number of errors on the incongruent condition compared to the congruent and neutral conditions as expected in a flanker task (see Figure 5(b)). Cumulative distribution function plots were derived and showed differences across the three conditions only in the range of the 60th to 90th percentile, which was not consistent with the mean RT performance, and showed less congruent RTs compared to neutral RTs and less neutral RTs compared to incongruent RT conditions (see Figure 5(c)). The trend of slower incongruent trials compared to congruent trials was also observed at the 5th percentile (fast trials) level.

MMH showed a 98.8% accuracy on the standard flanker task, demonstrating the expected congruency effect with faster RTs on congruent trials compared to the incongruent trials. According to the CDF analysis, a congruency effect was observed with respect to the neutral condition only on slow trials, indicating the involvement of reactive control (see Figures 6(a) and 6(b)). The CDF plots indicated that RTs for the neutral condition were faster than the incongruent condition throughout the distribution, which is suggestive of the presence of an interactive and efficient inhibitory control mechanism.

SC demonstrated a 67.2% accuracy on the nonlinguistic flanker task. However, all the errors were made on the incongruent trials. Thus, the flankers' identity was influencing

judgment more than the target's identity on the incongruent trials (see Figure 7(a)). The flanker effect was observed with slower RTs on incongruent trials compared to the congruent trials. RTs on incongruent trials were also compared with congruent and neutral conditions. And the RT distributions showed a uniform difference across conditions throughout the distribution (see Figure 7(b)). These results indicated that SC showed no difference between the slow versus fast trials on any of the conditions, demonstrating that both the proactive and reactive control mechanisms contributed to the flanker effects.

MU's performance on the nonlinguistic flanker task showed a congruency effect with respect to the mean RTs, although his performance on the neutral condition was exceptionally slow compared to the incongruent trials (see Figure 8(a)). CDF analysis showed that the congruency effect was absent (showing no difference between congruent and incongruent trials) on slow trials (i.e., 95th percentile and above), suggesting the involvement of proactive control mechanisms in the efficient performance, which was also highlighted by a high accuracy throughout the distribution (see Figure 8(b)). Uniformity was also observed in the distribution, which changed only in the slow trials, where the distribution shifted to its usual trend of differences across conditions.

Thus, performance on the flanker task with nonlinguistic stimuli showed a similar involvement of the reactive and proactive control mechanisms, contributing to the flanker effects for all four participants. All of the participants similarly showed conflict resolution and executive control effects on slow and fast trials, indicating the efficiency of the control processes in current trial inhibitory effects with nonlinguistic stimuli.

3.3. Flanker Task with Linguistic Stimuli. All of the participants performed the flanker task with linguistic stimuli with a fair amount of accuracy. Flanker effects with respect to the reaction times and accuracy on congruent and incongruent

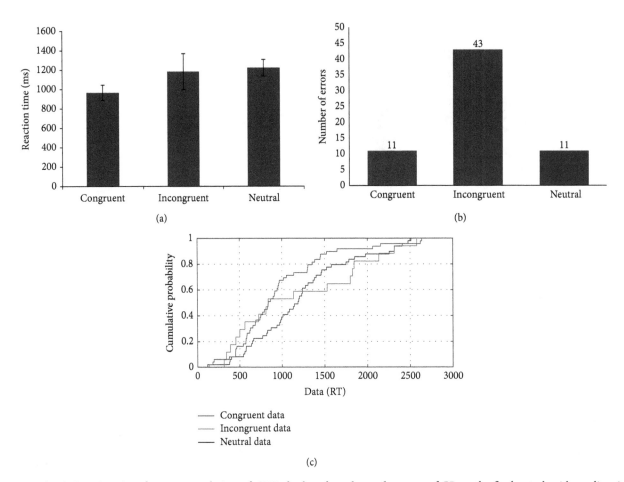

FIGURE 5: (a–c): Reaction time data, error analysis, and CDF plot based on the performance of CR on the flanker task with nonlinguistic stimuli.

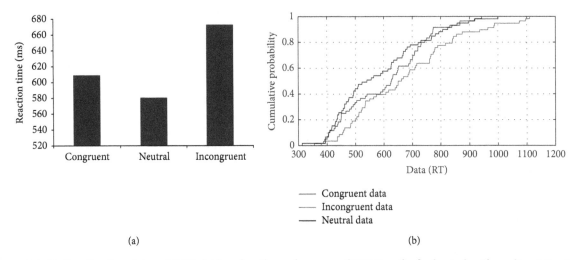

FIGURE 6: (a-b): Reaction time data and CDF plot based on the performance of MMH on the flanker task with nonlinguistic stimuli.

trials for L1 and L2 were observed, and the patterns of these effects on slow and fast trials were examined based on the CDF plots.

CR's performance on the linguistic flanker task showed a congruency effect for L2, whereas there was an absence of the congruency effect for L1 (see Figure 9(a)). The overall errors across all the conditions were greater for L1 compared to L2. L1 showed errors mostly on the congruent trials, whereas L2 showed a greater number of errors on the incongruent trials (see Figure 9(b)). For the language incongruent condition,

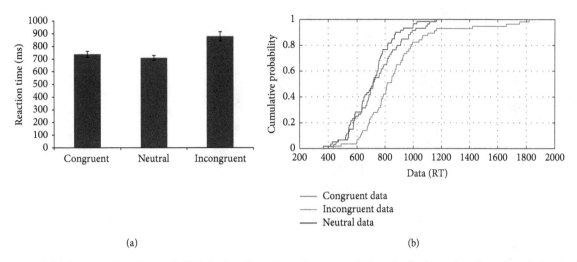

(a)

(b)

FIGURE 7: (a-b): Reaction time data and CDF plot based on the performance of SC on the flanker task with nonlinguistic stimuli.

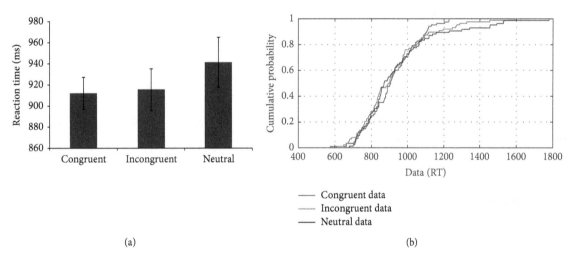

(a)

(b)

FIGURE 8: (a-b): Reaction time data and CDF plot based on the performance of MU on the flanker task with nonlinguistic stimuli.

the congruency effect was observed only for L2 throughout the distribution (see Figure 9(c)). Both L1 and L2 showed a flanker effect on the language incongruent condition on the fast (5th–20th percentile) and slow (70th–95th percentile) trials. Interestingly, similar patterns for the congruency effect for both L1 and L2 on the cross language incongruent condition were observed. The discrepancy in the mean scores for L1 versus L2 with respect to the congruency effect is suggestive of different underlying processes operating for L1 compared to L2. However, this difference was not explained by the CDF plots, which showed similar patterns of performance on the slow and fast trials for both languages (see Figures 9(c) and 9(d)).

MMH's performance on the linguistic flanker task showed a congruency effect for both types of incongruent conditions (i.e., IC within and IC across) for L2, whereas for L1, the flanker effect was absent in the within language condition (see Figure 10(a)). The CDF plots showed no difference in the pattern of RT distributions across the three conditions for L2, whereas for L1, the across language

incongruent trials showed a congruency effect between the 20th and 70th percentile, which was not observed for the within language incongruent condition (see Figure 10(b)). The congruency effect for the within language incongruent trials was observed only on the slow trials (see Figure 10(c)).

Unlike his performance on the flanker task with nonlinguistic stimuli, SC demonstrated a higher overall accuracy on the linguistic flanker task (92.69%), which supports our assumption with respect to his performance on the previous task; that is, the errors were not due to difficulties in the response selection. Although the differences in the mean reaction times were very small (see Table 4), there was a congruency effect for L1 only on the across language incongruent trials. However, the RT distributions of L1 showed an absence of a congruency effect on the fast trials for the across language incongruent condition (see Figure 11(b)). These results indicated that the interference caused by the flankers in L2 while attending to the target in L1 was resolved using proactive control mechanisms because the effect was not sustained throughout the distribution and was only present

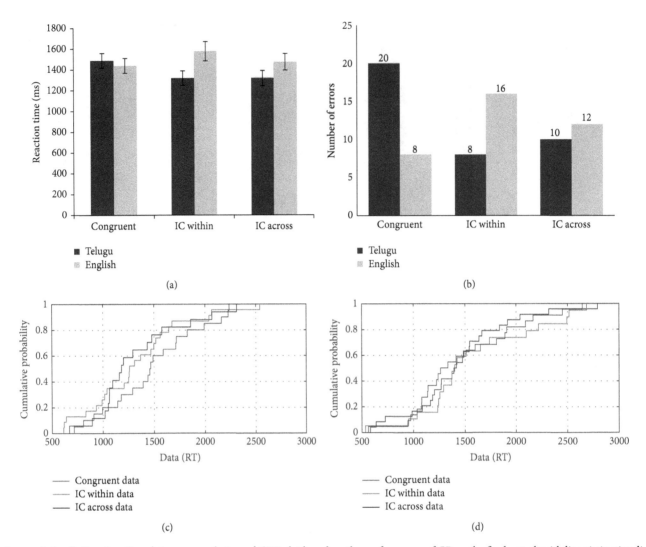

FIGURE 9: (a–d): Reaction time data, error analysis, and CDF plot based on the performance of CR on the flanker task with linguistic stimuli.

for the fast trials. For L2, CDF analysis showed a congruency effect on the within language incongruent condition, but only at the 5th percentile level (fast trials) and was not observed throughout the distribution (see Figure 11(c)). These results indicated a greater dependence on proactive control mechanisms because the difference between the congruent and incongruent trials within a particular language (L2) surfaced only on the fast trials.

MU's performance on this task showed a congruency effect for L1 and not for L2 with respect to the mean reaction time data (see Figure 12(a)). The flanker effect was present for L1 for the across language incongruent condition and not for the within language incongruent condition. These results indicated that the interference experienced was less when the flankers and the target were from the same language compared to the bilingual trials. Visual inspection of the CDF plots showed the presence of a congruency effect on the slow and fast trials, and these effects were absent only in the range of the 15th–50th percentile. CDF analysis of the across language congruency effect in L1 showed the

presence of a flanker effect throughout the distribution. CDF plots showed slowing on the across language incongruent condition compared to the congruent condition for L2 with RTs ranging from 75th to 95th percentiles (see Figure 12(b)). These results indicated an involvement of reactive control mechanisms in a more demanding situation where one needs to inhibit the flankers in L1 to attend to the targets in L2.

Thus, results based on the linguistic flanker task with respect to the within language and across language flanker effects for L1 and L2 indicated a greater variability in performance across the four participants as well as for each participant for L1 versus L2. Our results clearly show that in the case of bilingual language control, bilingual individuals with aphasia appear to show differences in the patterns of performance for L1 versus L2 as well as the recruitment of control mechanisms in resolving conflicts with linguistic stimuli. In addition, the flankers also greatly influenced inhibitory control processes compared to target processing of linguistic stimuli. Thus, it would be equally important to examine suppression-related mechanisms among individuals

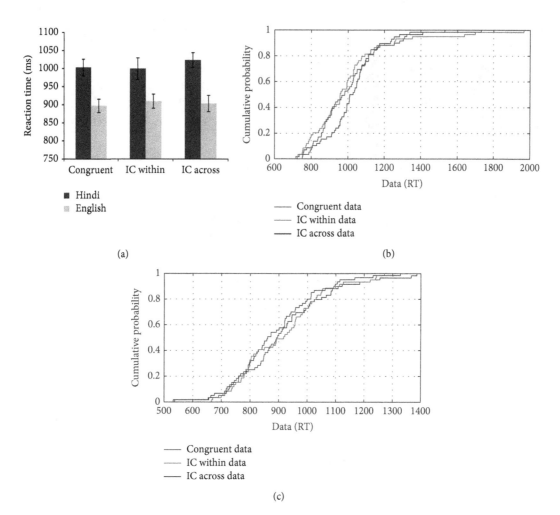

(a)

(b)

(c)

FIGURE 10: (a–c): Reaction time data and CDF plot based on the performance of MMH on the flanker task with linguistic stimuli.

with bilingual aphasia to investigate the activation-related mechanisms for languages affected in an individual with bilingual aphasia.

3.4. Correlation Analysis (Language History Variables and Performance on Control Tasks). Correlations were determined to examine the relationship between bilingualism-related factors, such as language use and self-rated language proficiency with the experimental task performance across the four participants. A bivariate correlation analysis was performed using two sets of variables: those related to the language background information (language use in L1 and L2, overall language proficiency in L1 and L2, proficiency in speaking, and understanding domain) and those pertaining to the control tasks (flanker effect for L1/L2 in the within language incongruent condition, flanker effect for L1/L2 in the across language incongruent condition, flanker effect for nonlinguistic stimuli, and a positive priming effect and negative priming effect on the negative priming task).

Language use did not show a significant correlation with performance on any of the control tasks. However, interesting trends were observed with respect to the relationship between L1 and L2 proficiency and control tasks, and specifically with

linguistic stimuli. Language proficiency in L1 was negatively correlated with the flanker effect of L2 in the within language incongruent condition ($r = -.970$, $p = .03$), whereas it was positively correlated with the flanker effect of L2 in the across language incongruent condition ($r = .979$, $p = .02$). L2 proficiency showed a negative correlation with the flanker effect of L1 and L2 across language incongruent condition ($r = -.986$, $p = .01$ and $r = .964$, $p = .03$, resp.). However, L2 proficiency was positively correlated with L2 within language incongruent condition ($r = .977$, $p = .02$). The observed correlations indicated that the relationship between proficiency and the control task performance among aphasic individuals emerged mostly in bilingual competition on the across language incongruent condition on the linguistic flanker task. When L1 proficiency is low or when L1 is the affected language in aphasia, the flanker effect would also be less on the across language incongruent condition in L2 because the competition/conflict from the weaker L1 flankers would be less. Second language proficiency has been reported to be enhanced compared to L1 by all participants. The negative correlation between L2 proficiency and the flanker effect for L1 and L2 on bilingual trials manifested differently across participants based on individual data. For

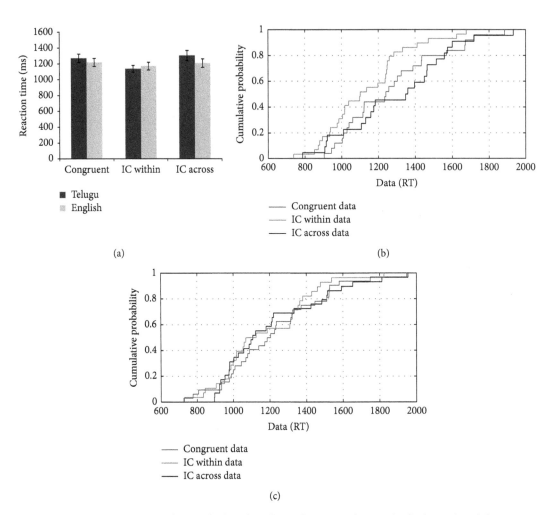

(a)

(b)

(c)

FIGURE 11: (a–c): Reaction time data and CDF plot based on the performance of SC on the flanker task with linguistic stimuli.

instance, CR showed a negative correlation in terms of a better L2 proficiency and reduced flanker effect for L1 on the L1 across language incongruent condition. However, for SC and MU, a lower L2 proficiency was correlated with greater flanker effects for L1 in the L1 across language incongruent condition. There was a near significant negative correlation between proficiency in the speaking/understanding domain in L1 and an inhibitory effect ($r = -.919$, $p = .08$) on the nonlinguistic negative priming task. These results suggested that the inhibitory effects on a nonlinguistic negative priming task might increase in lower L1 proficiency. This suggested a potential relationship between L1 proficiency and domain general inhibitory control.

Thus, results based on the correlation analysis suggested that a weaker or affected language in bilingual individuals with aphasia was not correlated with flanker effects in the weaker language compared to the L2 proficiency, which showed a significant relationship with flanker effects in L1 and L2. Inhibitory effects in L1 and L2 surfaced in bilingual competition and are more closely related to proficiency, particularly in the less affected language, which is L2 in most of the participants in the current study. These interesting trends in the current data should be further tested using a larger number of bilingual individuals with aphasia.

To summarise our results, all participants showed the presence of a facilitation effect, in the absence of an inhibitory effect (except for SC) on the negative priming task. CDF analysis showed the presence of an inhibitory effect only on the slow trials for CR, SC, and MU. SC also demonstrated inhibitory effects on fast trials. The flanker task with linguistic and nonlinguistic stimuli showed varying effects across the four participants. A congruency effect was evident on the nonlinguistic flanker task for all the participants with respect to the mean reaction times. CDF analysis revealed interesting patterns of performance. CR and SC showed a congruency effect throughout the distribution, whereas MMH showed a congruency effect only on the slow trials. Conversely, MU showed a congruency effect only on the fast trials. Thus, a rather complex picture emerged from the linguistic version of the flanker task, based on the mean reaction time data. A congruency effect was observed for L2 (i.e., while comparing the congruent condition with the incongruent within language and incongruent across language conditions) only for CR and MMH. However, SC and MU showed a congruency effect only for L1 compared to the congruent condition with the incongruent across language condition. CDF plots also showed varying patterns of performance across participants on the cross linguistic flanker task. CDF

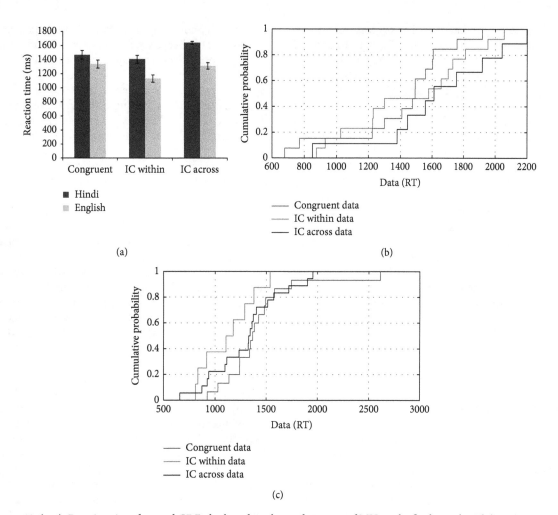

FIGURE 12: (a–c): Reaction time data and CDF plot based on the performance of MU on the flanker task with linguistic stimuli.

plots for L1 (compared to the congruent condition with the within language incongruent condition) showed an absence of a congruency effect except for MMH who showed a congruency effect on slow trials. Interestingly, the congruency effects for L1 (i.e., congruent condition versus incongruent across language condition) throughout the RT distribution of CR and MU on slow trials were observed. All participants showed different patterns of performance in their L2. Error analysis helped to understand the within subject variability in reaction times. However, the highly accurate performance of all the participants in different tasks limited our ability to draw any commonality among them.

4. Discussion

The findings of the current study are consistent with the view that the acquisition of another language involves an adaptation to an existing network. Different languages are represented in shared brain regions with common organising principles [36]. Specific patterns of deficits reflect problems of control rather than deficits of pure linguistic origin. Inferences drawn from deficits involve reverse extrapolation to a premorbid state of functioning. An influential aspect of this approach is that patterns of performance (both

intact and impaired) suggest selective damage to one or more components or processing pathways. The results of the current study suggest that although inhibitory control underlying selective attention may be impaired in participants with anterior aphasia. The ability to differentiate the target from the distracter may be preserved; thus, the presence of flanker effects in the flanker task. The flanker task and negative priming task are dependent on different processing mechanisms. The presence of positive priming in the absence of negative priming with respect to the RT data observed in our participants is suggestive of the dual route involved in the negative priming task. It has been postulated that positive priming is strongly affected by perception in contrast to negative priming, which emerges during selection [37]. We have found that such dissociations between positive and negative priming effects in the current study suggest difficulties with respect to selection as a component of control processes among bilingual individuals with aphasia.

Reactive and proactive control mechanisms underlying the performance on each task for each participant were explored using CDF analysis. All four participants showed a dependence on the reactive control mechanisms with specific variations observed between the two languages that were known by each of the four participants. For example, CR's congruency effect on the linguistic flanker task showed an interesting language specific variation. L2 (English) showed the involvement of reactive control, whereas L1 showed a reliance on proactive control mechanisms. MMH showed an L1 congruency effect only when L1 was flanked by L2 on slow trials, suggesting the involvement of reactive control. These effects were similar to those observed in CR's performance. An interesting observation was that MU showed greater interference from the same language (when flankers were in the same language as the target) compared to the condition that involved across language competition. However, this effect was only observed for L2, whereas L1 showed the congruency effect in across language conflict. The nonlinguistic flanker task showed the involvement of both proactive and reactive control mechanisms, except for MMH and MU. MMH showed an involvement of the reactive control mechanism and MU showed a reliance on proactive control. These two mechanisms are not mutually exclusive. Thus, it is possible that CR and SC showed the involvement of both mechanisms to resolve the conflict for efficient performance. CDF plots suggested that the magnitude of the effects was larger for facilitation or the positive priming effect on slow trials, and differences between the control condition and ignored repetition condition were more prominent on fast trials for MMH and MU on the negative priming task. In both cases, it is probable that the sustained activation of all four items (2 pictures from the prime trial and 2 from the probe trial) resulted in the slowing of the response in the control condition, due to a greater interference from unattended stimuli. There was an interesting dissociation observed in CR's performance, demonstrating an involvement of proactive control during facilitation and reactive control for inhibition. Such a tradeoff may be due to dual mechanisms involved in facilitation versus inhibition. The distinction between proactive and reactive control is useful in elucidating the variations in cognitive control mechanisms due to the influences from bilingualism-related factors, which need to be explicitly manipulated and examined in future research. As a result of their limited processing resources, the effective engagement of proactive control may be problematic for individuals with aphasia and may thus engage the reactive control mechanisms, which do not require the individual to sustain control over an extensive period of time [27].

Another interesting area to explore is the interaction of bilingual language control and general purpose cognitive control and thus, we compared the performance on linguistic and nonlinguistic flanker tasks. Performance-based differences were evident on flanker tasks with nonlinguistic versus linguistic stimuli. Interestingly, the variations in the performance of each participant surfaced to a greater degree in the linguistic stimuli for both L1 and L2. Except for CR, all of the other participants showed differences in their performance between the two tasks. For example, more reliance on reactive control mechanism in the performance of MMH on the nonlinguistic flanker task was observed, whereas the proactive control was predominant in the across language incongruent condition on the linguistic flanker task. This trend was reversed for MU.

Results obtained from the current study helped to form the stage for further studies to enhance our understanding of language control and cognitive control in bilingual aphasia as well as to improvise the rehabilitation process. This is supported by the fact that therapy in L2 was related to a better performance in L2 on the linguistic flanker task (in the case of CR and MMH), while therapy focusing predominantly on L1 resulted in a better performance in L1. Such a domain specific effect of therapy was also reported in a study by Abutalebi et al. [2], where improvement in the naming performance resulted in an improvement in the naming network only. Abutalebi and colleagues [2] also discussed the dissociation between the naming and control pathways, which was consistent with the observations of the present study with respect to the variations in performance between linguistic and nonlinguistic control tasks.

We also observed that individuals with better scores on the WAB did not show an involvement of the proactive control mechanism with the data based on the negative priming task. Thus, there is a need to perform both linguistic and nonlinguistic control tasks while profiling individuals with bilingual aphasia. It is possible that individuals with bilingual aphasia may respond to speech and language therapy and show an improvement in language skills in the affected language, but may still demonstrate problems with executive control. Another interesting relationship between subjective information (see Tables 1, 2, and 3) and task performance was via premorbid language use (in percentage) and the linguistic flanker task. Premorbid language use was the same for SC and MU, whereas for CR and MMH, L1 was the dominant language. This was translated to the performance on linguistic flanker task, where language was dominant premorbidly and was affected compared to the other language (in these cases L2). SC and MU with a similar dominance of language use premorbidly, showed an absence of the flanker effect in both languages. In contrast to CR and MMH, their L1 performance was better than L2. Although such links between language use and task performance are interesting, the extrapolation of such findings via only single case studies should be carefully performed. However, the descriptive account of language use and task performance shows a relationship between the two variables, but the correlation analysis did not show a statistically significant correlation with the performance on any of the control tasks, which could be due to the variance across participants with respect to language use.

Studies investigating the interaction between bilingualism and control processes have theoretical and clinical implications. The case study approach employed in the current study provided an individually specific profile of bilingual individuals with aphasia with respect to cognitive control processes and the nature of control mechanisms, which may influence the recovery patterns and could thus be considered during the rehabilitation process. This study also highlighted that the performance of no two bilingual aphasics was the same and thus required a detailed assessment of both language control and cognitive control processes particularly relevant for individuals with bilingual aphasia. It has been reported by Abutalebi and Green [2] that the effect of treatment in bilingual aphasia was dependent on the integrity of naming and control pathways, indicating the need to address both linguistic and control systems. Apart from providing insight into language control and cognitive control mechanisms, such a profile of individuals with aphasia may help to decide the language for therapy in bilingual aphasia. Although, the current data are limited in establishing such a claim, they open new avenues of research. Performance on the flanker task and negative priming task may indicate the use of selective language therapy or bilingual language therapy based on the level of interference. Apart from the treatment decisions, clinical implications of language control and cognitive control mechanisms may act as a main determinant of cognitive-linguistic recovery in aphasia [2].

Taken together, the variations observed in the performance of each participant across tasks and stimuli strongly suggested that there is dissociation between bilingual language control and general purpose cognitive control mechanisms. These observations were further strengthened by the findings based on the correlation analysis between bilingualism-related factors (language use and proficiency) and performance on control tasks, which showed that the relationship between proficiency and inhibitory effects in L1 and L2 surfaced primarily in case of bilingual competition. L1 proficiency with respect to the speaking/understanding domain was correlated with a sustained inhibitory control (negative priming effect with nonlinguistic stimuli) and L2 proficiency was correlated with cross-linguistic flanker effects for both L1 and L2, indicating a dissociation between the role of L1 versus L2 proficiency in domain general cognitive control and bilingual language control, respectively. These interesting trends in the current data need to be empirically tested further with explicit manipulations related to L1 and L2 proficiency using a larger group of individuals with bilingual aphasia and their performance on a range of control tasks.

5. Conclusion

The present study was designed to examine the performance of bilingual aphasics on executive control tasks that test the circuits implicated in language control and cognitive control. CDF analysis was a promising tool used to examine the variations in performance within and across individuals, tasks and stimuli. Current trial inhibitory effects were observed among individuals with bilingual aphasia, whereas a sustained inhibitory control (as assessed on the negative priming task with nonlinguistic stimuli) was found to be compromised. Interestingly, sustained inhibitory control was correlated with L1 proficiency. All the participants demonstrated the use of reactive control mechanisms to compensate for the limited resource system. We also found differences in the involvement of control mechanisms for linguistic stimuli between L1 and L2 with L1 depending more on proactive control and L2 depending more on the reactive control mechanisms. Importantly, these mechanisms were not mutually exclusive but interacted for efficient inhibitory control. The observations of the current investigation involved a series of four case studies, which provided valuable insight into the nature of the control mechanisms and were not limited to the task performance and deficits in cognitive abilities. A longitudinal study on individuals with bilingual aphasia helped to monitor the changes in cognitive control (which also appeared to be affected among bilingual aphasics). Control processes, such as selection, inhibition, and monitoring particularly sustained inhibitory control, appear to serve as the underlying resource systems for bilingual language control.

Acknowledgments

The authors are thankful to the Department of Science and Technology, Government of India, for funding this study as it is a part of their project on "Bilingualism and cognitive control" funded under the multi-institutional project on "Language and brain organization in normative multilingualism" under the Cognitive Science Research Initiative of the DST. They gratefully acknowledge their participants for their cooperation in the study. The authors would also like to thank All India Institute of Speech and Hearing and Sweekaar Academy of Rehabilitation Sciences for their support in the study.

References

[1] D. W. Green, "Mental control of the bilingual lexico-semantic system," *Bilingualism: Language and Cognition*, vol. 1, pp. 67–81, 1998.

[2] J. Abutalebi and D. Green, "Bilingual language production: the neurocognition of language representation and control," *Journal of Neurolinguistics*, vol. 20, no. 3, pp. 242–275, 2007.

[3] I. K. Christoffels, E. Formisano, and N. O. Schiller, "Neural correlates of verbal feedback processing: an fMRI study employing overt speech," *Human Brain Mapping*, vol. 28, no. 9, pp. 868–879, 2007.

[4] E. Bialystok, F. I. M. Craik, R. Klein, and M. Viswanathan, "Bilingualism, aging, and cognitive control: evidence from the Simon task," *Psychology and Aging*, vol. 19, no. 2, pp. 290–303, 2004.

[5] M. M. Martin-Rhee and E. Bialystok, "The development of two types of inhibitory control in monolingual and bilingual children," *Bilingualism: Language and Cognition*, vol. 11, no. 1, pp. 81–93, 2008.

[6] A. Costa, M. Hernández, and N. Sebastián-Gallés, "Bilingualism aids conflict resolution: evidence from the ANT task," *Cognition*, vol. 106, no. 1, pp. 59–86, 2008.

[7] M. Siegal, L. Iozzi, and L. Surian, "Bilingualism and conversational understanding in young children," *Cognition*, vol. 110, no. 1, pp. 115–122, 2009.

[8] E. Bialystok and X. Feng, "Language proficiency and its implications for monolingual and bilingual children," in *Challenges for Language Learners in Language and Literacy Development*, A. Durgunoglu, Ed., Guilford Press, 2009.

[9] E. Bialystok, F. I. M. Craik, and G. Luk, "Bilingualism: consequences for mind and brain," *Trends in Cognitive Sciences*, vol. 16, no. 4, pp. 240–250, 2012.

[10] J. F. Kroll, P. E. Dussias, C. A. Bogulski, and J. Valdes-Kroff, "Juggling two languages in one mind: what bilinguals tell us about language processing and its consequences for cognition," in *The Psychology of Learning and Motivation*, B. Ross, Ed., vol. 56, pp. 229–269, Academic press, San Diego, Calif, USA, 2012.

[11] P. A. Della-Rosa, G. Videsott, V. M. Borsa et al., "A interactive location for multilingual talent," *Cortex*, vol. 49, no. 2, pp. 605–608, 2012.

[12] E. Bialystok and M. M. Martin, "Attention and inhibition in bilingual children: evidence from the dimensional change card sort task," *Developmental Science*, vol. 7, no. 3, pp. 325–339, 2004.

[13] A. Costa, M. Hernández, J. Costa-Faidella, and N. Sebastián-Gallés, "On the bilingual advantage in conflict processing: now you see it, now you don't," *Cognition*, vol. 113, no. 2, pp. 135–149, 2009.

[14] M. Hernández, A. Costa, L. J. Fuentes, A. B. Vivas, and N. Sebastián-Gallés, "The impact of bilingualism on the executive control and orienting networks of attention," *Bilingualism: Language and Cognition*, vol. 13, no. 3, pp. 315–325, 2010.

[15] O. O. Adesope, T. Lavin, T. Thompson, and C. Ungerleider, "A systematic review and meta-analysis of the cognitive correlates of bilingualism," *Review of Educational Research*, vol. 80, no. 2, pp. 207–245, 2010.

[16] M. Calabria, M. Hernández, F. M. Branzi, and A. Costa, "Qualitative differences between bilingual language control and executive control: evidence from task-switching," *Frontiers in Psychology*, vol. 2, no. 399, pp. 1–10, 2011.

[17] E. K. Miller and J. D. Cohen, "An integrative theory of prefrontal cortex function," *Annual Review of Neuroscience*, vol. 24, pp. 167–202, 2001.

[18] J. Abutalebi, P. A. D. Rosa, M. Tettamanti, D. W. Green, and S. F. Cappa, "Bilingual aphasia and language control: a follow-up fMRI and intrinsic connectivity study," *Brain & Language*, vol. 109, no. 2-3, pp. 141–156, 2009.

[19] M. Purdy, "Executive function ability in persons with aphasia," *Aphasiology*, vol. 16, no. 4–6, pp. 549–557, 2002.

[20] J. Abutalebi, P. A. Della-Rosa, D. W. Green et al., "Bilingualism tunes the anterior cingulate cortex for conflict monitoring," *Cerrbral Cortex*, vol. 22, pp. 2076–2086, 2012.

[21] L. L. Murray, "Direct and indirect treatment approaches for addressing short-term or working memory deficits in aphasia," *Aphasiology*, vol. 26, no. 3-4, pp. 317–337, 2012.

[22] N. Helm-Estabrooks, "Cognition and aphasia: a discussion and a study," *Journal of Communication Disorders*, vol. 35, no. 2, pp. 171–186, 2002.

[23] M. van Mourik, M. Verschaeve, P. Boon, P. Paquier, and F. Van Harskamp, "Cognition in global aphasia: indicators for therapy," *Aphasiology*, vol. 6, no. 5, pp. 491–499, 1992.

[24] N. Helm-Estrabrook and N. B. Ratner, "Executive functions: what are they and why do they matter? Description disorders management," *Seminars in Speech and Language*, vol. 21, no. 2, pp. 91–92, 2000.

[25] C. Penn, T. Frankel, J. Watermeyer, and N. Russell, "Executive function and conversational strategies in bilingual aphasia," *Aphasiology*, vol. 24, no. 2, pp. 288–308, 2010.

[26] D. W. Green, A. Grogan, J. Crinion, N. Ali, C. Sutton, and C. J. Price, "Language control and parallel recovery of language in individuals with aphasia," *Aphasiology*, vol. 24, no. 2, pp. 188–209, 2010.

[27] T. S. Braver, "The variable nature of cognitive control: a dual mechanisms framework," *Trends in Cognitive Sciences*, vol. 16, no. 2, pp. 106–113, 2012.

[28] D. Vasanta, A. Suvarna, J. Sireesha, and S. Bapi Raju, "Language choice and language use patterns among Telugu-Hindi/Urdu-English speakers in Hyderabad, India," in *Proceedings of the International Conference on Language, Society, and Cul-ture in Asian Contexts*, pp. 57–67, Mahasarakam University, Mahasarakam, Thailand, 2010.

[29] T. Dash and B. R. Kar, "Characterizing language proficiency in Hindi and English language: implications for bilingual research," *International Journal of Mind Brain and Cognition*, vol. 3, no. 1, pp. 73–105, 2012.

[30] A. Kertesz, *Aphasia and Associated Disorders: Taxonomy Localization and Recovery*, Grune & Stratton, Orlando, Fla, USA, 1979.

[31] H. Goodglass and E. Kaplan, *The Assessment ofAphasia and Related Disorders*, Lea Febiger, Philadelphia, Pa, USA, 1983.

[32] S. P. Tipper, "Does negative priming reflect inhibitory mechanisms? A review and integration of conflicting views," *Quarterly Journal of Experimental Psychology A*, vol. 54, no. 2, pp. 321–343, 2001.

[33] J. Behrendt, H. Gibbons, H. Schrobsdorff, M. Ihrke, J. M. Herrmann, and M. Hasselhorn, "Event-related brain potential correlates of identity negative priming from overlapping pictures," *Psychophysiology*, vol. 47, no. 5, pp. 921–930, 2010.

[34] B. A. Eriksen and C. W. Eriksen, "Effects of noise letters upon the identification of a target letter in a nonsearch task," *Perception and Psychophysics*, vol. 16, no. 1, pp. 143–149, 1974.

[35] D. Vasanta, S. Bapi Raju, A. Suvarna et al., "Action verbs and body parts: a cross-linguistic study," *International Journal of Mind Brain and Cognition*, vol. 2, no. 1-2, pp. 19–38, 2011.

[36] D. W. Green, "Bilingual aphasia: adapted language networks and their control," *Annual Review of Applied Linguistics*, vol. 28, pp. 25–48, 2008.

[37] H. Schrobsdorff, M. Ihrke, J. Behrendt, J. M. Herrmann, and M. Hasselhorn, "Identity negative priming: a phenomenon of perception, recognition or selection?" *PLoS ONE*, vol. 7, no. 3, Article ID e32946, 2012.

6

Postoperative Cervical Haematoma Complicated by Ipsilateral Carotid Thrombosis and Aphasia after Anterior Cervical Fusion

Kingsley R. Chin,[1] **Jason Seale,**[2] **Veronica Butron,**[2] **and Vanessa Cumming**[3]

[1] *Charles E. Schmidt College of Medicine, Florida Atlantic University and Institute for Modern and Innovative Surgery (iMIS), 1100 W. Oakland Park Boulevard, Suite No. 3, Fort Lauderdale, FL 33311, USA*
[2] *iMIS Surgery, 1100 W. Oakland Park Boulevard, Suite No. 3, Fort Lauderdale, FL 33311, USA*
[3] *Less Exposure Surgery (LES) Society, 300 E. Oakland Park Boulevard, Suite 502, Fort Lauderdale, FL 33334, USA*

Correspondence should be addressed to Kingsley R. Chin; kingsleychin@gmail.com

Academic Editor: Aaron S. Dumont

Hematoma alone is the most common vascular complication reported after anterior cervical decompression and fusion (ACDF). We present this case to report the occurrence of postoperative cervical hematoma complicated by ipsilateral carotid thrombosis and aphasia after an uncomplicated C4–6 ACDF. This is a case of a 65-year-old woman who underwent revision fusions of the C4-5 and C6-7 levels complicated by postoperative cervical hematoma and carotid thrombosis. The patient's history, clinical examination, imaging findings, and treatment are reported. The revision fusions were performed and deemed routine. Approximately eight hours later 200 mL of blood was evacuated from a postoperative cervical hematoma. The patient became unresponsive and disoriented a few hours after evacuating the hematoma. Computed tomography and magnetic resonance imaging of the brain were normal, but magnetic resonance angiography demonstrated total occlusion of the left carotid artery. Thrombectomy was performed and the patient was discharged without residual deficits. At the latest followup she is fully functional and asymptomatic in her neck. We suggest, after evacuating a cervical hematoma, an evaluation of the carotids be made with MRA or cerebral angiography, as this may demonstrate a clot before the patient develops symptoms.

1. Introduction

Anterior cervical decompression and fusion (ACDF), a common treatment for cervical disc disease, is associated with good outcomes and low complication rates [1–5]. Complications can be devastating, especially hematoma, vascular injury, esophageal injury, neurological deficits, or graft dislodgement [4, 6–9]. Complications related to the carotid artery during ACDF are rare [10], and thrombosis has never been reported in association with a postoperative cervical hematoma, although interruption of laminar blood flow during retraction is documented [11].

We report a case of postoperative cervical hematoma complicated by ipsilateral carotid thrombosis and aphasia after a revision ACDF at C4-5 and C6-7 for adjacent segment disease. This case is presented to share the first documented case including this series of complications and to be instructive in sharing our management experience.

2. Case Presentation

A 65-year-old female patient with a body mass index of 19.2 kg/m^2 and past medical history including hepatitis C treated with interferon, Lyme disease, hypertension, osteoarthritis, lumbar laminectomy and fusion, C5-6 fusion, hysterectomy, and breast biopsy presented with multilevel spondylosis and adjacent level breakdown at C4-5 and C6-7.

She underwent revision fusions of C4-5 and C6-7 levels with interbody PEEK cage (Invibio PEEK Optima), demineralized bone matrix, and cervical plates (SpineFrontier Indus InVue cervical plate, Beverly, MA, USA). These procedures were completed via a left-sided approach. Hemostasis was achieved before closing the wound. This procedure was completed and was deemed routine without surgical, anesthetic, or cord monitoring complications.

Approximately 8 hours later swelling of the anterior neck was noted. This was assessed as a hematoma of the cervical spine causing airway compromise. Immediately the patient was returned to the operating suite for an urgent evacuation of the hematoma. Approximately 200 mL clotted blood was drained. Active oozing was noted from the muscles and cauterized. The wound was irrigated without force, then collagen sponge and gelatin matrix hemostatic sealant around the muscle areas were placed. After Penrose drain replacement and wound closure, excessive bleeding was noted, so the wound was reopened and more collagen sponge and thrombin were used along with cauterization. A bulb drain was placed with a 1/4 inch Penrose and the wound was closed.

Later that evening, the patient became increasingly disoriented and eventually unresponsive to commands. Clinically posterior fossa dysfunction was assessed with the patient obtunded and eyes gazing downward. The possibility of a cerebrovascular accident (CVA) in the posterior fossa was considered and computed tomography (CT) brain ordered. CT brain was normal and MRI demonstrated no acute infarct; however magnetic resonance angiography (MRA) revealed total occlusion of the left common carotid artery, including the bifurcation and external carotid artery with some reconstitution of the internal carotid at the level of the siphon from collateral blood flow (Figure 1). Therefore, without delay, vascular surgeons performed exploration and thrombectomy of the left carotid artery. The vascular surgeon commented only on the large size of the thrombus. There was no obvious intimal damage or arteriosclerosis as reported postoperatively. After all vascular clamps were released and good pulsations obtained in the entire common, external, and internal carotid arteries, the heparin injected prior to clamping was reversed with protamine sulfate and hemostasis was considered satisfactory. Another Penrose drain was left in the surgical bed.

Our patient's hospital stay was further complicated by an acute right brachial deep vein thrombosis secondary to a line *in situ*, and a heparin-induced thrombocytopenia. She also suffered a reactive leucocytosis immediately postoperatively and a nosocomial (MSSE) pneumonia. However, the patient was discharged from hospital on postoperative day 20 without any residual deficits, and at her latest followup at nine months she is fully functional and asymptomatic in her neck. Of note: our patient, since these reported procedures, had occipital and external carotid artery embolization performed, the coils and clips are obvious on X-ray (Figure 2). These procedures were completed by a separate team of vascular surgeons for discrete indications and are not directly related to the reported events herewith.

3. Discussion

Virchow's triad describes three broad categories which contribute to the development of thrombosis: stasis, endothelial

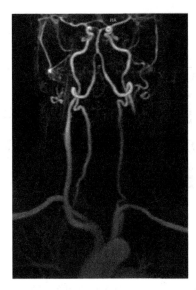

FIGURE 1: MRA postoperative day 2 demonstrates total occlusion of the left common carotid artery, including bifurcation and external carotid artery.

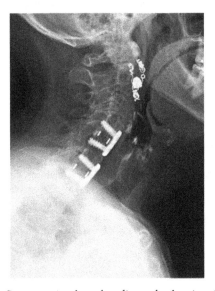

FIGURE 2: Postoperative lateral radiograph showing fixation at 9 months. (Please note: clips and coils postembolization of the occipital and external carotid arteries apparent in the anterolateral left neck.)

damage, and/or hypercoagulability. In this case our patient was not in a hypercoagulable state as evidenced by the hematoma and her normal liver function and bleeding indices, despite a history of hepatitis C [12]. No endothelial damage was identified at thrombectomy in this case, and considering that her aphasia developed after removal of the hematoma, it is our suspicion that the hematoma compressed the carotid artery enough to decrease laminar blood flow inducing stasis and providing a nidus for the development of a thrombus. Chronic long-term occlusion of the carotid may be another explanation of this patient's second event postoperatively certainly, but her medical history yielded no prior report of CVA-type events. This may have been masked, however, by compensatory mechanisms such as elevated oxygen extraction fraction improvement and/or improvements in blood flow with chronic occlusion [13].

It is unknown whether she would have developed aphasia from compression within the same time frame had we not removed the hematoma; nonetheless, our experience should raise awareness and prompt prophylactic action before evacuating a hematoma.

4. Conclusion

Our literature review yielded no prior cases detailing similar complications. This case documents perhaps the first report of this occurrence, is instructive, and raises awareness. We suggest after evacuating a cervical hematoma, especially in patients with risk factors, an evaluation of the carotids be made with MRA, Doppler ultrasonography, intraoperative pulse examination, or cerebral angiography as this may demonstrate a clot before the patient develops symptoms.

References

[1] L. Gebremariam, B. W. Koes, W. C. Peul, and B. M. Huisstede, "Evaluation of treatment effectiveness for the herniated cervical disk: a systematic review," *Spine*, vol. 37, no. 2, pp. E109–E118, 2012.

[2] M. J. Gray, A. Biyani, and A. Smith, "A retrospective analysis of patient perceived outcomes in patients 55 years and older undergoing anterior cervical discectomy and fusion," *Journal of Spinal Disorders and Techniques*, vol. 23, no. 3, pp. 157–161, 2010.

[3] P. G. Matz, T. C. Ryken, M. W. Groff et al., "Techniques for anterior cervical decompression for radiculopathy," *Journal of Neurosurgery*, vol. 11, no. 2, pp. 183–197, 2009.

[4] K. N. Fountas, E. Z. Kapsalaki, L. G. Nikolakakos et al., "Anterior cervical discectomy and fusion associated complications," *Spine*, vol. 32, no. 21, pp. 2310–2317, 2007.

[5] C. Cherry, "Anterior cervical discectomy and fusion for cervical disc disease," *AORN journal*, vol. 76, no. 6, pp. 998–1007, 1007-1008, 2002.

[6] A. H. Daniels, K. D. Riew, J. U. Yoo et al., "Adverse events associated with anterior cervical spine surgery," *Journal of the American Academy of Orthopaedic Surgeons*, vol. 16, no. 12, pp. 729–738, 2008.

[7] J. T. Liu, R. P. Briner, and J. A. Friedman, "Comparison of inpatient vs. outpatient anterior cervical discectomy and fusion: a retrospective case series," *BMC Surgery*, vol. 9, no. 1, article 3, 2009.

[8] N. H. Yu, T. A. Jahng, C. H. Kim, and C. K. Chung, "Life-threatening late hemorrhage due to superior thyroid artery dissection after anterior cervical discectomy and fusion," *Spine*, vol. 35, no. 15, pp. E739–E742, 2010.

[9] D. Daentzer, W. Deinsberger, and D. K. Böker, "Vertebral artery complications in anterior approaches to the cervical spine: report of two cases and review of literature," *Surgical Neurology*, vol. 59, no. 4, pp. 300–309, 2003.

[10] Y. C. Yeh, W. Z. Sun, C. P. Lin, C. K. Hui, I. R. Huang, and T. S. Lee, "Prolonged retraction on the normal common carotid artery induced lethal stroke after cervical spine surgery," *Spine*, vol. 29, no. 19, pp. E431–434, 2004.

[11] M. E. Pollard and P. W. Little, "Changes in carotid artery blood flow during anterior cervical spine surgery," *Spine*, vol. 27, no. 2, pp. 152–155, 2002.

[12] K. E. Sherman, "Advanced liver disease: what every hepatitis C virus treater should know," *Topics in Antiviral Medicine*, vol. 19, no. 3, pp. 121–125, 2011.

[13] C. P. Derdeyn, T. O. Videen, S. M. Fritsch, D. A. Carpenter, R. L. Grubb Jr., and W. J. Powers, "Compensatory mechanisms for chronic cerebral hypoperfusion in patients with carotid occlusion," *Stroke*, vol. 30, no. 5, pp. 1019–1024, 1999.

7

The Effectiveness of Transcranial Magnetic Stimulation (TMS) Paradigms as Treatment Options for Recovery of Language Deficits in Chronic Poststroke Aphasia

Anastasios M. Georgiou[1] and Maria Kambanaros[1,2]

[1]*The Brain and Neurorehabilitation Lab, Department of Rehabilitation Sciences, Cyprus University of Technology, Cyprus*
[2]*Allied Health and Human Performance, University of South Australia, Adelaide, Australia*

Correspondence should be addressed to Anastasios M. Georgiou; anastasios.georgiou@cut.ac.cy

Academic Editor: Efthymios Dardiotis

Background. In an effort to boost aphasia recovery, modern rehabilitation, in addition to speech and language therapy (SALT), is increasingly incorporating noninvasive methods of brain stimulation. The present study is aimed at investigating the effectiveness of two paradigms of neuronavigated repetitive transcranial magnetic stimulation (rTMS): (i) 1 Hz rTMS and (ii) continuous theta burst stimulation (cTBS) each as a standalone treatment for chronic aphasia poststroke. *Methods.* A single subject experimental design (SSED) trial was carried out in which six people with aphasia (PWA) were recruited, following a single left hemispheric stroke more than six months prior to the study. Three individuals were treated with 1 Hz rTMS, and the remaining three were treated with cTBS. In all cases, TMS was applied over the right pars triangularis (pTr). Language assessment, with standardized and functional measures, and cognitive evaluations were carried out at four time points: twice prior to treatment (baseline), one day immediately posttreatment, and at follow-up two months after treatment was terminated. Quality of life (QoL) was also assessed at baseline and two months posttreatment. In addition, one of the participants with severe global aphasia was followed up again one and two years posttherapy. *Results.* For all participants, both rTMS paradigms (1 Hz rTMS and cTBS) generated trends towards improvement in several language skills (i.e., verbal receptive language, expressive language, and naming and reading) one day after treatment and/or two months after therapy. Rated QoL remained stable in three individuals, but for the other three, the communication scores of the QoL were reduced, while two of them also showed a decline in the psychological scores. The participant that was treated with cTBS and followed for up to two years showed that the significant improvement she had initially exhibited in comprehension and reading skills two months after TMS (1st follow-up) was sustained for at least up to two years. *Conclusion.* From the current findings, it is suggested that inhibitory TMS over the right pTr has the potential to drive neuroplastic changes as a standalone treatment that facilitates language recovery in poststroke aphasia.

1. Introduction

To boost poststroke aphasia rehabilitation further, several noninvasive brain stimulation (NIBS) techniques have been applied to poststroke aphasia individuals over the past 20 years with promising results. Two of the most common methods that are being investigated are transcranial magnetic stimulation (TMS) and transcranial direct current stimulation (tDCS). The rationale behind their application is that both methods modulate neuronal plasticity and, in this way, facilitate language recovery.

Transcranial magnetic stimulation has shown exploratory potential to induce language recovery in aphasia poststroke [1]. Before 2014, only a few rTMS studies on poststroke aphasia recruited sufficiently large numbers of participants [2]. The majority of those studies explored the effects of low-frequency (LF) TMS over the contralesional inferior frontal gyrus (IFG) followed by speech and language therapy (SALT) in a clinically heterogeneous group of people with aphasia (PWA) at the postacute phase of recovery [3–6] with mixed results; hence, no conclusions could be drawn regarding the efficacy of LF rTMS over the contralesional IFG on recovery of poststroke aphasia [2]. After 2014, additional research with larger numbers of PWA has offered further insight on the possible effectiveness of rTMS on aphasia recovery in subacute aphasia [7, 8] and in the chronic stage [9–11]. The potential positive outcomes of rTMS on aphasia recovery poststroke have been further investigated by trials applying short rTMS burst protocols (e.g., theta burst stimulation (TBS)) with promising results [12–16]. For a review of TBS, see Huang and Rothwell [17] and Huang et al. [18]. Collective findings from LF rTMS in poststroke aphasia suggest that LF rTMS over the right IFG has the potential to reorganize the language networks and drive language improvement in people with poststroke aphasia. Nevertheless, with regard to high-frequency (HF) TMS, according to a recent review [2], no recommendations can be made for its use in poststroke aphasia rehabilitation.

Research on TMS aphasia rehabilitation is ongoing and promising but remains inconclusive for several reasons. For example, there are many inconsistencies between studies in several domains such as the following: (i) number of participants, (ii) paradigms employed (inhibitory vs. excitatory rTMS and inhibitory together with excitatory rTMS), (iii) anatomical sites of stimulation, (iv) methods of localization of stimulation sites (e.g., 10-20 international system vs. frameless stereotactic neuronavigation systems), (v) type and intensity of SALT, and (vi) the use of reliable outcome measures. With regard to SALT that is used as adjuvant to TMS, there are several studies that highlight major inconsistencies in SALT types and intensities. Examples of relevant randomized controlled trials include a study [7] in which a 45-minute SALT program was applied according to best-practice guidelines [19], a trial [20] in which a 30-minute SALT program focusing on language comprehension and expression was followed, a study [21] that used a 30-minute SALT regimen focusing on naming, another study [8] that applied a 45-minute SALT program aimed at reactivation of word retrieval, another trial [11] that used a 60-minute SALT program twice a week emphasising verbal expressive skills, five trials that followed a 45-minute SALT program focused on patient-specific language problems [3–5, 22, 23], and a study [6] that applied a 45-minute program focusing on expression and comprehension of spoken language. The wide variability in the reported studies and the absence of standardization of the SALT programs question their efficacy by not allowing the disentanglement of the beneficial effects of TMS from those of SALT. Therefore, the extent of the improvement on language abilities attributed to TMS cannot be evaluated.

The present study is aimed at measuring the effectiveness of rTMS as a standalone treatment for chronic stroke-induced aphasia. The objectives of the study were as follows:

(i) To explore whether continuous 1 Hz rTMS and cTBS (independent variables, IV) could modify performance on language tests (dependent variables,

DV) one day (short-term) and/or two months (long-term) posttreatment when administered for 10 consecutive days over the right pars triangularis (pTr) of individuals with chronic aphasia

(ii) To explore whether the above protocols (i.e., cTBS and 1 Hz rTMS) could bring about similar changes in language performance in the cohort of PWA under investigation

2. Materials and Methods

2.1. Bioethics Approval. Ethical approval for this study was obtained from the Cyprus National Bioethics Committee (CNBC) (ΕΕΒΚ/ΕΠ/2017/37).

2.2. Participants. A single-subject experimental design (SSED) trial was undertaken at the University Rehabilitation Clinic of the Department of Rehabilitation Sciences at the Cyprus University of Technology (CUT). Adults who had suffered a single left hemisphere stroke at least six months prior to participating in the study were actively sought for recruitment. The recruitment phase was open for 15 months. The inclusion criteria were as follows: (1) aged between 18 and 75 years of age, (2) native speakers of (Cypriot) Greek, (3) right-handed, (4) a diagnosis of a first ever left-sided middle cerebral artery (MCA) stroke verified by magnetic resonance imaging (MRI) or computerized tomography (CT), (5) chronic aphasia stage (>6 months poststroke), (6) no history of dementia or other neurological illnesses, and (7) no current participation in any type of language rehabilitation. Exclusion criteria included the following: (1) Greek not the mother tongue; (2) left-handedness; (3) prior stroke(s); (4) MRI and TMS exclusion criteria; (5) severe dysarthria affecting intelligibility; (6) any other neurological condition affecting the sensorimotor system (e.g., brain tumour); (7) medication that alerts brain excitability to avoid pharmacological influences on TMS, as there is evidence that the extent and direction of NIBS-induced plasticity can be significantly modulated by many neuropharmacological agents [24]; (8) cognitive disorders known before the stroke; and (9) involvement in behavioral language rehabilitation. Overall, 20 people were recruited but only eight actively took part and completed all phases of the study. Two participants were recruited to the pilot study (see [25]) and the remaining six to the main study (see Table 1 for demographics and clinical characteristics of the six participants and Figure 1 for brain MRIs). The remaining seven individuals from the initial cohort did not participate due to caregivers' reluctance/refusal because of time commitment to the study, and three PWA withdrew from the study during the TMS treatment stage while two more withdrew because of claustrophobia and subsequent failure to undergo an MRI scan.

2.3. Study Eligibility Measures. To determine eligibility for the study the following measures were carried out: (1) a detailed case history on demographics and health status, (2) a screening checklist for TMS eligibility, (3) the Hemispatial Neglect Test [26], and (4) the Handedness Inventory

TABLE 1: Demographics and clinical characteristics of the participants.

Participant	Sex	Age (years)	Handedness	Education (years)	Type of stroke	Months post stroke	Lesion site (left hemisphere)	Type of aphasia	Severity of aphasia	SALT prior to enrolment	Termination of SALT
1	F	74	Right	6	Ischemic	48	Diffuse frontal, parietal, and temporal (middle and superior gyri) lobes; insula; basal ganglia	Global	Severe	20 months–2 times per week–45 min of SALT	2 years before enrolment
2	M	61	Right	12	Ischemic	9	Broca's and Wernicke's areas; arcuate fasciculus; insula; inferior precentral gyrus; temporal pole	Anomic	Moderate-severe	6 months–2 times per week–45 min of SALT	2 months before enrolment
3	M	48	Right	15	Ischemic	11	IFG; internal capsule; insula; caudate nucleus; putamen; inferior precentral gyrus	Broca's	Moderate-severe	8 months–4 times per week–45 minutes	10 days before enrolment
4	F	72	Right	12	Ischemic	50	Broca's and Wernicke's areas; arcuate fasciculus; insula; superior posterior temporal gyrus; middle posterior temporal gyrus	Anomic	Moderate-severe	24 months–2 times per week–45 min of SALT	2 years before enrolment
5	M	55	Right	17	Ischemic	8	Precentral gyrus; postcentral gyrus; arcuate fasciculus; internal capsule; caudate nucleus; putamen	Global	Severe	4 months–4 times per week–45 minutes	10 days before enrolment
6	M	26	Right	16	Ischemic	109	IFG; MFG; SFG; insula; basal ganglia; arcuate fasciculus; internal capsule; anterior temporal lobe; Wernicke's area, anterior temporal lobe most likely due to an arachnoid cyst	Anomic	Mild	10 months–4 times per week–45 minutes	7 years before enrolment

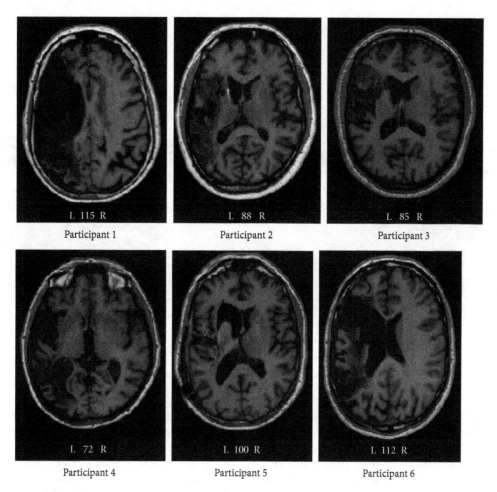

FIGURE 1: Brain MRI scans (axial plane) of the participants. Key: L: left hemisphere; R: right hemisphere; numbers indicate serial axial slice images.

(Edinburgh Handedness Inventory—Short Form [27]) to determine handedness.

2.4. Cognitive-Linguistic Measures Performed at Baseline, Posttreatment, and Follow-Up

2.4.1. The Greek Boston Diagnostic Aphasia Examination-Shortened Version (BDAE-SF). The Greek BDAE-SF [28] was used for language examination (i.e., oral and written language comprehension, expressive language, reading, and writing).

2.4.2. The Peabody Picture Vocabulary Test–Revised (PPVT-R). The short form (32 stimuli) of the Greek PPVT-R [29] was used to measure single word receptive vocabulary. The full and short versions of the PPVT-R are equivalent and constitute reliable and valid assessment tools of vocabulary for Greek students and immigrants who speak Greek [29].

2.4.3. The Greek Object and Action Test (GOAT). The Greek Object and Action Test (GOAT) is used to assess naming of nouns and verbs for assessment and/or research purposes in Greek speakers. It contains 84 coloured photographs measuring 42 actions and 42 objects. The test in total (production and comprehension subtests) takes under an hour to administer. The GOAT is reported in published studies investigating verb-noun grammatical dissociations across language-impaired populations [30]. For the purposes of this study, 19 informative verbs were used that distinguish language impaired from nonimpaired groups. This informative version was produced based on a new algorithm (ALNOVE) proposed to dismiss redundant/noninformative items from the tool [31].

2.4.4. The Multilingual Assessment Instrument for Narratives (MAIN). The Greek version of the Multilingual Assessment Instrument for Narratives (MAIN) [32] was used to evaluate production of narrative skills at the macro- and microstructure levels. In this study, the "Baby Goats" story, a story similar in concept to an Aesop fable, making it suitable for adult populations, was used.

2.4.5. The Raven's Coloured Progressive Matrices (RCPMs). The 36-item Raven's Coloured Progressive Matrix (RCPM) [33] was applied for problem-solving ability examination.

2.5. Quality of Life Measure: Used at Baseline and at Follow-Up

2.5.1. Stroke and Aphasia Quality of Life Scale-39 Item (SAQOL-39). The Greek version of the Stroke and Aphasia Quality of Life scale-39 item (SAQOL-39) [34] was applied for the assessment of TMS effects on QoL. The Greek

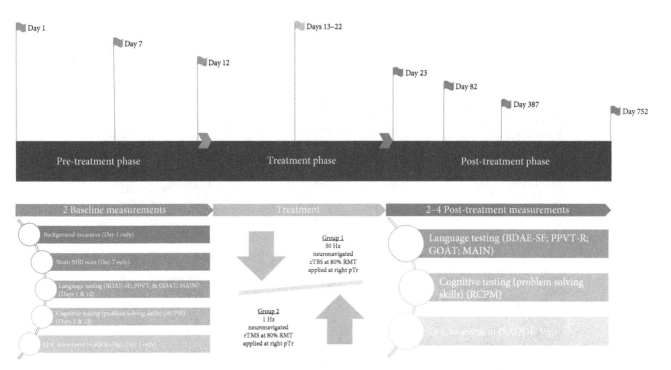

FIGURE 2: Experimental timeline of the study.

generic SAQOL-39 (SAQOL-39g) (i.e., the tool used in stroke patients without aphasia) is valid and reliable [35] and was used, and QoL was assessed using proxy ratings (caregivers) with all participants as three participants (P1, P4, and P5) struggled to respond to complex questions due to comprehension deficits.

2.6. Linguistic, Cognitive, and QoL Assessment and Analysis Procedures. All participants were assessed twice at baseline, one day posttreatment, and at two-month follow-up on all cognitive-linguistic measures. One participant (P1) was further assessed one and two years posttreatment. A schematic diagram illustrating the experimental timeline is shown in Figure 2. All participants did a brain MRI a week before therapy initiation. To ensure treatment fidelity, the Template for Intervention Description and Replication (TIDieR) [36] was used. A speech-language pathologist, blind to the study, performed all assessments and recorded the results in the project database. A second speech-language pathologist, also blind to the study, analyzed the responses. For the analysis of the MAIN, the Quantitative Production Analysis (QPA) protocol [37] as adopted for Greek [38] was applied by a linguist blind to the study protocol.

2.7. Repetitive TMS (rTMS) Procedures and Protocol. The six participants were randomly (via a computer-generated randomization schedule) allocated to two groups (three participants in each group) with each group (T1 or T2) receiving only one treatment type. To minimize placebo effects, the participants were informed that they had 50% chance to receive real treatment and 50% chance to receive sham treatment. Therefore, they were blinded to their status of TMS con-

ditioning (real vs. sham) until the end of the study. The treatment procedures that followed are described below.

2.8. Assessment of Resting Motor Threshold (RMT). The assessment of rest motor thresholds (RMTs) needed for determination of stimulation intensity was carried out for each participant using surface electromyography (EMG) [39]. After locating the "hot spot," for the appropriate RMT of the FDI, the standard stimulus magnitude used for mapping of the FDI was used and then the stimulus intensity was progressively reduced in 2% or 5% steps until the minimum single-pulse stimulator output intensity resulting in motor evoked potentials (MEPs) of at least $50\,\mu V$ peak-to-peak amplitude in $\geq 50\%$ of pursued trials was found. The rate of stimulation was more than 3 secs between consecutive stimuli. Motor threshold levels were used to determine stimulation parameters as they were considered as an indication of cortical excitability.

2.9. Repetitive TMS (rTMS) Stimulation Parameters. Participants underwent rTMS at 80% of their individual RMT, using the Magstim Rapid2® stimulator (Magstim Co., Wales, UK) connected to a 70 mm Double Air Film Coil. Stimulation parameters were in accordance with published guidelines [40]. The position of the coil was guided by a frameless stereotactic neuronavigation system (ANT NEURO) that uses the individual patients' MRI scan to precisely localize the target area for stimulation. Before stimulation, a T1-weighted MRI image was obtained from each patient to locate the optimal coil position.

2.9.1. Group T1: Continuous Theta Burst Stimulation (cTBS) over the Right Pars Triangularis (pTr). Participants in this group (P1, P2, and P3) received inhibitory rTMS (continuous theta burst stimulation paradigm, cTBS) to the pTr in the right inferior frontal gyrus (homologous BA45), following a published protocol [18].

2.9.2. Group T2: 1 Hz (Low Frequency) rTMS over the Right Pars Triangularis (pTr). Participants in this group (P4, P5, and P6) received 10 daily stimulation treatments of 1 Hz rTMS (1200 pulses in 20 minutes each) over the right pTr.

2.10. Statistical Analyses. To analyze data with categorical outcomes (e.g., correct/incorrect and target word naming), Weighted Statistics (WEST) ("West-Trend" and "West-ROC" (one tailed)) were applied (see [41] for a review and the algorithm that calculated the weighted factors). Such statistics offer a mean of analyzing single-case study data when multiple baselines have been undertaken. Functional language data are reported in detail according to the QPA protocol, and QoL findings are reported rounded to two decimal places.

3. Results

3.1. Categorical Language and Cognitive Outcomes. The interrater reliability agreement between the two speech and language pathologists who analyzed the data was above 95%. The weights used in this study for the testing schedule of baseline 1, baseline 2, posttreatment (i.e., one day posttreatment), and follow-up (i.e., two months posttreatment) were as follows: (i) −3, −1, 1, and 3 in order to evaluate the trend across the study (WEST-Trend) and (ii) 3, −4, −1, and 2 to compare the rates of change (ROCs) across treatment and no treatment phases (WEST-ROC). This was the main analysis for all participants (P1-P6). However, for participant 1 (P1), the testing schedule was different: baseline 1, baseline 2, posttreatment (i.e., one day posttreatment) follow-up 1 (i.e., two months posttreatment), follow-up 2 (i.e., one year posttreatment), and follow-up 3 (i.e., two years posttreatment). The WEST-Trend and WEST-ROC weights up to follow-up 2 period were −2, −1, 0, 1, and 2 and 2, −2, −1, 0, and 1, respectively. The WEST-Trend and WEST-ROC weights for periods follow-up 1, follow-up 2, and follow-up 3 were −2, 0, and 2 and 1, −2, and 1, respectively. In the last two analyses (up to follow-up 2 and follow-up 3 stages) for P1, WEST-ROC evaluated the rates of change in the short versus long-term periods to explore the possible long-term (i.e., one and two years posttreatment) effects of TMS therapy. Performance on categorical language and cognitive data for all participants is reported in Tables 2 and 3 and Figure 3. Data relating to short-term and long-term effects (up to one-year follow-up) for participant 1 (P1) have been also published previously [42].

3.1.1. Participant 1 (P1)

(1) Short-Term Effects (i.e., One Day Posttreatment) of cTBS (Pre-TMS 1–Pre-TMS 2–Post-TMS). P1 did not show any overall improvement in comprehension ($t(63) = 0.44$, $p = .32$), problem-solving skills, naming, or reading. However, she showed moderate improvement in expressive language ($t(25) = 1.79$, $p = .04$), but this improvement was not higher

in the treated (i.e., TMS period) versus the untreated periods (i.e., baseline periods) ($t(25) = 0.90$, $p = .19$).

(2) Long-Term Effects (i.e., Two Months Posttreatment) of cTBS (Pre-TMS 2–Post-TMS–Follow-Up 1). P1 did not show any overall improvement in expressive language ($t(25) = 0.57$, $p = .28$), problem-solving skills, or naming. However, she showed significant improvement in comprehension ($t(63) = 3.66$, $p < .001$) and moderate improvement in reading ($t(28) = 1.79$, $p = .04$), and such improvements were greater during the first follow-up period (i.e., two months post-TMS) compared to the short-term (i.e., one day post-TMS) for both language comprehension ($t(63) = 2.61$, $p < .01$) and reading ($t(28) = 1.79$, $p = .04$).

(3) Long-Term Effects (i.e., One Year Posttreatment) of cTBS (Post-TMS–Follow-Up 1–Follow-Up 2). P1 did not improve in expressive language ($t(25) = 0.76$, $p = .75$), cognition, and naming. However, she sustained significant improvement in comprehension ($t(63) = 2.80$, $p = .003$) and moderate improvement in reading ($t(28) = 2.11$, $p = .02$) up to one year post-TMS.

(4) Long-Term Effects (i.e., Two Years Posttreatment) of cTBS (Follow-Up 1–Follow-Up 2–Follow-Up 3). P1 did not show any downward trend in cognition ($t(35) = 1$, $p = .16$), expressive language abilities ($t(63) = 0$, $p = .5$), naming, comprehension ($t(63) = 0$, $p = .5$), and reading ($t(28) = −1$, $p = .84$), showing that language gains in comprehension and reading were sustained at least up to two years posttreatment.

3.1.2. Participant 2 (P2)

(1) Short-Term Effects (i.e., One Day Posttreatment) of cTBS (Pre-TMS 1–Pre-TMS 2–Post-TMS). P2 did not show any overall improvement in either cognition (problem-solving skills) ($t(35) = 0.32$, $p = .37$), comprehension ($t(63) = 1.52$, $p = .07$), expressive language ($t(25) = 0.46$, $p = .32$), or naming ($t(33) = −0.81$, $p = .79$). However, he showed an overall improvement in reading ($t(28) = 1.79$, $p = .04$), but this improvement was not higher in the treated (i.e., TMS period) versus the untreated periods (i.e., baseline periods) ($t(28) = 0.91$, $p = .187$).

(2) Long-Term Effects (i.e., Two Months Posttreatment) of cTBS (Pre-TMS 2–Post-TMS–Follow-Up 1). P2 did not show any overall improvement in either cognition (problem-solving skills) ($t(35) = 0.37$, $p = .35$), expressive language ($t(25) = 0.63$, $p = .27$), or reading ($t(28) = 0.81$, $p = .21$). However, he showed an overall improvement in comprehension ($t(63) = 1.76$, $p = .041$) and naming ($t(33) = 1.75$, $p = .04$), but such improvements were not higher during the first follow-up period (i.e., two months post-TMS) compared to short-term (i.e., one day post-TMS) for either comprehension ($t(63) = 0.12$, $p = .45$) or naming ($t(33) = 1.07$, $p = .14$).

3.1.3. Participant 3 (P3)

TABLE 2: Categorical language and cognitive scores at posttreatment and follow-up compared to baseline for P1, P2, and P3.

Participant item	P1						P2				P3			
	B1	B2	P-TMS	F1	F2	F3	B1	B2	P-TMS	F1	B1	B2	P-TMS	F1
Problem-solving skills	7/36	8/36	8/36	8/36	7/36	7/36	27/36	30/36	28/36	32/36	35/36	34/36	33/36	35/36
Auditory comprehension	12/64	13/64	13/64	26/64	24/64	24/64	18/64	18/64	21/64	24/64	31/64	29/64	30/64	31/64
Expressive language (Boston naming test—excluded)	0.5/26	0.5/26	2/26	1/26	1/26	1/26	4/26	4/26	5/26	6/26	13.5/26	13.5/26	13.5/26	15/26
Naming—accuracy	1/34	0/34	1/34	0/34	1/34	1/34	4/34	2/34	2/34	6/34	17/34	12/34	14/34	15.5/34
Reading skills	2/29	2/29	2/29	5/29	6/29	4/29	14/29	14/29	17/29	16/29	14/29	19/29	18/29	19/29

Key: P1: participant 1; P2: participant 2; P3: participant 3; B1: baseline 1; B2: baseline 2; P-TMS: post-TMS (1 day posttreatment); F1: follow-up 1 (2 months posttreatment); F2: follow-up 2 (1 year posttreatment); F3: follow-up 3 (2 years posttreatment).

TABLE 3: Categorical language and cognitive scores at posttreatment and follow-up compared to baseline for P4, P5, and P6.

Participant item	P4				P5				P6			
	B1	B2	P-TMS	F1	B1	B2	P-TMS	F1	B1	B2	P-TMS	F1
Problem-solving skills	17/36	22/36	21/36	16/36	33/36	32/36	34/36	34/36	32/36	32/36	32/36	34/36
Auditory comprehension	30/64	38/64	45/64	36/64	15/64	14/64	17/64	27/64	46/64	48/64	55/64	53/64
Expressive language (Boston naming test—excluded)	16.5/26	14.5/26	16.5/26	12.5/26	0/26	0/26	0/26	0/26	23.5/26	24.5/26	24.5/26	28.5/26
Naming—accuracy	4.5/34	5/34	9/34	4.5/34	0/34	0/34	0/34	0/34	25/34	25.5/34	25.5/34	28.5/34
Reading skills	23/29	21/29	23/29	25/29	8/29	9/29	11/29	9/29	24/29	26/29	28/29	27/29

Key: P4: participant 4; P5: participant 5; P6: participant 6; B1: baseline 1; B2: baseline 2; P-TMS: post-TMS (1 day posttreatment); F1: follow-up 1 (2 months posttreatment).

(1) Short-Term Effects (i.e., One Day Posttreatment) of cTBS (Pre-TMS 1–Pre-TMS 2–Post-TMS). P3 did not show any overall improvement in cognition (problem-solving skills) ($t(35) = -1.43$, $p = .91$), comprehension ($t(63) = 1.13$, $p = .13$), expressive language, or reading ($t(28) = 1$, $p = .17$). However, he showed an overall improvement in naming ($t(33) = 3.01$, $p < .01$), but this improvement was not higher in the treated (i.e., TMS period) versus the untreated periods (i.e., baseline periods) ($t(33) = -.55$, $p = .71$).

(2) Long-Term Effects (i.e., Two Months Posttreatment) of cTBS (Pre-TMS 2–Post-TMS–Follow-Up 1). P3 did not show any overall improvement in cognition (problem-solving skills) ($t(35) = 0.57$, $p = .28$), comprehension ($t(63) = 0.33$, $p = .37$), expressive language ($t(25) = 0.33$, $p = .37$), naming ($t(33) = 1.22$, $p < .01$), or reading ($t(28) = 0$, $p = .50$).

3.1.4. Participant 4 (P4)

(1) Short-Term Effects (i.e., One Day Posttreatment) of 1 Hz rTMS (Pre-TMS 1–Pre-TMS 2–Post-TMS). P4 did not show any overall improvement in cognition (problem-solving skills) ($t(35) = 1.07$, $p = .14$), expressive language ($t(25) = 0$, $p = .50$), or reading ($t(28) = 0$, $p = .50$). However, she showed an overall improvement in comprehension ($t(63) = 3.37$, $p < .001$) and naming ($t(33) = 2.31$, $p = 0.01$), but this improvement was not higher in the treated (i.e., TMS period) versus the untreated periods (i.e., baseline periods) for either comprehension ($t(63) = -.13$, $p = .55$) or naming ($t(25) = 1.09$, $p = .14$).

(2) Long-Term Effects (i.e., Two Months Posttreatment) of 1 Hz rTMS (Pre-TMS 2–Post-TMS–Follow-Up 1). P4 did not show any overall improvement in cognition (problem-solving skills) ($t(35) = -2.23$, $p = .98$), comprehension ($t(63) = -.046$, $p = .67$), expressive language ($t(25) = -1$, $p = .83$), naming ($t(33) = -0.29$, $p = .61$), or reading ($t(28) = 1.44$, $p = .08$).

3.1.5. Participant 5 (P5)

(1) Short-Term Effects (i.e., One Day Posttreatment) of 1 Hz rTMS (Pre-TMS 1–Pre-TMS 2–Post-TMS). P5 did not show any overall improvement in cognition (problem-solving skills) ($t(35) = 0.43$, $p = .33$), comprehension ($t(63) = 0.46$, $p = .32$), expressive language, naming, or reading ($t(28) = 1.36$, $p = .09$).

(2) Long-Term Effects (i.e., Two Months Posttreatment) of 1 Hz rTMS (Pre-TMS 2–Post-TMS–Follow-Up 1). P5 did not show any overall improvement in cognition (problem-solving skills) ($t(35) = 1$, $p = .16$), expressive language, naming, or reading ($t(28) = 0$, $p = .50$). However, he showed an overall improvement in comprehension ($t(63) = 2.72$, $p < .01$), but such improvement was not higher during the first follow-up period (i.e., two months post-TMS) compared to short-term (i.e., one day post-TMS) ($t(63) = 1.15$, $p = .12$).

3.1.6. Participant 6 (P6)

(1) Short-Term Effects (i.e., One Day Posttreatment) of 1 Hz rTMS (Pre-TMS 1–Pre-TMS 2–Post-TMS). P6 did not show any overall improvement in cognition (problem-solving

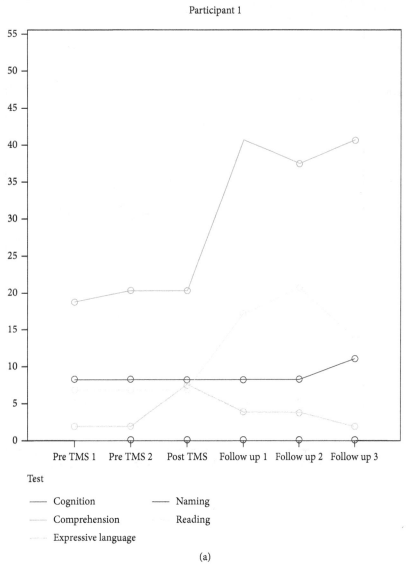

(a)

FIGURE 3: Continued.

Participant 2

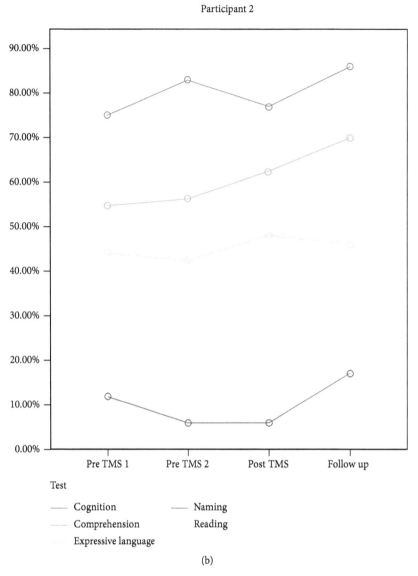

(b)

FIGURE 3: Continued.

Participant 3

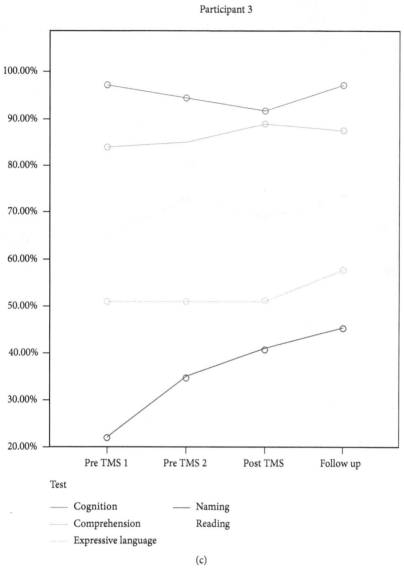

(c)

FIGURE 3: Continued.

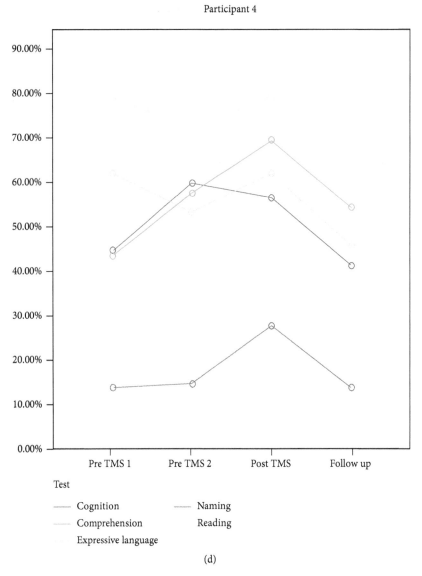

(d)

FIGURE 3: Continued.

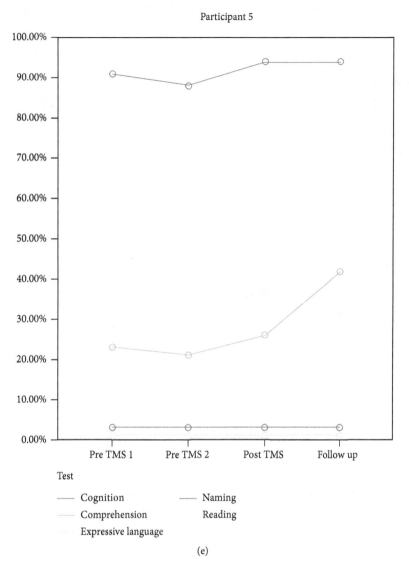

(e)

FIGURE 3: Continued.

Participant 6

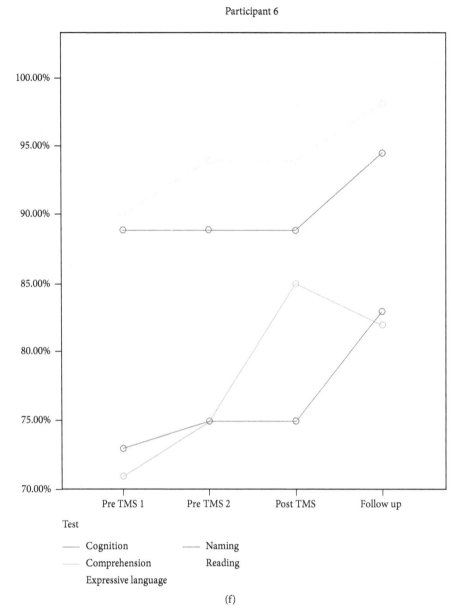

(f)

FIGURE 3: Short-term (one day posttreatment) and long-term (two months, one year, and two years posttreatment) effects of cTBS on cognitive and language performance for all 6 participants. The Y axis depicts relative values to demonstrate the magnitude of variation, if any, between assessments for each domain. Key: pre-TMS 1: baseline 1; pre-TMS 2: baseline 2; post-TMS: 1 day posttreatment; follow-up 1: 2 months posttreatment; follow-up 2: 1 year posttreatment; follow-up 3: 2 years posttreatment; follow-up: 2 months posttreatment.

skills) ($t(35) = 0$, $p = 0.5$), expressive language ($t(25) = 0.70$, $p = .25$), or naming ($t(33) = 0.37$, $p = .35$). However, he showed an overall improvement in comprehension ($t(63) = 2.60$, $p < .001$) and reading ($t(28) = 2.25$, $p = .02$), but such improvements were not higher in the treated (i.e., TMS period) versus the untreated periods (i.e., baseline periods) for either comprehension ($t(63) = 0.77$, $p = .21$) or reading ($t(28) = -0.15$, $p = .44$).

(2) Long-Term Effects (i.e., Two Months Posttreatment) of 1 Hz rTMS (Pre-TMS 2–Post-TMS–Follow-Up 1). P6 did not show any overall improvement in cognition (problem-

solving skills) ($t(35) = 1$, $p = .16$), expressive language ($t(25) = 1$, $p = .16$), naming ($t(33) = 1.49$, $p = .07$), or reading ($t(28) = .44$, $p = .33$). However, he showed an overall improvement in comprehension ($t(63) = 1.69$, $p = .04$), but such improvement was not higher during the first follow-up period (i.e., two months post-TMS) compared to short-term (i.e., one day post-TMS) ($t(63) = -1.58$, $p = .93$).

3.2. Functional Language Outcomes. P1 and P5 had global aphasia and did not produce any narratives. A baseline average score was calculated for each linguistic index for each of the remaining participants (P2, P3, P4, and P6) individually.

But for this study analyses, both baseline measurements were taken into account as they provided information on the range of microstructure performance.

3.2.1. Participant 2 (P2)

(1) Short-Term Outcomes (i.e., One Day Posttreatment). P2 produced a significantly higher number of narrative words (mostly adverbs and verbs) in the posttreatment assessment phase compared to baseline. Sentence productivity remained stable, and grammatical accuracy remained stable with an exception in the proportion of sentences with verbs that increased. The number and types of errors also remained stable. Results from the short-term microstructure analysis of the MAIN for P2 are shown in Table 4.

(2) Long-Term Outcomes (i.e., Two Months Posttreatment). At follow-up, P2 reverted to baseline with regard to the total number of narrative words. This was the case for all lexical categories except pronouns that increased. Sentence productivity also remained stable. With regard to grammatical accuracy, the proportion of sentences with verbs reverted to baseline and well-formed utterances showed a downward trend. The number and types of errors remained stable. Results from the long-term microstructure analysis of the MAIN for P2 are shown in Table 4.

3.2.2. Participant 3 (P3)

(1) Short-Term Outcomes (i.e., One Day Posttreatment). P3 produced the same number of narrative words in the posttreatment assessment period compared to baseline. Sentence productivity remained stable. Grammatical accuracy also remained stable with the exception of the proportion of well-formed utterances that showed trends for improvement. With regard to error types and numbers, phonological errors and neologism showed a decreasing trend. Results from the short-term microstructure analysis of the MAIN for P3 are shown in Table 5.

(2) Long-Term Outcomes (i.e., Two Months Posttreatment). At follow-up, P3 produced more narrative words (closed class words and nouns) compared to baseline. Sentence productivity remained stable, but the embedding index showed a declining trend. With regard to grammatical accuracy, the participant showed trends for improvement in the proportion of sentences with verbs and the proportion of well-formed utterances remained increased compared to baseline. With regard to error types and numbers; the number of phonological errors reverted to baseline, but neologisms retained the downward trend that was also exhibited in the short-term. Overall, the percentage of errors retained the downward trend that was also exhibited in the short-term. Results from the long-term microstructure analysis of the MAIN for P3 are shown in Table 5.

3.2.3. Participant 4 (P4)

(1) Short-Term Outcomes (i.e., One Day Posttreatment). No differences in the number of narrative words in the short-term were observed with the exception of closed class words

that showed an upward trend. With regard to sentence productivity, MLU showed a trend of increase. In terms of grammatical accuracy, the proportion of well-formed utterances showed a declining trend, but no single word utterances were produced. As for error types and numbers, the participant made more phonological and lexical errors. Results from the short-term microstructure analysis of the MAIN for P4 are shown in Table 6.

(2) Long-Term Outcomes (i.e., Two Months Posttreatment). At follow-up, P4 produced an overall lower number of narrative words compared to baseline. This was the case for closed class words and nouns. On the other hand, she produced more prepositions compared to baseline. Sentence productivity was similar to that of baseline. The overall percentage of errors and error types reverted to baseline. Results from the long-term microstructure analysis of the MAIN for P4 are shown in Table 6.

3.2.4. Participant 6 (P6)

(1) Short-Term Outcomes (i.e., One Day Posttreatment). P6 produced a higher number of narrative words in the posttreatment assessment compared to baseline. This was mainly the case for closed class words and adjectives. Sentence productivity increased significantly mainly in the MLU. Grammatical accuracy remained stable in all aspects except for the proportion of well-formed utterances that showed a declining trend. The proportion and types of errors remained stable. Results from the short-term microstructure analysis of the MAIN for P6 are shown in Table 7.

(2) Long-Term Outcomes (i.e., Two Months Posttreatment). At follow-up, P6 retained the increasing trend he exhibited in the short-term with regard to the number of narrative words. This was mainly the case for closed class words, adjectives, and prepositions. Regarding sentence productivity, MLU and embedding indices remained increased compared to baseline, while the elaboration index decreased. Grammatical accuracy and the proportion and types of errors remained stable. Results from the long-term microstructure analysis of the MAIN for P6 are shown in Table 7.

3.3. Quality of Life Outcomes. Quality of life was assessed once at baseline (i.e., day 1 of study) and at follow-up (i.e., two months posttreatment) in all participants. However, P1 was further assessed at one- and two-year follow-ups. Results from the SAQOL-39g assessment are rounded to two decimal places and reported in Table 8. The observed score fluctuations in QoL domains for P1, P4, P5, and P6 were insignificant. However, P2 showed a moderate decline in the communication score and moderate-significant decline in the psychosocial score at two months posttreatment. P3 showed a moderate decline in the psychosocial score at two months posttreatment.

4. Discussion

This study set out to investigate the effectiveness of two rTMS paradigms (i.e., 1 Hz rTMS and cTBS) as standalone

Table 4: Short-term (one day posttreatment) and long-term (two months posttreatment) effects of cTBS on narration outcomes (i.e., functional communication) for participant 2.

Category	Participant 2				
Lexical selection	Pre-TMS 1	Pre-TMS 2	Baseline	Post-TMS	Follow-up
Closed class	10	21	15.50	20	10
Nouns	3	3	3.00	4	1
Adjectives	4	7	5.50	11	4
Prepositions	4	7	5.50	6	1
Adverbs	1	4	2.50	16	5
Pronouns	11	8	9.50	14	18
Verbs	18	21	19.50	31	18
Sentence productivity					
MLU	2.55	4.44	3.49	3.40	3.17
Elaboration index	1.06	1.75	1.40	1.21	1.53
Embedding index	0.00	0.31	0.16	0.10	0.17
Discourse productivity					
Narrative words	51	71	61.00	102	57
Grammatical accuracy					
Prop of S with V	18	16	17.00	29	15
Prop of U w/o V	2	0	1.00	0	2
Prop of single word U	0	0	0.00	1	1
Prop of well-formed U	0.94	0.75	0.85	0.79	0.33
AUX complexity index	1.06	1.07	1.06	1.00	1.00
Error types					
Phonological	1	1	1.00	2	2
Morphosyntactic	2	0	1.00	2	1
Semantic	1	0	0.50	0	1
Lexical	2	2	2.00	3	3
Neologisms	0	0	0.00	0	0
Circumlocution	0	1	0.50	0	1
Phonological %	0.02	0.01	0.02	0.02	0.04
Morphosyntactic %	0.04	0.00	0.02	0.02	0.02
Semantic %	0.02	0.00	0.01	0.00	0.02
Lexical %	0.04	0.03	0.03	0.03	0.05
Neologisms %:	0.00	0.00	0.00	0.00	0.00
Circumlocution %	0.00	0.01	0.01	0.00	0.02
All errors %	0.12	0.06	0.08	0.07	0.14

Key: prop: proportion; s: sentences; V: verbs; U: utterances; w/o: without.

treatments for chronic poststroke aphasia in six individuals. Acute and subacute aphasia were both excluded from this study since only in chronic aphasia is there a remarkable slowing in the rate of spontaneous functional recovery [43].

The rationale behind the decision of using rTMS as a standalone treatment was based on (i) previous evidence suggesting that rTMS alone can lead to long-term language recovery in chronic aphasia poststroke [44–46] and (ii) the inconsistencies in SALT approaches (type and intensity) amongst several TMS aphasia studies [3–8, 20–23].

The decision to use two rTMS paradigms (i.e., cTBS and 1 Hz rTMS) was made in order to explore whether such protocols would induce similar changes in language performance in the sample under investigation, since both neuromodulation paradigms exert the same neurophysiological effects on the human brain (i.e., suppression of neuronal activity) even though they differ in the duration of TMS conditioning.

The trial followed a single study experimental design (SSED) in which all participants underwent two baseline measurements, then received 10 daily sessions of rTMS, and were reassessed one day and two months posttreatment. Participant 1 was further reassessed one- and two years posttreatment. The rest of the participants were not reassessed after the two-month follow-up period for several reasons (P3, P4, and P5 started one-to-one speech therapy; P2 lost interest as he did not observe any functional improvement; P6 started group aphasia therapy). More recently, it was

TABLE 5: Short-term (one day posttreatment) and long-term (two months posttreatment) effects of cTBS on narration outcomes (i.e., functional communication) for participant 3.

| Category | | | Participant 3 | | |
Lexical selection	Pre-TMS 1	Pre-TMS 2	Baseline	Post-TMS	Follow-up
Closed class	21	22	21.50	25	33
Nouns	17	19	18.00	21	29
Adjectives	4	2	3.00	1	5
Prepositions	5	5	5.00	7	7
Adverbs	3	2	2.50	0	2
Pronouns	6	8	7.00	4	8
Verbs	19	19	19.00	19	23
Sentence productivity					
MLU	5.36	6.42	5.89	6.42	5.35
Elaboration index	2.31	2.92	2.61	2.67	2.25
Embedding index	0.36	0.58	0.47	0.58	0.15
Discourse productivity					
Narrative words	75	77	76.00	77	107
Grammatical accuracy					
Prop of S with V	13	12	12.50	12	20
Prop of U w/o V	1	0	0.50	0	0
Prop of single word U	0	0	0.00	0	0
Prop of well-formed U	0.38	0.42	0.40	0.75	0.60
AUX complexity index	1.07	1.00	1.04	1.17	1.05
Error types					
Phonological	26	25	25.50	21	28
Morphosyntactic	3	2	2.50	4	5
Semantic	0	1	0.50	0	0
Lexical	4	0	2.00	0	3
Neologisms	4	4	4.00	0	0
Circumlocution	0	0	0.00	0	2
Phonological %	0.35	0.32	0.34	0.27	0.26
Morphosyntactic %	0.04	0.03	0.03	0.05	0.05
Semantic %	0.00	0.01	0.01	0.00	0.00
Lexical %	0.05	0.00	0.03	0.00	0.03
Neologisms %	0.05	0.05	0.05	0.00	0.00
Circumlocution %	0.00	0.00	0.00	0.00	0.02
All errors %	0.49	0.42	0.45	0.32	0.36

Key: prop: proportion; s: sentences; V: verbs; U: utterances; w/o: without.

alleged that two pretherapy probes can track the level of performance and rate of change [41]. In the present study, two baseline measurements were applied to lessen concerns that the observed effects may be due to random variation in subject performance and also to minimize placebo effects [42]. Furthermore, participants were blind to their status of TMS conditioning (real vs. sham) until the end of the study. Crucially, none of the six participants experienced any side effects during or after TMS conditioning.

Results from the present study corroborate findings from other studies that have successfully used TBS paradigms [13, 14, 16] revealing that cTBS and 1 Hz rTMS bring about comparable changes in language performance. In the short-term (i.e., one day posttreatment), all participants but one

(P5 with global aphasia) showed trends towards improvement in several language skills. In the long-term (i.e., two months posttreatment), three participants showed trends towards improvement in various language skills. All three participants with anomic aphasia exhibited trends of improvement in comprehension (one in the short-term, one in the long-term, and one in the short- and long-term); two showed trends of improvement in reading (one in the short-term and one in the short- and long-term), and two showed trends towards improvement in naming (one in the short-term and one in the long-term). One participant (P1 with global aphasia) showed overall improvements in comprehension and reading at two months and at one-year follow-up [42] that were sustained two years posttreatment as well. Notably, this was the

TABLE 6: Short-term (one day posttreatment) and long-term (two months posttreatment) effects of 1 Hz rTMS on narration outcomes (i.e., functional communication) for participant 4.

Category Lexical selection	Pre-TMS 1	Pre-TMS 2	Participant 4 Baseline	Post-TMS	Follow-up
Closed class	15	21	18.00	26	7
Nouns:	11	21	16.00	20	6
Adjectives	0	7	3.50	2	0
Prepositions	0	1	0.50	1	6
Adverbs	1	1	1.00	0	0
Pronouns	14	8	11.00	6	13
Verbs	11	17	14.00	12	10
Sentence productivity					
MLU	3.50	4.00	3.75	4.86	3.23
Elaboration index	2.38	1.53	1.95	1.64	1.60
Embedding index	0.14	0.05	0.10	0.07	0
Discourse productivity					
Narrative words	52	76	64,00	68	42
Grammatical accuracy					
Prop of S with V	8	15	11.50	11	10
Prop of U w/o V	3	2	2.50	3	1
Prop of single word U	3	2	2.50	0	2
Prop of well-formed U	0.50	0.27	0.38	0.09	0.50
AUX complexity index	1.00	1.00	1.00	0.90	1.00
Error types					
Phonological	0	2	1.00	6	1
Morphosyntactic	3	14	8.50	14	2
Semantic	0	5	2.50	4	3
Lexical	0	1	0.50	3	2
Neologisms	1	1	1.00	0	1
Circumlocution	0	0	0.00	1	0
Phonological %	0.00	0.03	0.02	0.09	0.02
Morphosyntactic %	0.06	0.18	0.13	0.21	0.05
Semantic %	0.00	0.07	0.04	0.06	0.07
Lexical %	0.00	0.01	0.01	0.04	0.05
Neologisms %	0.02	0.01	0.02	0.00	0.02
Circumlocution %	0.00	0.00	0.00	0.01	0.00
All errors %	0.08	0.30	0.21	0.41	0.21

Key: prop: proportion; s: sentences; V: verbs; U: utterances; w/o: without.

oldest participant who exhibited severe global aphasia resulting from diffuse left hemispheric lesions that also had the least years of education (i.e., six) compared to the other participants. No decline in linguistic and cognitive performance compared to baseline was observed in any participant. Also, none of the participants showed any (trend towards) improvement in the control variable (i.e., problem-solving skills). The control variable was assessed at baseline as many times (i.e., two) as the dependent language variables (i.e., comprehension, expression, reading, and naming accuracy) in all participants, and as it remained stable in all participants, it was assumed that (i) the chances that TMS led to language specific gains were increased and (ii) the possibilities for the placebo and training effects were reduced.

To date, three studies have shown that 1 Hz (LF) rTMS as a standalone therapy can lead to language gains in some PWA. In particular, one study [44] investigated the effects of 1 Hz rTMS on naming performance and noticed immediate and long-lasting improvements (6 months posttreatment) in nine individuals with mild-to-moderate chronic nonfluent aphasia. In the present study, along with two participants that had anomic aphasia and exhibited trends towards improvement in naming, the participant with Broca's aphasia also showed a trend of improvement in naming, however only in the short-term. In another study, improvements in several language skills (i.e., naming, repetition, picture description tasks, and length of utterances) were observed that lasted up to 12 months post (1 Hz)-rTMS

TABLE 7: Short-term (one day posttreatment) and long-term (two months posttreatment) effects of 1 Hz rTMS on narration outcomes (i.e., functional communication) for participant 6.

Category Lexical selection	Pre-TMS 1	Pre-TMS 2	Participant 6 Baseline	Post-TMS	Follow-up
Closed class	22	30	26.00	41	41
Nouns	17	26	21.50	27	24
Adjectives	3	3	3.00	10	12
Prepositions	6	6	6.00	8	13
Adverbs	3	3	3.00	3	2
Pronouns	4	5	4.50	4	3
Verbs	14	21	17.50	23	22
Sentence productivity					
MLU	6.56	6.00	6.28	9.67	8.83
Elaboration index	3.33	2.93	3.13	4.17	1.83
Embedding index	0.5	0.38	0.44	0.92	0.85
Discourse productivity					
Narrative words	69	94	81.5	116	117
Grammatical accuracy					
Prop of S with V	9	15	12	11	12
Prop of U w/o V	1	1	1	1	1
Prop of single word U	0	0	0	0	0
Prop of well-formed U	0.89	0.93	0.91	0.73	0.83
AUX complexity index	1.11	1.07	1.09	1.00	1.00
Error types					
Phonological	4	0	2.00	0	0
Morphosyntactic	3	0	1.50	1	2
Semantic	0	3	1.50	0	4
Lexical	1	2	1.50	2	2
Neologisms	0	0	0.00	0	0
Circumlocution	0	0	0.00	1	0
Phonological %	0.06	0.00	0.02	0.00	0.00
Morphosyntactic %	0.04	0.00	0.02	0.01	0.02
Semantic %	0.00	0.03	0.02	0.00	0.03
Lexical %	0.01	0.02	0.02	0.02	0.02
Neologisms %	0.00	0.00	0.00	0.00	0.00
Circumlocution %	0.00	0.00	0.00	0.01	0.00
All errors %	0.12	0.05	0.08	0.03	0.07

Key: prop: proportion; s: sentences; V: verbs; U: utterances; w/o: without.

in six people with chronic nonfluent aphasia poststroke [45]. In the present study, one participant with severe global aphasia showed sustained improvements in comprehension and reading two months, one year, and two years posttreatment. In another trial [46], an increase in the number of closed-class words of discourse productivity was noticed in 10 individuals with chronic nonfluent aphasia two months posttreatment with 1 Hz rTMS. In our study, the analysis of narratives yielded mixed results. With regard to error types and percentages, the participant with Broca's aphasia (P3) exhibited less phonological errors and neologisms in the short-term and less neologisms in the long-term. On the other hand, one of the participants with moderate-severe anomic aphasia (P4) made more phonological and

lexical errors in the short-term but reverted to baseline performance in the long-term. Discourse productivity increased in the short-term in one participant with moderate-severe anomic aphasia (P2) and in the long-term in the participant with Broca's aphasia (P3). The participant with mild anomic aphasia (P6) showed improvement in the short-term that was also sustained in the long-term. Finally, one of the participants with moderate-severe anomic aphasia (P4) showed a declining trend only in the long-term. Interestingly, the participant with mild anomic aphasia (P6) manifested an increase in his MLU both in the short- and long-term.

Up until now, several TMS randomized controlled trials (RCTs) have indicated that 1 Hz rTMS over the contralesional IFG in conjunction with SALT has the potential to

TABLE 8: Quality of life at the pretreatment (baseline) stage and at 2 months follow-up using the SAQOL-39g for all participants and at baseline, at 2 months follow-up, at 1 year follow-up, and at 2 years follow-up for participant 1.

Item (maximum score: 5)	Participant 1				Participant 2		Participant 3		Participant 4		Participant 5		Participant 6	
	Baseline	2 months post-TMS	1 year post-TMS	2 years post-TMS	Baseline	2 months post-TMS	Baseline	2 months post-TMS	Baseline	2 months post TMS	Baseline	2 months post TMS	Baseline	2 months post TMS
SAQOL-39g mean score	2.05	2.18	2.12	1.9	3.57	3.1	4.03	3.82	3.32	3.2	1	1	4.24	4.28
Physical score	2.38	2.44	2.25	2.1	4.62	4.43	5	5	4.68	4.5	1	1	4.75	4.81
Communication score	1.57	1.72	1.85	1.6	2.71	2.28	3.28	3.14	2.42	2.1	1	1	4.71	4.71
Psychosocial score	2.2	2.38	2.25	2	3.37	2.56	3.81	3.31	2.87	3	1	1	3.25	3.31

drive change in various language domains in at least some people with subacute [3–5, 8, 22, 23] and chronic aphasia [11, 21]. Nonetheless, there are several inconsistencies in those studies concerning the site of stimulation within the homologue of Broca's area; the methods of localization of the stimulation site; the ingredients, dosage, and intensity of the adjunct SALT; the number and types of language outcomes measures; and the number and duration of follow-up assessments. In addition, not all studies have reported positive outcomes. For example, a most recent RCT [47] did not find any beneficial add on effects of 1 Hz rTMS to SALT in chronic poststroke aphasia rehabilitation. Another study raises concerns about applying LF TMS over the right pTr in patients with apraxia of speech (AoS) [48]. In this study, the researchers demonstrated that a 69-year-old individual with AoS due to a left first ever small ischemic stroke of the left precentral gyrus deteriorated after one session of real cTBS over the contralesional precentral gyrus and improved after sham cTBS over the same area according to both objective and subjective evaluations. The findings of those trials highlight the possible impact of lesion location on noninvasive neuromodulation response and point towards the development of individualized rTMS aphasia rehabilitation protocols by considering individual-intrinsic variables (age at the time of stroke, lesion volume and location, white matter integrity, and cognitive-linguistic impairment) and individual extrinsic variables (e.g., environment, treatment mode, language, and brain recovery) [49], rather than providing a "one-size fits all" neuromodulation approach. Furthermore, such findings imply that expressive language processes rely on cortical networks that involve both hemispheres.

In addition to RCTs supporting the potential benefit of LF rTMS on aphasia rehabilitation poststroke, some systematic reviews with/without meta-analyses are also supportive [50–53]. However, other recent work has indicated that the quality of the conduct of reviews 50–53 is low, and therefore, more research is needed [54]. More recently, a meta-analysis of RCTs and randomized cross-over trials [55] found a moderate long-term effect size of rTMS effects in language gains especially in naming in both subacute and chronic patients with aphasia. In this review, five studies applied LF rTMS, one study combined LF with HF rTMS, and one study compared LF with HF and sham TMS (see [55] and references within).

Overall, research in the field of 1 Hz rTMS to the contralesional IFG in aphasia recovery is ongoing but is also parallel to trials investigating the effects of different paradigms, either in terms of stimulation sites and/or TMS paradigms per se. For example, an emerging number of studies have started exploring inhibitory cTBS over the contralesional IFG [15, 25, 56], excitatory iTBS over perilesional areas of the left hemisphere [12, 13, 16], and sequential cTBS and iTBS [14].

Aphasia-related TMS research is flourishing, and TMS technology has now become a mainstream application in many aphasia labs worldwide. The challenge researchers are facing is the unravelment of the mechanisms of TMS-induced language recovery and the understanding of why some people respond (more or less) whilst others do not respond to this neuromodulation technique. Despite numerous clinical studies that have explored the therapeutic potential of rTMS in several neurological disorders, the cellular and molecular mechanisms responsible for the after-effects of rTMS are largely unknown. The mixture of LTD and LTP effects on synapses measured by MEP behavioral changes is highly variable across individuals, showing that it would be an oversimplification to describe the rTMS after-effects as LTD or LTP-like plasticity solely based on MEP modifications [57]. Additional research is needed to elucidate how structural and functional properties of individual neurons and local networks are related to the effects of single pulse rTMS [58]. Beyond the molecular mechanisms underlying behavioral recovery, a few insightful accounts about the underpinnings of the observed TMS-induced language improvement, that also explain the rationale behind the application of various aphasia TMS protocols, have been suggested and are based in principle on models of brain reorganization after a stroke.

The first account is related to stroke-induced disruption of the interhemispheric balance. This disruption leads to reduced inhibition from the affected to the unaffected hemisphere and to increased and deleterious inhibition of the affected from the unaffected hemisphere [59]. This process is considered maladaptive for language recovery as it blocks the dominant hemisphere, where language processes are established, from resuming their role in language processes [60]. The decision of applying LF rTMS over the contralesional hemisphere in this research was motivated by the hypothesis that by inhibiting the right hemisphere, residual language supported by the left hemisphere is released from transcallosal inhibitory input by the intact right hemisphere [61].

A second possible scenario is that language gains are associated with recruitment of regions of the right hemisphere that are homotopic to the damaged components of the left language network [62]. A third account is based on the increasingly accepted theory that language processes rely on highly localized brain regions and bilaterally distributed brain networks [63], and language reorganization poststroke is based on domain-specific and domain-general network processes [64]. The hypothesis that the suppression of a hyperactive right pTr with LF rTMS modulates the right pars opercularis (pOp), and in turn, other right brain regions may explain the results of the present study.

In addition to the unravelment of the neural mechanisms of TMS-induced language recovery, cognitive and psycholinguistic analyses demonstrating which cognitive processes are implicated in language facilitation and where in the language system, rTMS induces language improvements, may provide researchers with an insight into the issue of candidacy for and responsiveness to TMS. On this basis, research is poor as most clinical aphasia studies focus on the mechanistic aspects of recovery (i.e., neuroanatomical and behavioral changes). Some explanations however provide evidence on how the language system is reorganized post-TMS. It is postulated that the observed improvement in discourse productivity in chronic nonfluent aphasia may be explained by TMS-induced improved lexical-semantic access allowing retrieval of word- and word meaning representations [46]. This could explain the noticeable improvement in accessing words in several categories and no improvement in grammatical complexity or sentence construction [46]. In the present study, there was only one participant with nonfluent aphasia who showed improvement in discourse productivity in the long-term and the above account may explain his performance.

The current study has several strengths as follows. First, we suggest adopting an SSED methodology in aphasia research and using WEST statistics to measure treatment change as such statistics are suitable for studies with small numbers of participants and nonhomogenous profiles. Second, we performed follow-up assessments to investigate the long-term effects of TMS treatment. In fact, one participant was followed up for two years posttreatment and demonstrated sustained language gains in comprehension and reading skills in that period. The findings corroborate prior evidence that TMS can lead to sustained language changes without any additional behavioral therapy [44–46]. Third, this study employed an ecologically valid measure to assess functional communication which is related to phrase and sentence production and narration and not experimental language tasks. Finally, as stroke affects health-related QoL [65], the effects of treatment on the QoL of the participants were also assessed. Proxy ratings were used as three participants struggled to respond to questions due language comprehension problems. Existing evidence supports that proxies exaggerate QoL problems of patients [66]. Hence, caution is needed when proxies contribute to QoL assessments. Nonetheless, when patient reports cannot be obtained, proxies can be helpful [67]. In the current study, the findings indicated that QoL did not significantly change in three participants because of the treatment. For the remaining participants, posttreatment communication scores showed a declining trend in three participants and the psychological scores dropped for two others. Such findings clearly capture the difference between statistical and clinical significance. Statistical significance is important for researchers and service providers but is of little value to patients and their families. Clinical significance is vital for the person with communication problems and their caregivers. Based on the results from the QoL measure, treatment results failed to meet the needs and expectations of the participants and their families. Therefore, we strongly recommend that future TMS aphasia studies are also aimed at capturing the clinical significance of this type of treatment using relevant tools.

Despite the promising results of this study, there are several limitations that warrant discussion. First, the sample size was small, and the participants had various clinical profiles. This compromises the generalizability of our findings, but on the other hand, this clinical profile heterogeneity can be seen as advantageous as it is typical of what is observed in clinical settings. Also, the fact that the TMS protocol was the same for all participants (i.e., inhibitory rTMS) allowed insight into who may benefit more from this particular protocol. It seems, for example, that it could prove beneficial for global aphasia on the grounds of diffuse left hemisphere damage. However, as direct measurements of

brain activation and connectivity were not obtained, no hypotheses could be formulated regarding which model(s) of brain-reorganization best explain(s) the findings. In TMS aphasia research, direct measures of brain activation and connectivity are needed to help with the elucidation of the neuroplastic effects of treatments [42]. Realistically though, individual fMRI localization is expensive, time consuming, and not available in all aphasia labs.

We suggest that to enhance the effectiveness of rTMS in aphasia rehabilitation, future studies should systematically document all their data in an Aphasia TMS Database similar to the PLORAS (predicting language outcome and recovery after stroke) project [68]. In particular, with regard to participants' intrinsic factors, parameters such as age, lesion location and size, vascular perfusion, brain connectivity and integrity of white matter, genetics, body mass indices, sex, handedness, education, type of aphasia, and its severity should all be documented as there is robust evidence that they all affect aphasia recovery. For instance, with regard to age, there is evidence that young people with aphasia improve more compared to older individuals [69]. Regarding lesion location, some studies suggest that lesions involving the left STG (superior temporal gyrus) and Wernicke's area are associated with poor aphasia improvement [70]. With regard to lesion magnitude, even though large left hemisphere lesions are typically associated with poorer recovery [71], in a recent study, patients with larger stroke volumes showed greater aphasia improvements regardless of the involvement of the language areas [72]. This could explain the findings from the current study in which the only participant who showed statistically significant improvements had diffuse and large brain lesions in the left hemisphere. In addition, several studies have shown shifts in vascular perfusions poststroke [73, 74], but the extent to which such alterations influence recovery of the neural networks for language is unknown [49]. Furthermore, the degree of white matter integrity in the infarcted hemisphere together with the integrity of white matter tracts in the contralesional hemisphere is also likely to be linked to recovery ([49] and references within). Research on the role of BDNF (brain-derived neurotrophic factor) variants on language recovery poststroke is emerging, and several studies have demonstrated that it influences recovery [75, 76]. Also, through univariate analysis, it has been shown that total lean body mass—not adipose tissue—may be a positive factor for predicting aphasia improvement [72]. Lastly, evidence in relation to the impact of sex [77], handedness, and educational background [78] on language recovery is controversial.

Aphasia severity has been shown to be a good predictor of recovery of both short- [79] and long-term outcomes [80]. It is postulated that all the above biological (intrinsic) factors have a synergistic effect on language recovery poststroke, and this can be verified by the observed variability in progression of aphasia and recovery even between people with the same type of aphasia. In addition, TMS parameters (e.g., type of coil, stimulation site, duration, dosage, intensity, and frequency of the stimulation) also affect outcomes. In particular, the amount of surface charge produced and thus the extent of action of the current in the brain tissue depend on many biological and physical parameters such as the magnetic pulse waveform, the intensity, frequency and pattern of stimulation, the type and orientation of coil, the distance between coil and brain, and the respective orientation of the current lines and excitable neuronal elements into the brain [43]. For example, if the handle of f8c is oriented parallel to the interhemispheric midline (posteroanterior direction), motor cortex TMS activates the pyramidal tract only indirectly through interneurons [81]. When the handle of an f8c is oriented perpendicular to the interhemispheric midline (lateromedial direction), both interneurons and pyramidal neurons are activated [82]. The lowest intensity threshold to elicit MEPs in the M1 is achieved when the stimulus creates a posteroanterior current that is orthogonal to the central sulcus (i.e., the handle of the f8c oriented 45° posteriorly and laterally) [83], but the reverse orientation (anteroposterior) makes the latency time increase by several milliseconds [43] and is considered better for inducing motor cortex plasticity [84]. To optimize the effects of TMS, it is suggested that the strength of the electric field perpendicular to the targeted area (for all cortical surface areas) is maximised [85]. Also, even though MEP measurements in healthy individuals have led to the consensus that low-frequency stimulation (≤ 1 Hz) induces inhibition, whereas high frequencies (≥ 5 Hz) induce excitation [43], both conditions may lead to mixed effects [86]. By doubling, for example, the duration of stimulation on the motor cortex inhibition may reverse to excitation and vice versa [87]. Moreover, SALT is the gold standard in aphasia rehabilitation [88], and the above discussion demonstrates the high variability and lack of standardization of SALT approaches in the field of aphasia rehabilitation [89]. The effectiveness of SALT approaches first needs to be evaluated against standards of evidence-based practice (EBP). Until then, researchers are prompted to use structured aphasia programs as adjuncts to TMS based on the evidence that this leads to neuroplastic changes that support aphasia recovery.

5. Conclusion

The advent of modern noninvasive brain stimulation techniques has shifted the attention of aphasia rehabilitation scientists to additional ways that could enhance plasticity in the lesioned language brain network. Even though the number of studies that have applied TMS in poststroke aphasia rehabilitation is increasing, results remain controversial. From the current findings, it can be concluded that inhibitory TMS over the right pTr has the potential to drive neuroplastic changes that facilitate language recovery in chronic poststroke aphasia. However, to elucidate the precise mechanisms of action that TMS exerts in the lesioned language network, researchers are urged to experiment with different protocols and follow up their participants for potential long-term and generalization effects. The importance of the clinical relevance of therapies urges future researchers to include ecological outcome measures that capture the effects of TMS aphasia treatment on everyday communication.

Acknowledgments

This work was cofunded by the European Regional Development Fund and the Republic of Cyprus through the Research and Innovation Foundation (Project: EXCELLENCE/1216/0517). We thank Mr. Karayiannis Demetris, clinical linguist (M.Sc., B.A.), for his contribution to the analysis of linguistic data.

References

[1] Z. Keser and G. E. Francisco, "Neuromodulation for post-stroke aphasia," *Current Physical Medicine and Rehabilitation Reports*, vol. 4, no. 3, pp. 171–181, 2016.

[2] J. P. Lefaucheur, A. Aleman, C. Baeken et al., "Evidence-based guidelines on the therapeutic use of repetitive transcranial magnetic stimulation (rTMS): an update (2014-2018)," *Clinical Neurophysiology*, vol. 131, no. 2, pp. 474–528, 2020.

[3] W. D. Heiss, A. Hartmann, I. Rubi-Fessen et al., "Noninvasive brain stimulation for treatment of right- and left-handed poststroke aphasics," *Cerebrovascular Diseases*, vol. 36, no. 5-6, pp. 363–372, 2013.

[4] J. Seniów, K. Waldowski, M. Leśniak, S. Iwański, W. Czepiel, and A. Członkowska, "Transcranial magnetic stimulation combined with speech and language training in early aphasia rehabilitation: a randomized double-blind controlled pilot study," *Topics in Stroke Rehabilitation*, vol. 20, no. 3, pp. 250–261, 2013.

[5] A. Thiel, A. Hartmann, I. Rubi-Fessen et al., "Effects of noninvasive brain stimulation on language networks and recovery in early poststroke aphasia," *Stroke*, vol. 44, no. 8, pp. 2240–2246, 2013.

[6] K. Waldowski, J. Seniów, M. Leśniak, S. Iwański, and A. Członkowska, "Effect of Low-Frequency Repetitive Transcranial Magnetic Stimulation on Naming Abilities in Early-Stroke Aphasic Patients: A Prospective, Randomized, Double- Blind Sham-Controlled Study," *The Scientific World Journal*, vol. 2012, Article ID 518568, 8 pages, 2012.

[7] A. Zumbansen, S. Black, J. L. Chen, and A. Thiel, "P240 Comparing the effectiveness of rTMS and tDCS for aphasia recovery after stroke," *Clinical Neurophysiology*, vol. 131, no. 4, pp. e153–e154, 2020.

[8] I. Rubi-Fessen, A. Hartmann, W. Huber et al., "Add-on effects of repetitive transcranial magnetic stimulation on subacute aphasia therapy: enhanced improvement of functional communication and basic linguistic skills. A randomized controlled study," *Archives of Physical Medicine and Rehabilitation*, vol. 96, no. 11, pp. 1935-1944.e2, 2015.

[9] T. H. Yoon, S. J. Han, T. S. Yoon, J. S. Kim, and T. I. Yi, "Therapeutic effect of repetitive magnetic stimulation combined with speech and language therapy in post-stroke non-fluent aphasia, *Neuro Rehabilitation.*, vol. 36, no. 1, pp. 107–114, 2015. "

[10] P. Y. Tsai, C. P. Wang, J. S. Ko, Y. M. Chung, Y. W. Chang, and J. X. Wang, "The persistent and broadly modulating effect of inhibitory rTMS in nonfluent aphasic patients: a sham-controlled, double-blind study," *Neurorehabilitation and Neural Repair*, vol. 28, no. 8, pp. 779–787, 2014.

[11] C. P. Wang, C. Y. Hsieh, P. Y. Tsai, C. T. Wang, F. G. Lin, and R. C. Chan, "Efficacy of synchronous verbal training during

repetitive transcranial magnetic stimulation in patients with chronic aphasia," *Stroke*, vol. 45, no. 12, pp. 3656–3662, 2014.

[12] J. P. Szaflarski, J. Griffis, J. Vannest et al., "A feasibility study of combined intermittent theta burst stimulation and modified constraint-induced aphasia therapy in chronic post-stroke aphasia," *Restorative Neurology and Neuroscience*, vol. 36, no. 4, pp. 503–518, 2018.

[13] J. C. Griffis, R. Nenert, J. B. Allendorfer, and J. P. Szaflarski, "Interhemispheric plasticity following intermittent theta burst stimulation in chronic poststroke aphasia," *Neural Plasticity*, vol. 2016, Article ID 4796906, 16 pages, 2016.

[14] J. Vuksanović, M. B. Jelić, S. D. Milanović, K. Kačar, L. Konstantinović, and S. R. Filipović, "Improvement of language functions in a chronic non-fluent post-stroke aphasic patient following bilateral sequential theta burst magnetic stimulation," *Neurocase*, vol. 21, no. 2, pp. 244–250, 2015.

[15] J. Kindler, R. Schumacher, D. Cazzoli et al., "Theta burst stimulation over the right Broca's homologue induces improvement of naming in aphasic patients," *Stroke*, vol. 43, no. 8, pp. 2175–2179, 2012.

[16] J. P. Szaflarski, J. Vannest, S. W. Wu, M. W. DiFrancesco, C. Banks, and D. L. Gilbert, "Excitatory repetitive transcranial magnetic stimulation induces improvements in chronic post-stroke aphasia," *Medical Science Monitor: International Medical Journal Of Experimental And Clinical Research*, vol. 17, no. 3, pp. CR132–CR139, 2011.

[17] Y.-Z. Huang and J. C. Rothwell, "Theta burst stimulation," in *Transcranial magnetic stimulation for treatment of psychiatric disorders*, Advances in Biological Psychiatry, M. A. Marcolin and F. Padberg, Eds., pp. 187–203, Karger, Basel, Switzerland, 2007.

[18] Y. Z. Huang, M. J. Edwards, E. Rounis, K. P. Bhatia, and J. C. Rothwell, "Theta burst stimulation of the human motor cortex," *Neuron*, vol. 45, no. 2, pp. 201–206, 2005.

[19] D. Hebert, M. P. Lindsay, A. McIntyre et al., "Canadian stroke best practice recommendations: stroke rehabilitation practice guidelines, update 2015," *International Journal of Stroke*, vol. 11, no. 4, pp. 459–484, 2016.

[20] C. Ren, G. Zhang, X. Xu et al., "The effect of rTMS over the different targets on language recovery in stroke patients with global aphasia: a randomized sham-controlled study," *BioMed Research International*, vol. 2019, Article ID 4589056, 7 pages, 2019.

[21] X. Y. Hu, T. Zhang, G. B. Rajah et al., "Effects of different frequencies of repetitive transcranial magnetic stimulation in stroke patients with non-fluent aphasia: a randomized, sham-controlled study," *Neurological Research*, vol. 40, no. 6, pp. 459–465, 2018.

[22] M. Haghighi, M. Mazdeh, N. Ranjbar, and M. A. Seifrabie, "Further evidence of the positive influence of repetitive transcranial magnetic stimulation on speech and language in patients with aphasia after stroke: results from a double-blind intervention with sham condition," *Neuropsychobiology*, vol. 75, no. 4, pp. 185–192, 2017.

[23] N. Weiduschat, A. Thiel, I. Rubi-Fessen et al., "Effects of repetitive transcranial magnetic stimulation in aphasic stroke: a randomized controlled pilot study," *Stroke*, vol. 42, no. 2, pp. 409–415, 2011.

[24] M. C. Ridding and U. Ziemann, "Determinants of the induction of cortical plasticity by non-invasive brain stimulation in healthy subjects," *Journal of Physiology*, vol. 588, no. 13, pp. 2291–2304, 2010.

[25] A. Georgiou, N. Konstantinou, I. Phinikettos, and M. Kambanaros, "Neuronavigated theta burst stimulation for chronic aphasia: two exploratory case studies," *Clinical Linguistics & Phonetic*, vol. 33, no. 6, pp. 532–546, 2019.

[26] M. L. Albert, "A simple test of visual neglect," *Neurology*, vol. 23, no. 6, pp. 658–664, 1973.

[27] J. F. Veale, "Edinburgh Handedness Inventory-Short Form: a revised version based on confirmatory factor analysis," *Laterality*, vol. 19, no. 2, pp. 164–177, 2014.

[28] L. Messinis, E. Panagea, P. Papathanasopoulos, and A. Kastellakis, *Boston Diagnostic Aphasia Examination-Short Form in Greek Language*, Gotsis, Patras, 2013.

[29] P. G. Simos, D. G. Sideridis, A. Protopapas, and A. Mouzaki, "Psychometric evaluation of a receptive vocabulary test for Greek elementary students," *Assessment for Effective Intervention*, vol. 37, no. 1, pp. 34–49, 2011.

[30] M. Kambanaros and K. K. Grohmann, "Grammatical class effects across impaired child and adult populations," *Frontiers in Psychology*, vol. 6, p. 1670, 2015.

[31] I. Phinikettos and M. Kambanaros, "An algorithm for noun and verb ranking in linguistic data (ALNOVE)," *Archives of Applied Science Research*, vol. 9, pp. 16–29, 2017.

[32] N. Gagarina, D. Klop, S. Kunnari et al., *MAIN: Multilingual Assessment Instrument for Narratives [Part I]/Download Materials to Be Used for Assessment (IIa) Pictorial Stimuli; (IIb) Adaption of MAIN in Different Languages: Guidelines for Assessment; Protocols, Scoring Sheets for Cat, Dog, Baby Birds, Baby Goats; Background Questions; Story Scripts [Part II] (ZAS Papers in Linguistics 56)*, ZAS, Berlin, 2012.

[33] J. Raven, J. C. Raven, and J. H. Court, *Manual for Raven's Progressive Matrices and Vocabulary Scales. Section 2: The Coloured Progressive Matrices*, Harcourt Assessment, San Antonio, TX, 1998.

[34] A. Kartsona and K. Hilari, "Quality of life in aphasia: Greek adaptation of the stroke and aphasia quality of life scale -39 item (SAQOL-39)," *Eura Medicophys*, vol. 43, no. 1, p. 2735, 2007.

[35] E. A. Efstratiadou, E. N. Chelas, M. Ignatiou, V. Christaki, I. Papathanasiou, and K. Hilari, "Quality of life after stroke: evaluation of the Greek SAQOL-39g," *Folia Phoniatrica et Logopaedica*, vol. 64, no. 4, pp. 179–186, 2012.

[36] T. C. Hoffmann, P. P. Glasziou, I. Boutron et al., "Better reporting of interventions: template for intervention description and replication (TIDieR) checklist and guide," *BMJ*, vol. 348, article g1687, 2014.

[37] E. M. Saffran, R. S. Berndt, and M. F. Schwartz, "The quantitative analysis of agrammatic production: procedure and data," *Brain and Language*, vol. 37, no. 3, pp. 440–479, 1989.

[38] M. Varkanitsa, "Quantitative and error analysis of connected speech: evidence from Greek-speaking patients with aphasia and normal speakers," in *Current Trends in Greek Linguistics*, G. Fragaki, A. Georgakopoulos, and C. Themistocleous, Eds., pp. 313–338, Cambridge Scholars Publishing, Cambridge, 2012.

[39] J. C. Rothwell, M. Hallett, A. Berardelli, A. Eisen, P. Rossini, and W. Paulus, "Magnetic stimulation: motor evoked potentials. The International Federation of Clinical Neuro-

physiology," *Electroencephalography and clinical neurophysiology. Supplement*, vol. 52, pp. 97–103, 1999.

[40] E. M. Wassermann, "Risk and safety of repetitive transcranial magnetic stimulation: report and suggested guidelines from the International Workshop on the Safety of Repetitive Transcranial Magnetic Stimulation, June 5-7, 1996," *Electroencephalography and Clinical Neurophysiology/Evoked Potentials Section*, vol. 108, no. 1, pp. 1–16, 1998.

[41] D. Howard, W. Best, and L. Nickels, "Optimising the design of intervention studies: critiques and ways forward," *Aphasiology*, vol. 29, no. 5, pp. 526–562, 2015.

[42] A. M. Georgiou, I. Phinikettos, C. Giasafaki, and M. Kambanaros, "Can transcranial magnetic stimulation (TMS) facilitate language recovery in chronic aphasia post-stroke? Evidence from a case study," vol. 55, Article ID 100907, Journal of Neurolinguistics, 2020.

[43] J. P. Lefaucheur, N. André-Obadia, A. Antal et al., "Evidence-based guidelines on the therapeutic use of repetitive transcranial magnetic stimulation (rTMS)," *Clinical Neurophysiology*, vol. 125, no. 11, pp. 2150–2206, 2014.

[44] D. Y. Harvey, J. Podell, P. E. Turkeltaub, O. Faseyitan, H. B. Coslett, and R. H. Hamilton, "Functional reorganization of right prefrontal cortex underlies sustained naming improvements in chronic aphasia via repetitive transcranial magnetic stimulation," *Cognitive and behavioral Neurology*, vol. 30, no. 4, pp. 133–144, 2017.

[45] C. H. Barwood, B. E. Murdoch, S. Riek et al., "Long term language recovery subsequent to low frequency rTMS in chronic non-fluent aphasia," *Neuro Rehabilitation*, vol. 32, no. 4, pp. 915–928, 2013.

[46] J. Medina, C. Norise, O. Faseyitan, H. B. Coslett, P. E. Turkeltaub, and R. H. Hamilton, "Finding the right words: transcranial magnetic stimulation improves discourse productivity in non-fluent aphasia after stroke," *Aphasiology*, vol. 26, no. 9, pp. 1153–1168, 2012.

[47] P. H. Heikkinen, F. Pulvermüller, J. P. Mäkelä et al., "Combining rTMS with intensive language-action therapy in chronic aphasia: a randomized controlled trial," *Frontiers in Neuroscience*, vol. 12, p. 1036, 2019.

[48] B. C. Kaufmann, M. Pastore-Wapp, M. Lübeck et al., "cTBS over contralesional homologue areas deteriorates speech output in isolated apraxia of speech after stroke," *Brain Stimulation: Basic, Translational, and Clinical Research in Neuromodulation*, vol. 12, no. 4, pp. 1069–1071, 2019.

[49] S. Kiran and C. K. Thompson, "Neuroplasticity of language networks in aphasia: advances, updates, and future challenges," *Frontiers in Neurology*, vol. 10, p. 295, 2019.

[50] L. Sebastianelli, V. Versace, S. Martignago et al., "Low-frequency rTMS of the unaffected hemisphere in stroke patients: a systematic review," *Acta Neurologica Scandinavica*, vol. 136, no. 6, pp. 585–605, 2017.

[51] C. D. Gadenz, T. Moreira, D. M. Capobianco, and M. Cassol, "Effects of repetitive transcranial magnetic stimulation in the rehabilitation of communication and deglutition disorders: systematic review of randomized controlled trials," *Folia Phoniatrica et Logopaedica*, vol. 67, no. 2, pp. 97–105, 2016.

[52] Y. Li, Y. Qu, M. Yuan, and T. Du, "Low-frequency repetitive transcranial magnetic stimulation for patients with aphasia after stoke: a meta-analysis," *Journal of Rehabilitation Medicine*, vol. 47, no. 8, pp. 675–681, 2015.

[53] C. L. Ren, G. F. Zhang, N. Xia et al., "Effect of low-frequency rTMS on aphasia in stroke patients: a meta-analysis of randomized controlled trials," *PLoS One*, vol. 9, no. 7, article e102557, 2014.

[54] A. M. Georgiou, E. Lada, and M. Kambanaros, "Evaluating the quality of conduct of systematic reviews on the application of transcranial magnetic stimulation (TMS) for post-stroke aphasia rehabilitation," *Aphasiology*, vol. 34, no. 5, pp. 540–556, 2020.

[55] M. Bucur and C. Papagno, "Are transcranial brain stimulation effects long-lasting in post-stroke aphasia? A comparative systematic review and meta-analysis on naming performance," *Neuroscience & Biobehavioral Reviews*, vol. 102, pp. 264–289, 2019.

[56] D. Y. Harvey, J. A. Mass, P. P. Shah-Basak et al., "Continuous theta burst stimulation over right pars triangularis facilitates naming abilities in chronic post-stroke aphasia by enhancing phonological access," *Brain and Language*, vol. 192, pp. 25–34, 2019.

[57] M. Hamada and J. C. Rothwell, "Neurophysiology of rTMS: Important Caveats When Interpreting the Results of Therapeutic Interventions," in *Therapeutic rTMS in Neurology*, T. Platz, Ed., Springer, Cham, 2016.

[58] M. Lenz, F. Müller-Dahlhaus, and A. Vlachos, "Cellular and Molecular Mechanisms of rTMS-induced Neural Plasticity," in *Therapeutic rTMS in Neurology*, T. Platz, Ed., pp. 11–22, Springer, Charm, 2016.

[59] F. Fregni and A. Pascual-Leone, "Technology insight: noninvasive brain stimulation in neurology-perspectives on the therapeutic potential of rTMS and tDCS," *Nature Clinical Practice Neurology*, vol. 3, no. 7, pp. 383–393, 2007.

[60] A. Thiel and A. Zumbansen, "The pathophysiology of post-stroke aphasia: a network approach," *Restorative Neurology and Neuroscience*, vol. 34, no. 4, pp. 507–518, 2016.

[61] M. A. Naeser, P. I. Martin, M. Nicholas et al., "Improved picture naming in chronic aphasia after TMS to part of right Broca's area: an open-protocol study," *Brain and Language*, vol. 93, no. 1, pp. 95–105, 2005.

[62] S. C. Blank, H. Bird, F. Turkheimer, and R. J. Wise, "Speech production after stroke: the role of the right pars opercularis," *Annals of Neurology*, vol. 54, no. 3, pp. 310–320, 2003.

[63] E. Fedorenko and S. L. Thompson-Schill, "Reworking the language network," *Trends in Cognitive Sciences*, vol. 18, no. 3, pp. 120–126, 2014.

[64] J. S. Siegel, L. E. Ramsey, A. Z. Snyder et al., "Disruptions of network connectivity predict impairment in multiple behavioral domains after stroke," *Proceedings of the National Academy of Sciences of the United States of America*, vol. 113, no. 30, pp. E4367–E4376, 2016.

[65] A. Towfighi and J. L. Saver, "Stroke declines from third to fourth leading cause of death in the United States: historical perspective and challenges ahead," *Stroke*, vol. 42, no. 8, pp. 2351–2355, 2011.

[66] J. A. Pinkney, G. Gayle, K. Mitchell-Fearon, and J. Mullings, "Health-related quality of life in stroke survivors at the University Hospital of the West Indies," *Journal of Neurology Research*, vol. 7, no. 3, pp. 46–58, 2017.

[67] M. Ignatiou, V. Christaki, E. V. Chelas, E. A. Efstratiadou, and K. Hilari, "Agreement between people with aphasia and their proxies on health-related quality of life after stroke, using the Greek SAQOL-39g," *Psychology*, vol. 3, no. 9, pp. 686–690, 2012.

[68] M. L. Seghier, E. Patel, S. Prejawa et al., "The PLORAS database: a data repository for predicting language outcome and recovery after stroke," *Neuroimage*, vol. 124, Part B, pp. 1208–1212, 2016.

[69] S. K. Ghotra, J. A. Johnson, W. Qiu, A. Newton, C. Rasmussen, and J. Y. Yager, "Age at stroke onset influences the clinical outcome and health-related quality of life in pediatric ischemic stroke survivors," *Developmental Medicine & Child Neurology*, vol. 57, no. 11, pp. 1027–1034, 2015.

[70] R. E. Hanlon, W. E. Lux, and A. W. Dromerick, "Global aphasia without hemiparesis: language profiles and lesion distribution," *Journal of Neurology, Neurosurgery, and Psychiatry*, vol. 66, no. 3, pp. 365–369, 1999.

[71] T. M. Hope, M. L. Seghier, A. P. Leff, and C. J. Price, "Predicting outcome and recovery after stroke with lesions extracted from MRI images," *NeuroImage: clinical*, vol. 2, pp. 424–433, 2013.

[72] K. A. Kim, J. S. Lee, W. H. Chang et al., "Changes in language function and recovery-related prognostic factors in first-ever left hemispheric ischemic stroke," *Annals of Rehabilitation Medicine*, vol. 43, no. 6, pp. 625–634, 2019.

[73] C. K. Thompson, M. Walenski, Y. Chen et al., "Intrahemispheric perfusion in chronic stroke-induced aphasia," *Neural Plasticity*, vol. 2017, Article ID 2361691, 15 pages, 2017.

[74] K. P. Brumm, J. E. Perthen, T. T. Liu, F. Haist, L. Ayalon, and T. Love, "An arterial spin labeling investigation of cerebral blood flow deficits in chronic stroke survivors," *Neuro Image*, vol. 51, no. 3, pp. 995–1005, 2010.

[75] S. Kristinsson, G. Yourganov, F. Xiao et al., "Brain-derived neurotrophic factor genotype-specific differences in cortical activation in chronic aphasia," *Journal of Speech, Language, and Hearing Research*, vol. 62, no. 11, pp. 3923–3936, 2019.

[76] R. de Boer, K. Spielmann, M. H. Heijenbrok-Kal, R. van der Vliet, G. M. Ribbers, and W. van de Sandt-Koenderman, "The role of the BDNF Val 66Met polymorphism in recovery of aphasia after stroke," *Neurorehabilitation and Neural Repair*, vol. 31, no. 9, pp. 851–857, 2017.

[77] F. Sohrabji, M. J. Park, and A. H. Mahnke, "Sex differences in stroke therapies," *Journal of Neuroscience Research*, vol. 95, no. 1-2, pp. 681–691, 2017.

[78] I. Henseler, F. Regenbrecht, and H. Obrig, "Lesion correlates of patholinguistic profiles in chronic aphasia: comparisons of syndrome-, modality- and symptom-level assessment," *Brain*, vol. 137, no. 3, pp. 918–930, 2014.

[79] A. Osa García, S. M. Brambati, A. Brisebois et al., "Predicting early post-stroke aphasia outcome from initial aphasia severity," *Frontiers in Neurology*, vol. 11, p. 120, 2020.

[80] A. Kertesz and P. McCabe, "Recovery patterns and prognosis in aphasia," *Brain*, vol. 100, no. 1, pp. 1-18, 1977.

[81] K. Sakai, Y. Ugawa, Y. Terao, R. Hanajima, T. Furubayashi, and I. Kanazawa, "Preferential activation of different I waves by transcranial magnetic stimulation with a figure-of-eight-shaped coil," *Experimental Brain Research*, vol. 113, no. 1, pp. 24–32, 1997.

[82] V. di Lazzaro, A. Oliviero, F. Pilato et al., "Descending volleys evoked by transcranial magnetic stimulation of the brain in conscious humans: effects of coil shape," *Clinical Neurophysiology*, vol. 113, no. 1, pp. 114–119, 2002.

[83] V. Di Lazzaro, U. Ziemann, and R. N. Lemon, "State of the art: physiology of transcranial motor cortex stimulation," *Brain Stimulation*, vol. 1, no. 4, pp. 345–362, 2008.

[84] M. Sommer, A. Alfaro, M. Rummel et al., "Half sine, monophasic and biphasic transcranial magnetic stimulation of the human motor cortex," *Clinical Neurophysiology*, vol. 117, no. 4, pp. 838–844, 2006.

[85] A. M. Janssen, T. F. Oostendorp, and D. F. Stegeman, "The coil orientation dependency of the electric field induced by TMS for M1 and other brain areas," *Journal of Neuroengineering and Rehabilitation*, vol. 12, no. 1, p. 47, 2015.

[86] E. Houdayer, A. Degardin, F. Cassim, P. Bocquillon, P. Derambure, and H. Devanne, "The effects of low- and high-frequency repetitive TMS on the input/output properties of the human corticospinal pathway," *Experimental Brain Research*, vol. 187, no. 2, pp. 207–217, 2008.

[87] O. L. Gamboa, A. Antal, V. Moliadze, and W. Paulus, "Simply longer is not better: reversal of theta burst after-effect with prolonged stimulation," *Experimental Brain Research*, vol. 204, no. 2, pp. 181–187, 2010.

[88] M. C. Brady, H. Kelly, J. Godwin, P. Enderby, and P. Campbell, "Speech and language therapy for aphasia following stroke," *Cochrane Database of Systematic Reviews*, no. 6, article CD000425, 2016.

[89] RELEASE Collaboration, "Communicating simply, but not too simply: reporting of participants and speech and language interventions for aphasia after stroke," *International Journal of Speech Language Pathology*, vol. 22, no. 3, pp. 302–312, 2020.

8

Evaluating the Long-Term Efficacy of Acupuncture Therapy for Subacute Poststroke Aphasia: Study Protocol for a Randomized, Blinded, Controlled, Multicentre Trial

Xiaolin Li[1], Ying Gao,[1,2] Chi Zhang,[1] Qingsu Zhang,[3] Xiyan Xin,[4] Zhongjian Tan,[1] Binlong Zhang,[5] Ruiwen Fan,[1] Xing Huang,[1] Minjie Xu,[1] Xin Shu,[1] Heming Yan,[1] Changming Li,[1] Qiao Kong,[1] Shuren Li,[6] and Jingling Chang[1]

[1]*Department of Neurology, Dongzhimen Hospital, Beijing University of Chinese Medicine, Beijing 100700, China*
[2]*Institute for Brain Disorders, Beijing University of Chinese Medicine, Beijing 100700, China*
[3]*Hearing and Speech Rehabilitation Department, China Rehabilitation Research Center, Beijing 100068, China*
[4]*Traditional Chinese Medicine Department, Peking University Third Hospital, Beijing 100191, China*
[5]*Guang'anmen Hospital, China Academy of Chinese Medical Sciences, Beijing 100053, China*
[6]*Division of Nuclear Medicine, Department of Biomedical Imaging and Image-guided Therapy, Medical University of Vienna, Vienna, Austria*

Correspondence should be addressed to Jingling Chang; ear6979@163.com

Academic Editor: Haroon Khan; hkdr2006@gmail.com

Background. Poststroke aphasia (PSA) is a disabling condition that decreases the quality of life, and the duration of the disease harms the quality of life of PSA patients. Acupuncture has been widely employed for PSA. There is some evidence for the immediate treatment efficacy of acupuncture for PSA; however, long-term results after acupuncture may be poorer. *Methods.* This is a multicentre, randomized, blinded, nonacupoint (NA) acupuncture controlled, multimodal neuroimaging clinical trial. A total of 48 subjects with subacute PSA will be randomly assigned to an acupoint group or an NA control group. The acupoint group will receive acupuncture with normal needling at DU20, EX-HN1, HT5, GB39, EX-HN12, EX-HN13, and CV23. The NA control group will receive acupuncture in locations not corresponding to acupuncture points as sham acupoints. Both groups will receive identical speech and language therapy thrice a week for four weeks. The primary outcome will be the change in the aphasia quotient (AQ) score measured by the Western Aphasia Battery (WAB) test during the 12th week after randomization. Participants will be blindly assessed at prerandomization (baseline) and 4 weeks, 12 weeks, and 24 weeks after randomization. The secondary outcomes include the Boston Diagnostic Aphasia Examination (BDAE) score, the Disease Prognosis Scale score for ischaemic stroke, etc. Magnetic resonance imaging (MRI) and electroencephalogram (EEG) will also be performed at 4-time intervals as secondary outcomes. All scores and image evaluations will be taken at the same point as the linguistic evaluation. The multilevel evaluation technique will be used to assess the long-term efficacy of acupuncture therapy. MRI scans and EEG will be used to assess acupuncture-related neuroplasticity changes. *Discussion.* The results from our trial will help to supply evidence for the long-term acupuncture effects for PSA over a long follow-up period. It will provide valuable information for future studies in the field of PSA treatment. The trial was registered at the Chinese Clinical Trial Registry on 16 March 2020 (ChiCTR2000030879).

1. Introduction

Stroke is a leading cause of mortality and disability globally [1]. Poststroke aphasia (PSA) is one of the most devastating symptoms in stroke survivors [2], who rarely spontaneously recover in the ensuing time. Approximately 30% of stroke patients suffer from aphasia [3], 50% of stroke survivors are still aphasic one year after stroke, and residual symptoms may persist for many years [4]. It can impact an individual's ability to speak, comprehend spoken language, read, and write [5]. Basic requirements of daily life that rely on communication are affected, and social participation can be dramatically impaired. A large-scale survey investigated the relationship between the presence or absence of 75 diseases and the quality of life scores. The highest negative correlation is aphasia [6]. Aphasia rehabilitation has been listed as one of the top 10 research priorities related to life after aphasia [2]. Patients with PSA experience longer hospitalization stays and need more healthcare support, so studying the long-term curative effect of acupuncture treatment on PSA is conducive to maximizing of medical resources.

A review of clinical trials for PSA over the past 5 years revealed that a multitude of interventions can be beneficial in improving language and functional outcomes for patients with PSA [5], with the majority of high-quality clinical research focusing on the chronic phase of aphasia [7–9]. Language disorders are diverse and can change over time. The clinical symptoms may be different in the subacute phase as well as in the chronic phase [10]. Only a few randomized studies ($n = 12$–30) have examined the efficacy of PSA treatment in the subacute phase [11–13]. Research on the subacute period is therefore relatively scarce.

Effective therapies focusing on improving speech and language in patients with PSA are essential. At present, considerable evidence has suggested that treatment with speech and language therapy (SLT) is effective in improving communication and quality of life in individuals with aphasia. These studies have provided evidence of the effectiveness of SLT for people with aphasia following stroke in terms of improved functional communication, reading, writing, and expressive language compared with no therapy [14]; however, the effect sizes of SLT are moderate, potentially reflecting a physiological limit of training-induced progress, the treatment is costly, and progress is often slow. One of the studies also stated that SLT for more than 2 hours a day provided no added value on PSA [15]. It is certain that the various stages of PSA are associated with varying degrees of language recovery, but recovery requires a large number of therapy sessions. It remains a challenge to optimize the effect of aphasia therapy. As a result, an increasing amount of research has been devoted to alternative methods to improve the effectiveness of aphasia treatment, generally by increasing the total amount of treatment achieved [16].

Acupuncture is an easy-to-use, low-cost adjunct to traditional SLT to enhance language outcomes in individuals with PSA. It is one of the main treatments of traditional Chinese medicine (TCM) and has been used for thousands of years. During the past decade, the results of several meta-analyses have concluded that acupuncture after stroke seems to be effective in improving PSA functional communication and language function [17, 18]; however, most of the studies did not assess therapeutic effects over extended periods. For acupuncture treatment, long-term efficacy is considered one of the most important therapeutic effects, which has been suggested by numerous clinical studies [19–25]. It represents the cumulative effect of positive achievements [16]. Long-term efficacy will allow the patient's therapeutic effects to accumulate ("more is better"). Our previous studies on the

effects of acupuncture on PSA have shown that participants in the acupuncture group had lower severity than the control group in week 4, but the difference was not significant; however, a significant reduction in PSA severity during weeks 5 to 12 was noted [26]. In addition, we explored the traditional Chinese medical theory and acupuncture technique of this acupuncture programme [27, 28]. Acupuncture has also been shown to have long-term efficacy in chronic pain and tinnitus, which has shown effective therapeutic results [29, 30]. Therefore, we speculate that the long-term therapeutic effect for PSA will also be well maintained; however, the long-term efficacy of acupuncture compared with the placebo effect in patients with PSA has not been investigated.

In terms of the current state of evaluation of aphasia, the requirements for a comprehensive evaluation of PSA have not yet been fully implemented. One of the important means was to evaluate the language characteristics of PSA, which is the major part of the evaluation; however, to date, this single evaluation approach is often insufficient. As such, neuropsychological tests in conjunction with in vivo measures may be more sensitive than neuropsychological tests alone in the assessment of brain structure and electrophysiology [31–33]. We introduce MRI and EEG for evaluation of the objective characteristics of PSA because the multimodal assessment of brain structure and function allows for a more objective evaluation of the recovery characteristics of patients with aphasia. Based on the previous study [34], we conducted a TCM syndrome evaluation of PSA patients and confirmed the relationship between linguistic features and TCM syndrome. Therefore, in this study, we have also introduced the evaluation of TCM syndrome to provide more comprehensive evidence of efficacy based on the combined evaluation of Chinese and Western medicine. For the reasons above, we propose to investigate whether acupuncture treatment on PSA has the value of maintaining long-term efficacy through this randomized controlled trial (RCT) with multimodal evaluation.

We designed an assessor- and participant-blinded RCT with PSA patients. Using NA acupuncture as a control, the trial aims to identify the efficacy of acupuncture by answering two questions: (1) what is the long-term efficacy and reliability of acupuncture as an intervention for PSA compared with the placebo effect? and (2) what interactions will be observed through an integrated evaluation of linguistic features, brain function, and TCM syndrome?

2. Methods and Analysis

2.1. Study Design. This is a multicentre, randomized, assessor- and participant-blinded, NA acupuncture controlled, multimodal neuroimaging clinical trial. It aims to compare the long-term efficacy of the acupoint group and NA control group (in locations not corresponding to acupuncture points). In all groups, participants will receive identical SLT but will be permitted to use medications for the basic internal medicine treatment of stroke. The type, dose, and time of administration of the agent will be recorded in the case report form. The trial design is depicted by the flow diagram in Figure 1. The timeline for study enrolment, intervention, and assessment is illustrated in Table 1. We designed this acupuncture research at full length following the Standard Protocol Items: Recommendations for Interventional Trials (SPIRIT) 2013 statement [35]. The design and reporting of the study will follow the Consolidated Standards of Reporting Trials (CONSORT) statement for non-pharmacological interventions [36] (http://www.consort-statement.org/home/).

2.2. Randomization and Blinding.

Eligible patients will be randomly assigned to the acupoint group or NA control group with a 1:1 ratio. The randomization sequence will be generated by a third-party professional statistician using a computer-generated randomization digital table using SAS V.9.4 software (SAS Institute Inc., North Carolina, USA). An independent assessor will interview the participants and carry out the screening. Random numbers and group assignments will be confirmed immediately through short message service to the practitioners who conduct acupuncture. All participants will be blinded to the types of acupuncture. An independent, blinded assessor who does not know the group assignment will conduct the outcome evaluation after the treatment. The researcher who will oversee the statistical analysis will also be blinded, with the treatment for each group remaining unknown; however, it is impossible to blind practitioners who conduct acupuncture. The practitioner will be forbidden from discussing the type of acupuncture with the participants. We will endeavour to ensure that subjects begin the trial with similar expectations of efficacy by informing them that the provided treatments are effective. In this study, participants, assessors, and statisticians will be blinded to treatment allocation. Participants will receive treatments alone at different times to avoid communication with each other. An eye patch will be applied to patients during the acupuncture treatment. To minimize the unintentional physical cues and bias in this trial, acupuncturists will be required to emulate the same procedure for the nonacupoint control group. In addition, participants will be asked to answer the following question during week 4 to test the blinding effect: "Do you think you have received real acupuncture treatment?" The participants can choose "yes" or "no" as an answer [37, 38]. The percentage of participants who answered "yes" in both groups after the final treatment will be analyzed. If the results show no significant difference in the response to this question between the two groups, they could suggest that the blinding effect is sufficient.

2.3. Setting and Recruitment.

Participants who meet the inclusion and exclusion criteria will be recruited from the inpatients in the Dongzhimen Hospital affiliated to Beijing University of Chinese Medicine (BUCM), China Rehabilitation Research Center, and Peking University Third Hospital. Participating institutions and the level of the institution are listed in Table 2. The study will be advertised through the Internet and posters in communities and hospitals. The inpatients and potential participants will call an investigator and be prescreened for eligibility and will learn how to participate in this clinical trial through visits or telephone calls to our hospital. During visits to the clinical research centre of Dongzhimen Hospital affiliated to BUCM, China Rehabilitation Research Center, and Peking University Third Hospital, the accessors will explain the study to the patients, who will be asked to sign an informed consent form before voluntary participation. The participants of this study will be selected from the applicants who meet all the inclusion criteria but do not meet any of the exclusion criteria. To facilitate participation in this study, the accessors will properly adjust the evaluation and treatment schedule of the enrolled participants. Therefore, the enrolled participant will be able to complete the treatment and evaluation. Every time the enrolled participant visits, the accessors will inform the participant of the next scheduled visit, and the day before the visit, the accessors will remind the enrolled participant of the schedule by telephone.

2.4. Eligibility Criteria

2.4.1. Inclusion Criteria. Participants meeting all of the following criteria will be included in this trial: (1) diagnosed as stroke through computed tomography (CT) or MRI, 1 to 6 months after stroke onset; (2) 30 to 80 years of age (After the expert discussion and the actual situation of our country, the age range has been adjusted), the native language is Chinese, and right-handed; (3) primary school and above education with no serious heart, liver, or kidney diseases; (4) clear consciousness and no cognitive impairment; (5) normal language function before the stroke onset and dominant language dysfunction with mild limb dysfunction; (6) specific aphasia syndrome diagnosed as motor aphasia by the WAB; (7) BDAE score of 2 to 4; and (8) able to cooperate for the 30-minute MRI examination.

2.4.2. Exclusion Criteria. The exclusion criteria are as follows: (1) received pacemaker surgery, coronary intervention, or coronary artery bypass surgery or have other metal products in the body; (2) language dysfunction caused by congenital or childhood diseases; (3) language dysfunction caused by mental disturbance and normal mental retardation; (4) severe dysarthria and hearing impairment; (5) superficial sensation abnormalities in the neurological examination, and (6) participation in other studies.

2.5. Interventions.

Acupuncture will be performed by registered acupuncturists with over 2 years of experience who will be trained in the standardization of the acupuncture scheme. Only sterile, stainless steel, disposable acupuncture needles (size 0.25 mm × 40 mm, product no. 20182270011; ANDE Acupuncture, Guizhou ANDE Medical Equipment, China) will be used. Both acupuncture and sham acupuncture points will be located in the limbs and head. All the participants will receive 3 treatment sessions per week (alternate days) for 4 consecutive weeks, resulting in a total of 12 sessions. Each treatment will be administered for

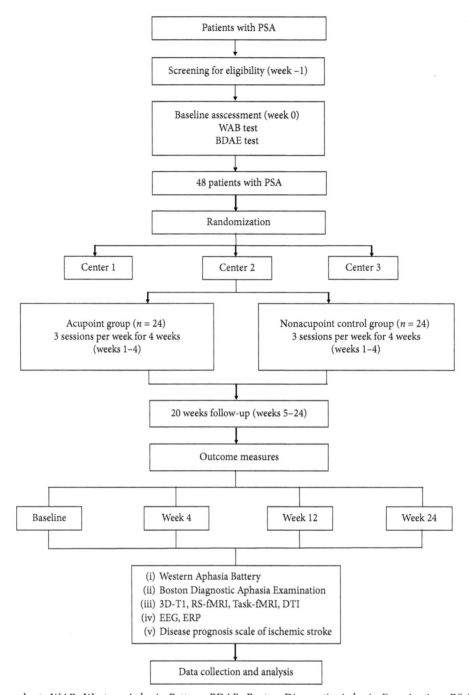

FIGURE 1: Trial flow chart. WAB, Western Aphasia Battery, BDAE, Boston Diagnostic Aphasia Examination; RS-fMRI, resting-state functional magnetic resonance imaging; Task-fMRI, task functional magnetic resonance imaging; DTI, diffusion tensor imaging; EEG, electroencephalogram; ERP, event-related potential.

30 minutes. The acupuncture and sham acupuncture interventions will be performed by a consensus of acupuncture experts. To ensure strict adherence to the study protocol, the experts will receive training together and use the same techniques. The details of the acupuncture treatment are described in the Standards for Reporting Interventions in Clinical Trials of Acupuncture (STRICTA [39]) checklist in Table 3.

2.5.1. Acupoint Group. Participants in the acupoint group will receive acupuncture at bilateral Tongli (HT5) and Xuanzhong (GB39) limb acupuncture points. After skin disinfection, acupuncture needles will be inserted through the skin and approximately 0.5 cun [≈10 mm] into the skin. Needle insertion will follow an angle of 90° in an inferomedial direction for the two points. Following needle insertion, small, equal manipulations of twirling and thrusting

TABLE 1: Study design schedule.

Period	Screening and baseline	Treatment (w1–4)				Follow-up (w5–12)	Follow-up (w13–24)
Week (W)	W −1	W1	W2	W3	W4	W12	W24
Eligibility	×						
CT or MRI	×						
General information	×						
Physical examination	×			×		×	×
Medical history and demography	×						
Informed consent	×						
WAB		×			×	×	×
BDAE		×			×	×	×
Disease Prognosis Scale of ischaemic stroke		×			×	×	×
MRI (3D-T1, RS-fMRI, Task-fMRI, DTI)		×			×	×	×
EEG		×			×	×	×
ERP		×			×	×	×
Discomfort and acceptance of acupuncture		×	×	×	×	×	×
Assessment of blind method		×					
Adverse event			×	×	×	×	×
Compliance			×	×	×	×	×

CT, computed tomography; MRI, magnetic resonance imaging; WAB, Western Aphasia Battery; BDAE: Boston Diagnostic Aphasia Examination; RS-fMRI, resting-state functional magnetic resonance imaging; DTI, diffusion tensor imaging; EEG, electroencephalogram; ERP, event-related potentials.

TABLE 2: List of participating institutions and level of the institution.

Participating centre	Level of the institution
Dongzhimen Hospital Affiliated to Beijing University of Chinese Medicine	Tertiary A hospital
China Rehabilitation Research Center	Tertiary A hospital
Peking University Third Hospital	Tertiary A hospital

will be performed on all needles to reach de qi (a composite of sensations including numbness, distention, soreness, and heaviness that is an important indicator of successful acupuncture treatment), which is believed to be an essential component for acupuncture efficacy. The needles placed in HT5 and GB39 will be manually stimulated every 10 minutes. The acupuncture points on the head are Lianquan (RN23), Jinjin (EX-HN12), Yuye (EX-HN13), Baihui (DU20), and Sishencong (EX-HN1). For RN23, acupuncture needles will be inserted through the skin and approximately 1 cun [≈20 mm] into the skin. Following needle insertion, small, equal manipulations will be performed on the needles to reach numbness. EX-HN12 and EX-HN13 will be quickly inserted for bloodletting. DU20 and EX-HN1 will be inserted through the skin approximately 0.5 cun. Needle insertion will follow an angle of 15° in an inferomedial direction for the two points (for details, see Table 4 and Figure 2).

2.5.2. NA Control Group. Participants in the NA control group will receive sham acupuncture with real needles on an NA. NA 1 will be 0.5 cun (≈10 mm) lateral to HT5. NA 2 will be 0.5 cun (≈10 mm) horizontal to GB39, and NA 3 will be 0.5 cun (≈10 mm) lateral to ST8 (for details, see Table 5 and Figure 3). Procedures and other treatment settings will be the same as in the acupoint group but with no needle manipulation for de qi. In both groups, the needles will be retained for 30 minutes for each treatment session. The

participants will be treated with acupuncture three times a week, on alternate days, for 4 successive weeks, resulting in a total of 12 sessions for each patient.

2.5.3. Permitted and Prohibited Concomitant Treatments. All the participants will receive identical SLT. The treatment period is 4 weeks (3 treatment sessions per week, alternate days), resulting in a total of 12 sessions. Speech therapy will be performed by an experienced language therapist who received standardized training in language rehabilitation.

The language rehabilitation training method will be as follows: first, the patients will be assessed for their language function and scored, and then a training plan and training principles will be formulated according to the type of aphasia and language ability; the training is progressively followed by targeted strengthening exercises. The main content includes motor training of pronunciation organs, oral pronunciation training, naming, intonation, etc. (1) Mouth shape and voice training: at the beginning of the training, patients will be taught to control their lip and tongue movements through mouth shape and voice control to practice pronunciation. The patients will practice the rhymes and consonants first and then gradually transition to the differentiation of approximate sounds. (2) Use of language training equipment (cell phones, iPads, etc.): patients can use phrases and sentences from daily life to make audio files that are suitable for reading. The patients will practice the phrases first, and then, the sentences. (3) Training the pronunciation muscles:

TABLE 3: Revised standards for reporting intervention in clinical trials of acupuncture (STRICTA [39]]).

Item	Item criteria	Description
(1) Acupuncture rationale	(1a) Style of acupuncture	Traditional Chinese medicine therapy
	(1b) Reasoning for treatment provided, based on historical context, literature sources, and/or consensus methods, with references where appropriate	(i) Reasoning for treatment provided—based on historical context, literature sources, and traditional Chinese medicine (consensus) (ii) Reasoning for treatment provided—based on historical context, literature [27,28], selection of treatment regions based on related papers, expert experience, and textbooks
	(1c) Extent to which treatment varied	Standardized treatment
(2) Details of needling	(2a) Number of needle insertions per subject per session (mean and range where relevant)	10 or 12
	(2b) Names (or location if no standard name) of points used (unilateral/bilateral)	DU20 (Baihui), EX-HN1 (Sishencong), HT5 (Tongli), GB39 (Xuanzhong), EX-HN12 (Jinjin), EX-HN13 (Yuye), CV23 (Lianquan)
	(2c) Depth of insertion, based on a specified unit of measurement or a particular tissue level	Needle insertion will follow an angle of 90°in an inferomedial direction for the two points (HT5, GB39). Depth: 0.5 cun [≈10 mm]. Needle insertion followed an angle of 15° in an inferomedial direction for the two points (DU20, EX-HN1). Depth: 0.5 cun. For RN23, the angle is 90° and the depth is 1 cun [≈20 mm]. EX-HN12 and EX-HN13 were quickly inserted for bloodletting
	(2d) Responses sought	Following needle insertion, small, equal manipulations of twirling and thrusting will be performed on all needles to reach de qi
	(2e) Needle stimulation	Small, equal manipulations of twirling and thrusting will be performed on the needles of HT5 and GB39
	(2f) Needle retention time	30 min per session
	(2g) Needle type	Sterile, stainless, disposable acupuncture needles (size 0.25 mm × 40 mm, product no. 20182270011; ANDE Acupuncture, Guizhou ANDE Medical Equipment, China)
(3) Treatment regimen	(3a) Number of treatment sessions	12
	(3b) Frequency and duration of treatment sessions	3 times/week, 30 min per session, on alternate days, for 4 successive weeks
(4) Other components of treatment	(4a) Details of other interventions administered to the acupuncture group	None
	(4b) Setting and context of treatment, including instructions to practitioners, and information and explanations to patients	The study will be conducted in the Dongzhimen Hospital affiliated to BUCM, China Rehabilitation Research Center, and Peking University Third Hospital, and all information will be provided to the subjects
(5) Practitioner background	(5a) Description of participating acupuncturists	The chief physician of Dongzhimen Hospital, Ph.D., 11 years of formal university training in traditional Chinese medicine, with qualifications for practising doctors stipulated in the law
(6) Control or comparator interventions	(6a) rationale for the control or comparator in the context of the research question, with sources that justify the choice	The nonacupoint control group will receive sham acupuncture with real acupuncture needles at nonacupoint locations. Through such an approach, the self-perception of placebo effects in the nonacupoint control group is difficult to distinguish from the real acupoints
	(6b) Precise description of the control or comparator; details for items 1–3 with the use of sham acupuncture or any other type of acupuncture-like control	Participants in the nonacupoint control group received sham acupuncture with a pragmatic placebo needle on a sham acupoint. The needles used are the same as the acupoint group. Procedures and other treatment settings will be the same as in the acupoint group but with no needle manipulation for de qi

patients with aphasia may have different degrees of wasting atrophy of the pronunciation-related muscles, which results in slurred speech. During training, patients are instructed to practice tonal movements of the tongue and oral muscles to promote accurate pronunciation. (4) Regular check-ups and weakness reinforcement exercises: weaknesses in

TABLE 4: Location of acupoints used in the acupuncture group.

Acupoints	Location
DU20 (Baihui)	On the median line of the head, 5 cun superior to the anterior hairline, at about the middle on the connecting line between the two auricular tips
EX-HN1 (Sishencong)	On the vertex, 1 cun from the front, back, left, and right to DU20 (Baihui), common 4 points
HT5 (Tongli)	On the palmar side of the forearm, 1 cun superior to the transverse crease of the wrist, at the radial border of the ulnar carpal flexor muscular tendon
GB39 (Xuanzhong)	On the lateral side of the leg, 3 cun directly above the tip of lateral malleolus at the anterior border of the fibula
EX-HN12 (Jinjin)	In the mouth, EX-HN12 (Jinjin) is located with tongue furled, on the vein on the left side of the frenulum of the tongue
EX-HN13 (Yuye)	EX-HN13 (Yuye) is located on the vein on the right side of the frenulum of the tongue
CV23 (Lianquan)	In the neck, on the anterior midline, above the laryngeal protuberance, in the depression of the superior border of the hyoid bone

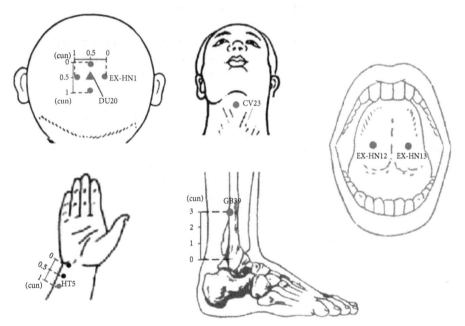

FIGURE 2: Locations of acupoints.

TABLE 5: Location of sham acupoints used in the NA group.

Nonacupoint (NA)	Location
NA 1	0.5 cun lateral to HT5 (Tongli)
NA 2	0.5 cun horizontal to GB39 (Xuanzhong)
NA 3	0.5 cun lateral to ST8 (Touwei)

pronunciation for targeted exercises will be identified, and individual reinforcement training for patients will be provided if necessary.

2.6. Sample Size Calculation. No large RCTs have been carried out within the field examining the long-term effects of acupuncture on PSA. Previous studies have used interventions not applicable to the current protocol and have been of varying quality and used small sample sizes. We were, therefore, unable to calculate the prior accurate sample size. Thus, our RCT will support a more accurate sample size estimate and inform a definitive trial examining the long-term effectiveness of acupuncture for aphasia. The study involves the experimental study

of functional magnetic resonance imaging (fMRI) and EEG for language tasks, which falls under the scope of experimental psychology. Taking into account individual psychological differences, it is expected that the PSA patients to be included will be divided into 2 groups. The number of patients to be included in the statistics in each group will be 20. Considering a drop-out rate of 20%, the target recruitment number is 48 participants (24 per group).

2.7. Multimodal Data Acquisition

2.7.1. MRI Data Acquisition. Patients will undergo brain MRI at prerandomization (baseline) and 4 weeks, 12 weeks, and 24 weeks after randomization. MRI scans will be performed with a 3.0-T MR scanner (Siemens AG, Germany) in the Dongzhimen Hospital affiliated to BUCM. The parameters of the sequences to be employed in this study are provided by the China Association of Brain Imaging. Sagittal structural images will be acquired using a magnetization-prepared rapid gradient-echo three-dimensional (3D) T1-

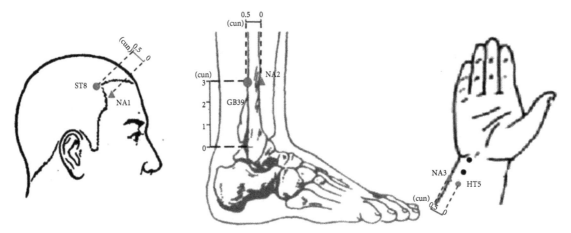

FIGURE 3: Locations of nonacupoints. NA, nonacupoint.

weighted sequence with the following parameters: repetition time (TR)/echo time (TE) = 1900/2.13 ms, flip angle = 9°, inversion time = 1100 ms, resolution = 256 × 256, voxel size: 1.0 × 1.0 × 1.0, 1-mm slice thickness without slice gap.

RS-fMRI and task-fMRI will be performed using an echo-planar imaging (EPI) sequence with the following parameters: TR/TE = 2000/30 ms, flip angle = 90°, resolution = 64 × 64, FOV = 225 × 225, bandwidth = 2520, slice thickness = 3.5 mm with 0.7 mm slice gap, 31 axial slices, and voxel size: 3.5 × 3.5 × 3.5.

Diffusion tensor imaging (DTI) will be acquired with a diffusion-weighted, single-shot, spin-echo, echo-planar imaging sequence that uses 30 directions with $b = 0$ s/mm^2 and $b = 1000$ s/mm^2, slice thickness: 2 mm, gap = 0 mm, slices = 65, TR: 11000 ms, TE: 94 ms, matrix: 128 × 128, FOV: 256 × 256, and phase encode direction: $A >> P$.

All scans will be qualitatively reviewed by two radiologists to screen for possible brain lesions or structural abnormalities. fMRI data will be collected during the word-picture judgement task and at rest. fMRI data will be performed with the SPM12 (https://www.fil.ion.ucl.ac.uk/spm/software/spm12/) for MATLAB. Brain activation and connectivity changes will be compared between the two groups.

2.7.2. EEG Data Acquisition. The 64-channel EEG recording and analysis system produced by the Neuroscan of Australia, E-prime 2.0 stimulation display software, scan data analysis software, SYNAMPS EEG amplifier, Fastrak 3D imaging digital instrument, Quick-Cap electrode cap, recording electrode, electrode paste, and Curry multichannel neuroimaging software will be used to collect EEG signals. EEG data in the resting state will be collected for 8 minutes, and event-related potentials (ERPs) will be collected during language task assessment for 8 minutes. The same word-picture judgement task used for the MRI will be applied to ERP collection. Patients will undergo an EEG at a different time on the same day as the MRI scan.

2.7.3. Word-Picture Judgement Task. The patients will be trained before entering the fMRI scanner. They will complete a practice version of the word-picture judgement task

paradigm in the computer. They need to perform the task and reach an accuracy criterion of 90% to ensure that the patients understand how to do the task in the scanner. Patients will view black and white line pictures and Chinese high-frequency nouns. The patients are required to press a mouse button when the picture and the noun appear on a white background. The patients are asked to press the left button if the picture and the noun express the same meaning; otherwise, they should right-click. The stimuli are presented in 60 blocks on a computer using E-prime 2.0. In the ERP experiment, there will be 120 blocks. Trial types within blocks are presented in a pseudorandomized order. During the MRI scanning, all patients are asked to lie quietly in the scanner with their eyes open, trying to avoid systematic thinking, and moving as little as possible. In task-state fMRI scanning, the patients are instructed to maintain a central view and try to not think of other things. During ERP testing, patients are asked to sit in front of the computer, and the surroundings will be kept quiet (Figure 4).

2.8. Outcome Measures

2.8.1. Clinical Outcome Assessments. The primary outcome will be the change in the AQ score during the 12th week after randomization. For the assessment of language functioning, the WAB with the subtests spontaneous speech, auditory comprehension, repetition, and naming is included in the test battery. The WAB test will be conducted based on a previous study [40]. Secondary outcomes include four items, the details of which are listed in Table 1.

2.8.2. Neuroplasticity Assessments. In this study, neuroplasticity changes between the two groups will be measured by MRI. Before acupuncture treatment, patients will complete the fMRI scan within 3 days. They will also have a follow-up fMRI scan within 3 days after the completion of their intervention and at 8 weeks and 16 weeks after the intervention (Figure 1). Brain activity and functional connectivity will be assessed under a resting state and a word-picture judgement task. Group differences in white matter integrity will be assessed using DTI.

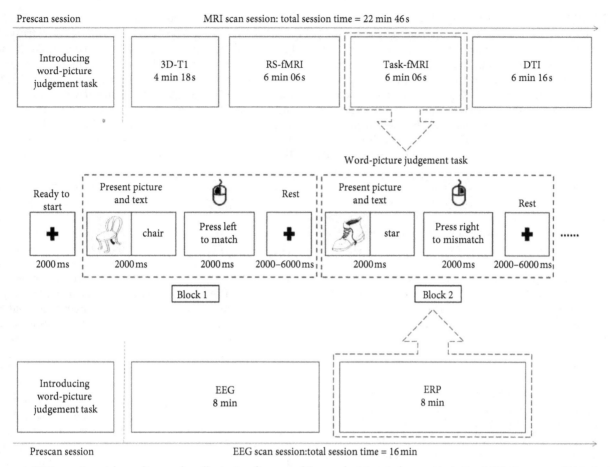

FIGURE 4: MRI experimental paradigm and an illustrative diagram of the word-picture judgement task. For fMRI, there were 60 blocks. For ERP, 60 blocks. When presenting the task, the word is displayed in Chinese.

2.8.3. Assessment of Acupuncture Safety. Acupuncture is considered to be a generally safe procedure [41–43]; however, all adverse events will be recorded in every detail. In this study, acupuncture-related adverse events would mainly refer to broken needles, fainting due to the needling procedure, local infection, hematoma, and other events that can be caused by acupuncture (such as headache, dizziness, and insomnia).

2.8.4. Quality Control. All practitioners will conduct the study according to the standard operating procedure of the study. We will conduct several simulations for our volunteers before the start of the study. During the study, regular meetings will be held to discuss issues raised by researchers or participants, the need to improve protocols, the side effects, and participant recruitment.

2.9. Statistical Analysis

2.9.1. Clinical Data Analysis. All statistical analyses will be performed by a statistician from the Clinical Evaluation and Analysis Centre of Dongzhimen Hospital affiliated to BUCM using Statistical Package for the Social Sciences (SPSS) V.22.0. The statistician will be blinded to the allocation of groups. The level of significance is established at $\alpha < 0.05$ with a two-tailed test. The main objective is to compare the change in the AQ score at week 12 from baseline between the acupoint group and the NA control group. The null hypothesis is that the acupoint group will show the same change as the NA control group, while the alternative hypothesis is that the acupoint group shows a greater improvement. Categorical data will be represented by percentages, whereas continuous data will be represented by the average, standard deviation, median, minimum value, and maximum value. For comparison with the baseline, a t-test or nonparametric test will be used for continuous data and nonparametric tests for categorical data. For comparison of two independent samples, if the residuals are normally distributed, the analysis of covariance (ANCOVA) will be used for the primary outcome and subgroup analysis stratified by aphasia severity, t-tests for other continuous data, and chi-square tests for categorical data; if the residuals are non-normally distributed, a nonparametric test will be used for both the continuous and categorical data. The results of the intention-to-treat (ITT) analysis will be used to assess the validity of the study as a whole. The ITT analysis will collect data from all the participants in this trial, and for those lost to follow-up, the last observation carried forward method will be implemented.

2.9.2. MRI Data Analysis. For imaging, data will be analyzed using the Data Processing & Analysis for (Resting-State) Brain Imaging (DPABI) toolbox [44] performed on MATLAB V.8.6 (MathWorks) to detect any changes in brain function due to acupuncture treatment. Lesion symptom mapping was demarcated on T1-weighted images manually using MRIcroGL (http://www.cabiatl.com/mricrogl/) in native space by neurologists who were blinded to the participants' language scores. DTI images will be analyzed using MATLAB (https://www.mathworks.com/) and FMRIB Software Library (http://www.fmrib.ox.ac.uk/fsl). After data preprocessing, some data-driven approaches will be performed to investigate neuroplasticity between the two groups, such as the amplitude of the low-frequency fluctuation, regional homogeneity, and voxel-wise degree centrality. A two-sample *t*-test will be conducted to investigate the differences in brain regions between the acupoint group or NA control group in the DPABI software. Multiple comparisons will be used to better control for a highly inflated false positivity rate. Pearson's correlation analysis will be performed to examine the association between the fMRI data and clinical variables.

2.9.3. EEG Data Analysis. EEG data will be preprocessed by NeuroScan software, and electrocardiogram, ophthalmic, and myoelectric artefacts will be removed by independent component analysis (ICA). eLORETA software will be used to extract the characteristic indexes of the brain network. The electric current sources in different brain regions will be accurately and intuitively calculated, and the functional network characteristics of the brain in different frequency bands will be analyzed.

2.9.4. ERP Data Analysis. Using the threshold selection method based on a small-world network across different thresholds to build a functional brain network, analyses will be conducted to examine the network topological structure of the brain under the different thresholds, build different threshold brain networks, and use the theory of the complex network diagram analysis method to calculate the weighted aggregation coefficient, weighted characteristic path length, and small-world network features.

3. Discussion

PSA has proven to be difficult to treat. There is a degree of spontaneous recovery in the subacute phase, so there are few studies on the subacute phase of PSA. However, the subacute phase also requires treatment. The extant literature shows that acupuncture is probably effective for PSA [18, 45–47]. We intend to evaluate the long-term efficacy of acupuncture in maintaining speech production function. One common problem is the lack of standardization of acupoint selection, needle retention time, number of needles used, needling depth, and needle manipulation in acupuncture research.

From 2006 to now, we attempted to explore the general acupuncture scheme based on syndrome differentiation. In our PSA acupuncture treatment programme, DU20 is located in the area at the top of the head and is particularly closely related to the regulation of brain speech activity. The EX-HN1 are the acupuncture points around the DU20, both of which are used together to benefit the brain and promote speech rehabilitation. The treatment of PSA by EX-HN12 and EX-HN13 bloodletting has a theoretical basis in TCM and unique clinical efficacy. CV23 is mainly used for the treatment of speechlessness, stabbing into the skin towards the root of the tongue, and has the effect of restoring speech. The acupuncture theory of HT5 and GB39 to be used in our study is different from the traditional meaning of these points. FMRI can help us evaluate the changes of needle-related neuroplasticity, so we have conducted fMRI experiments based on this pair of effective points for aphasia. Electroacupuncture at HT5 and GB39 may modulate language and cognition function through a complex network formed by an extensive area of the brain cortex. It is beneficial to the recovery of language function [47]. In previous studies, we have demonstrated that this acupuncture protocol has shown significant improvements in auditory comprehension, reading, and dictation in patients with subacute PSA after 4 weeks of treatment. Therefore, we would like to know more about whether this treatment programme has long-term effects in these areas and observe the association with overall linguistic changes.

Regarding the study design, we developed an assessor- and participant-blinded design to minimize bias. The specific effects are thought to be generated by needling the acupoint with the appropriate manipulation. The nonspecific effects are due to other aspects of the therapy, such as the expectations of the patient, which might influence the treatment outcome. To recognize the specific effects, a placebo is needed. Among acupuncture research, placebo controls for acupuncture studies have been difficult to select. To maximally exclude the placebo effect, rigorous methodological designs are followed. In our study, control conditions involve being punctured with real acupuncture needles at NA locations. Thus, the self-perception of placebo effects in the NA control group is difficult to distinguish from the real acupoints. Additional needle manipulations will not be used in the NA control group. De qi is a characteristic constellation of sensations felt by patients during acupuncture needling. It has been regarded as an important factor related to clinical effects; however, we do not pursue this kind of sensation in the NA control group. By following these methods, participants can be successfully blinded, and the efficacy of acupuncture could be confirmed if the results of the acupoint group prove superior to those of the NA control group.

We will assess patients with PSA on multiple levels, including multiple neuropsychological tests, functional and structural brain alterations, and TCM syndrome evaluation. This multidomain assessment will be used to identify possible biomarkers involved in the effects of acupuncture in PSA.

It is worth mentioning that functional and structural brain alterations will be used as outcome measures. MRI allows for noninvasive evaluations of neural functional changes [48]. fMRI studies use two modalities, task-related and resting-state methods [49]. Task-related fMRI has revealed functional disturbances in individuals with aphasia. MRI may be more sensitive to smaller treatment effects. It can be used as a tool to assess the efficacy of acupuncture in treating aphasia. These analyses may identify whether neural efficiency is improved or the brain connectome is reorganized to achieve language enhancement. Electrophysiological methods, such as intracranially recorded EEG or ERP, are particularly promising to offer a mechanistic understanding of language formation processes. Compared with the language scales alone, the combination of in vivo measures of brain alterations in this study will be more sensitive in detecting acupuncture efficacy [50].

Therefore, this study can provide clinical evidence on the long-term efficacy of our acupuncture programme in patients with PSA and explore biomarkers for the recovery of function and the efficacy of acupuncture in patients with PSA through a multidimensional evaluation. This trial will fill the gaps in the evidence on the long-term efficacy of acupuncture for aphasia and provide a model for the multimodal evaluation of PSA.

Abbreviations

PSA:	Poststroke aphasia
AQ:	Aphasia quotient
WAB:	Western Aphasia Battery
BDAE:	Boston Diagnostic Aphasia Examination
MRI:	Magnetic resonance imaging
EEG:	Electroencephalogram
SLT:	Speech and language therapy
TCM:	Traditional chinese medicine
RCT:	Randomized controlled trial
SPIRIT:	Standard Protocol Items: Recommendations for Interventional Trials
CONSORT:	Consolidated Standards of Reporting Trials
BUCM:	Beijing University of Chinese Medicine
CT:	Computed tomography
STRICTA:	Standards for Reporting Interventions in Clinical Trials of Acupuncture
NA:	Nonacupoint
RS-fMRI:	Resting-state functional magnetic resonance imaging
DTI:	Diffusion tensor imaging
ERP:	Event-related potentials.

Consent

All participants gave their written informed consent to the research assistant before joining the RCT. The purpose, procedures, confidentiality, and potential risks of the RCT were explained clearly to the participants.

Disclosure

The trial results will be published through publication in scientific papers and posters or oral presentations at conferences. The funding source has no role in the study design and do not have any role during the execution, analyses, interpretation of the data, or decision to submit results.

Authors' Contributions

The trial was designed and developed by JLC and YG. The manuscript was prepared by XLL. CZ and SRL revised carefully the protocol and provided methodological support. JLC and XLL registered the protocol in the Chinese Clinical Trial Registry and obtained ethical approval. XLL and CML prepared the tables and figures. QSZ and XYX contributed to recruitment. ZJT and BLZ are responsible for image parameter setting and data acquisition. RWF, XH, MJX, XS, HMY, and QK are the coordinators and responsible for the screening and enrolment of patients. All authors read and approved the final manuscript.

Acknowledgments

This work was supported by the Beijing Natural Science Foundation (Funding no. 7181005). This work was also supported by the Special Funds for Basic Scientific Research in the Central Universities of China (Funding no. 2020-JYB-ZDGG-110-2).

References

[1] Global, Regional, and National Burden of Stroke, "1990-2016: a systematic analysis for the Global Burden of Disease Study 2016," *Lancet Neurology*, vol. 18, no. 5, pp. 439–458, 2019.

[2] A. Pollock, B. St George, M. Fenton, and L. Firkins, "Top ten research priorities relating to life after stroke," *The Lancet Neurology*, vol. 11, no. 3, p. 209, 2012.

[3] L. Worrall and A. Foster, "Does intensity matter in aphasia rehabilitation?" *The Lancet*, vol. 389, no. 10078, pp. 1494-1495, 2017.

[4] H. El Hachioui, H. F. Lingsma, M. W. M. E. van de Sandt-Koenderman, D. W. J. Dippel, P. J. Koudstaal, and E. G. Visch-Brink, "Long-term prognosis of aphasia after stroke," *Journal of Neurology, Neurosurgery & Psychiatry*, vol. 84, no. 3, pp. 310–315, 2013.

[5] S. Berube and A. E. Hillis, "Advances and innovations in aphasia treatment trials," *Stroke*, vol. 50, no. 10, pp. 2977–2984, 2019.

[6] J. M. C. Lam and W. P. Wodchis, "The relationship of 60 disease diagnoses and 15 conditions to preference-based health-related quality of life in ontario hospital-based long-term care residents," *Medical Care*, vol. 48, no. 4, pp. 380–387, 2010.

[7] C. Breitenstein, T. Grewe, A. Floel et al., "Intensive speech and language therapy in patients with chronic aphasia after stroke: a randomised, open-label, blinded-endpoint, controlled trial in a health-care setting," *Lancet*, vol. 389, no. 10078, pp. 1528–1538, 2017.

[8] J. Fridriksson, C. Rorden, J. Elm, S. Sen, M. S. George, and L. Bonilha, "Transcranial direct current stimulation vs sham stimulation to treat aphasia after stroke," *JAMA Neurology*, vol. 75, no. 12, pp. 1470–1476, 2018.

[9] R. Palmer, M. Dimairo, C. Cooper et al., "Self-managed, computerised speech and language therapy for patients with chronic aphasia post-stroke compared with usual care or attention control (Big CACTUS): a multicentre, single-blinded, randomised controlled trial," *The Lancet Neurology*, vol. 18, no. 9, pp. 821–833, 2019.

[10] A. M. Raymer and L. J. G. Rothi, "Aphasia syndromes: introduction and value in clinical practice," 2017.

[11] E. M. Khedr, N. Abo El-Fetoh, A. M. Ali et al., "Dual-hemisphere repetitive transcranial magnetic stimulation for rehabilitation of poststroke aphasia," *Neurorehabilitation and Neural Repair*, vol. 28, no. 8, pp. 740–750, 2014.

[12] M. Haghighi, M. Mazdeh, N. Ranjbar, and M. A. Seifrabie, "Further evidence of the positive influence of repetitive transcranial magnetic stimulation on speech and language in patients with aphasia after stroke: results from a double-blind intervention with sham condition," *Neuropsychobiology*, vol. 75, no. 4, pp. 185–192, 2017.

[13] I. van der Meulen, W. M. E. van de Sandt-Koenderman, M. H. Heijenbrok-Kal, E. G. Visch-Brink, and G. M. Ribbers, "The efficacy and timing of melodic intonation therapy in subacute aphasia," *Neurorehabilitation and Neural Repair*, vol. 28, no. 6, pp. 536–544, 2014.

[14] M. C. Brady, H. Kelly, J. Godwin et al., "Speech and language therapy for aphasia following stroke," *Cochrane Database System Reviews*, vol. 6, 2016.

[15] B. Stahl, B. Mohr, V. Büscher, F. R. Dreyer, G. Lucchese, and F. Pulvermüller, "Efficacy of intensive aphasia therapy in patients with chronic stroke: a randomised controlled trial," *Journal of Neurology, Neurosurgery & Psychiatry*, vol. 89, no. 6, pp. 586–592, 2018.

[16] M. Bucur and C. Papagno, "Are transcranial brain stimulation effects long-lasting in post-stroke aphasia? A comparative systematic review and meta-analysis on naming performance," *Neuroscience & Biobehavioral Reviews*, vol. 102, pp. 264–289, 2019.

[17] B. Zhang, Y. Han, X. Huang et al., "Acupuncture is effective in improving functional communication in post-stroke aphasia: a systematic review and meta-analysis of randomized controlled trials," *Wiener Klinische Wochenschrift*, vol. 131, no. 9-10, pp. 221–232, 2019.

[18] H. Y. Tang, W. Tang, F. Yang et al., "Efficacy of acupuncture in the management of post-apoplectic aphasia: a systematic review and meta-analysis of randomized controlled trials," *BMC Complement Alternative Medicine*, vol. 19, no. 1, p. 282, 2019.

[19] Y. Li, H. Zheng, C. M. Witt et al., "Acupuncture for migraine prophylaxis: a randomized controlled trial," *Canadian Medical Association Journal*, vol. 184, no. 4, pp. 401–410, 2012.

[20] B. Brinkhaus, M. Ortiz, C. M. Witt et al., "Acupuncture in patients with seasonal allergic rhinitis," *Annals of Internal Medicine*, vol. 158, no. 4, pp. 225–234, 2013.

[21] R. S. Hinman, P. McCrory, M. Pirotta et al., "Acupuncture for chronic knee pain," *Jama*, vol. 312, no. 13, pp. 1313–1322, 2014.

[22] S. Zhang, B. Wu, M. Liu et al., "Acupuncture efficacy on ischemic stroke recovery," *Stroke*, vol. 46, no. 5, pp. 1301–1306, 2015.

[23] C. Ee, C. Xue, P. Chondros et al., "Acupuncture for menopausal hot flashes," *Annals of Internal Medicine*, vol. 164, no. 3, pp. 146–154, 2016.

[24] Z. Liu, Y. Liu, H. Xu et al., "Effect of electroacupuncture on urinary leakage among women with stress urinary incontinence," *Jama*, vol. 317, no. 24, pp. 2493–2501, 2017.

[25] J. W. Yang, L. Q. Wang, X. Zou et al., "Effect of acupuncture for postprandial distress syndrome A randomized clinical trial," *Annals of Internal Medicine*, vol. 1, 2020.

[26] J. L. Chang, Y. Gao, S. L. Li et al., "Effect of acupuncture and speech rehabilitation on motor aphasia after stroke," *China Journal of Rehabilitation Theory Practise*, vol. 16, no. 1, pp. 58-59, 2010.

[27] J. L. Chang, X. Huang, T. L. Lv et al., "Theoretical connotations on arousing brain and nourishing marrow method for post-stroke aphasia," *World Chinese Medicine*, vol. 12, no. 7, pp. 1487–1490, 2017.

[28] M. J. Xu, X. Shu, X. L. Li et al., "Discussion on the application of centro-square needling in post-stroke aphasia treatment from the prospective of cognitive neuropsychology of traditional Chinese medicine," *Global Traditional Chinese Medicine*, vol. 12, no. 10, pp. 1495–1498, 2019.

[29] S. W. Jeon, K. S. Kim, and H. J. Nam, "Long-term effect of acupuncture for treatment of tinnitus: a randomized, patient- and assessor-blind, sham-acupuncture-controlled, pilot trial," *The Journal of Alternative and Complementary Medicine*, vol. 18, no. 7, pp. 693–699, 2012.

[30] M. Xu, S. Yan, X. Yin et al., "Acupuncture for chronic low back pain in long-term follow-up: a meta-analysis of 13 randomized controlled trials," *The American Journal of Chinese Medicine*, vol. 41, no. 1, pp. 1–19, 2013.

[31] M. Yang, P. Yang, Y.-S. Fan et al., "Altered structure and intrinsic functional connectivity in post-stroke aphasia," *Brain Topography*, vol. 31, no. 2, pp. 300–310, 2018.

[32] Y. Zhao, M. A. Lambon Ralph, and A. D. Halai, "Relating resting-state hemodynamic changes to the variable language profiles in post-stroke aphasia," *NeuroImage: Clinical*, vol. 20, pp. 611–619, 2018.

[33] D. Wu, J. Wang, and Y. Yuan, "Effects of transcranial direct current stimulation on naming and cortical excitability in stroke patients with aphasia," *Neuroscience Letters*, vol. 589, pp. 115–120, 2015.

[34] J. L. Chang, A. Q. Wang, S. L. Li et al., "Exploration of Chinese medical evidence and clinical symptoms of post-stroke aphasia under comprehensive rehabilitation intervention in Traditional Chinese medicine," *Global Traditional Chinese Medicine*, vol. 9, no. 8, pp. 1020–1023, 2016.

[35] A.-W. Chan, J. M. Tetzlaff, D. G. Fau Altman, D. G. Altman et al., "SPIRIT 2013 statement: defining standard protocol items for clinical trials," *Annals of Internal Medicine*, vol. 158, no. 3, pp. 200–207, 2013.

[36] I. Boutron, D. G. Altman, D. Moher, K. F. Schulz, and P. Ravaud, "CONSORT statement for randomized trials of nonpharmacologic treatments: a 2017 update and a

CONSORT extension for nonpharmacologic trial abstracts," *Annals of Internal Medicine*, vol. 167, no. 1, pp. 40–47, 2017.

[37] Z. Qin, Y. Ding, J. Wu et al., "Efficacy of acupuncture for degenerative lumbar spinal stenosis: protocol for a randomised sham acupuncture-controlled trial," *BMJ Open*, vol. 6, no. 11, 2016.

[38] Z. Liu, H. Xu, Y. Chen et al., "The efficacy and safety of electroacupuncture for women with pure stress urinary incontinence: study protocol for a multicenter randomized controlled trial," *Trials*, vol. 14, no. 1, p. 315, 2013.

[39] H. MacPherson, D. G. Altman, R. Hammerschlag et al., "Revised STandards for reporting interventions in clinical trials of acupuncture (STRICTA): extending the CONSORT statement," *PLoS Medicine*, vol. 7, no. 6, 2010.

[40] C. M. Shewan, "The language quotient (LQ): a new measure for the western aphasia battery," *Journal of Communication Disorders*, vol. 19, no. 6, pp. 427–439, 1986.

[41] L. Lao, G. R. Hamilton, J. Fu et al., "Is acupuncture safe? A systematic review of case reports," *Alternative Theory Health Medicine*, vol. 9, no. 1, pp. 72–83, 2003.

[42] X. F. Zhao, Y. Du, P. G. Liu, and S. Wang, "Acupuncture for stroke: evidence of effectiveness, safety, and cost from systematic reviews," *Topics in Stroke Rehabilitation*, vol. 19, no. 3, pp. 226–233, 2012.

[43] L.-X. Li, K. Deng, and Y. Qu, "Acupuncture treatment for post-stroke dysphagia: an update meta-analysis of randomized controlled trials," *Chinese Journal of Integrative Medicine*, vol. 24, no. 9, pp. 686–695, 2018.

[44] C.-G. Yan, X.-D. Wang, X.-N. Zuo, and Y.-F. Zang, "DPABI: data processing & analysis for (Resting-State) brain imaging," *Neuroinformatics*, vol. 14, no. 3, pp. 339–351, 2016.

[45] Q. Wu, X. Hu, X. Wen, F. Li, and W. Fu, "Clinical study of acupuncture treatment on motor aphasia after stroke," *Technology and Health Care*, vol. 24, no. s2, pp. S691–S696, 2016.

[46] J. Chang, H. Zhang, Z. Tan et al., "Effect of electroacupuncture in patients with post-stroke motor aphasia: neurolinguistic and neuroimaging characteristics," *Wiener Klinische Wochenschrift*, vol. 129, no. 3-4, pp. 102–109, 2017.

[47] J. Xiao, H. Zhang, J.-L. Chang et al., "Effects of electroacupuncture at Tongli (HT 5) and Xuanzhong (GB 39) acupoints from functional magnetic resonance imaging evidence," *Chinese Journal of Integrative Medicine*, vol. 22, no. 11, pp. 846–854, 2016.

[48] B.-Y. Park, K. Byeon, and H. Park, "FuNP (fusion of neuroimaging preprocessing) pipelines: a fully automated preprocessing software for functional magnetic resonance imaging," *Frontiers in Neuroinformatics*, vol. 13, p. 5, 2019.

[49] R. Achalia, A. Jacob, G. Achalia, A. Sable, G. Venkatasubramanian, and N. Rao, "Investigating spontaneous brain activity in bipolar disorder: a resting-state functional magnetic resonance imaging study," *Indian Journal of Psychiatry*, vol. 61, no. 6, pp. 630–634, 2019.

[50] C.-Q. Yan, P. Zhou, X. Wang et al., "Efficacy and neural mechanism of acupuncture treatment in older adults with subjective cognitive decline: study protocol for a randomised controlled clinical trial," *BMJ Open*, vol. 9, no. 10, 2019.

9

Orthographic Visualisation Induced Brain Activations in a Chronic Poststroke Global Aphasia with Dissociation between Oral and Written Expression

Jurgita Usinskiene ⬡,[1] Michael Mouthon,[2] Chrisovalandou Martins Gaytanidis,[3] Agnes Toscanelli,[2,4] and Jean-Marie Annoni ⬡[2]

[1]National Cancer Institute; Faculty of Medicine, Vilnius University, Vilnius, Lithuania
[2]Neurology Unit, Department of Neuro and Movement Sciences, Faculty of Science and Medicine, Fribourg University, Switzerland
[3]Fribourg Cantonal Hospital, Switzerland
[4]Cabinet de Logopédie du Sonnenberg, Fribourg, Switzerland

Correspondence should be addressed to Jurgita Usinskiene; jurgita.usinskiene@gmail.com

Academic Editor: Peter Berlit

We propose a method of orthographic visualisation strategy in a poststroke severe aphasia person with dissociation between oral and written expression. fMRI results suggest that such strategy may induce the engagement of alternative nonlanguage networks and visual representations may help improving oral output. This choice of rehabilitation method can be based on the remaining capacities and, therefore, on written language. Most notably, no study so far addressed how orthographic visualisation strategy during speech rehabilitation might influence clinical outcomes in nonfluent aphasia and apraxia patients.

1. Introduction

While many studies have examined poststroke functional reorganization of language brain networks in aphasic patients with left hemispheric damage [1, 2], the behavioural and functional effects of teaching patients to implement new compensatory cognitive strategies in their language impairments remain underexplored [3]. Such speech therapies can indeed be very effective through spontaneously evolved suboptimal strategies [4]. For example, speech and language therapeutic strategies shown to improve recovery of identifying an object or entity [5] may include teaching the patient to utilize visual recognition (access to structural description), use semantic representation, learn pronunciation (phonologic representation), and employ motor planning (articulation) [6]. It is typically as reported in chronic left hemispheric aphasic patients who correctly identify a subject involving left IFG, left TG, SMA, and right IFG [7, 8]. Verbally identifying objects has also been demonstrated to be mediated by a brain network independent of the classical network [9].

2. Materials and Methods

The present study focuses on an 18-month rehabilitation program of patients' ability to correctly name objects in a rare case of chronic severe nonfluent aphasia with severe apraxia of speech (AOS) following a large left hemisphere stroke. The therapy consisted of training articulatory movements using visual support, then teaching the patient to visualise the orthographic form of the word before pronunciation. The strategy suggested to the patient was to retrieve simultaneously the visual mental representations of the articulatory movement for a given phoneme, as well as the corresponding grapheme; then, the orthography of the word allowed to deconstruct the words into phonemes that would be subsequently enunciated [10]. To investigate the functional consequences of this therapeutic approach, we recorded at the end of therapy fMRI the poststroke participant performing a task of naming objects from their pictures with success measured by correct application of the taught orthographic visualisation technique. We hypothesised that using the visual word

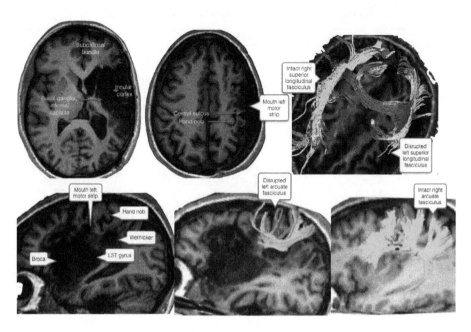

FIGURE 1: Poststroke brain lesions are shown in 3T MRI.

imagery strategy might help access to phonological/phonetic stores for allowing word production [11]. At the brain functional level, we predicted that the orthographic strategy could be associated with nontraditional language areas which had been destroyed in the patients in our study. We also expected activations related to visual form processing cortex activation due to orthographic word visualisation strategy.

2.1. Case Report. A 29-year-old female (T.W.), a native French speaker, suffered from global aphasia and right hemiplegia following a left hemispheric stroke (NIHS 18/42), due to a dissection of the left internal carotid artery. The stroke involved the left cortico–subcortical frontotemporoparietal areas. Lesion included 44 – Broca's, 22 – Wernicke's, 4 – motor cortex areas, insular cortex, basal ganglia, the most medial and rostral portion of the subcallosal fasciculus, the periventricular white matter near the body of the lateral ventricle, deep to the lower motor/sensory cortex area for the mouth and disrupted left arcuate fasciculus (see Figure 1).

T.W. was a governess by profession, right-handed, and an active smoker. For 9 to 12 months following the stroke, she was practically mute and could not pronounce a single word. On first language examination two weeks after the stroke, she was diagnosed with global aphasia with AOS, buccofacial apraxia and oral suppression, agraphia, oral and written comprehension impairment, and executive dysfunction. She underwent intensive inpatient neurorehabilitation for four months then was discharged with ambulatory speech therapy, physiotherapy, and ergotherapy. She started to walk in the city (with a stick) accompanied by her family and her boyfriend; she also resumed listening to music and watching movies. However, the severe AOS remained. Nine months after the stroke, she was still nearly mute, with no oral functional output, only the capacity to repeat some isolated phonemes (/a/, /ou/, /m/, /f/, /n/) and syllables (*mamama, nanana,*

moumoumou), and could whisper "no". She had necessitated an explicit control for every phoneme output. However, her written production improved and she started to write words and small sentences with her left hand. T.W. communicated essentially by gestures during the first months. At home, she began to use some written support to communicate, either with a pencil in her left hand or with a speech program named I-Word Q, which allowed her to write. She could also use a selected written vocabulary on her iPad. Nine months after the stroke, despite some residual difficulties in finding written words, she could take advantage of her written communication ability for her daily messages, particularly with smartphone messages. Language and neuropsychological performances of T.W. at the different postonset times and steps of speech rehabilitation are demonstrated in Table 1. The following tests were acquired: (1) for language evaluation – Montréal-Toulouse 86 (MT-86) [12]; (2) for description of a picture – Nicholas & Brookshire (1993) [13]; (3) for writing – Croisiles battery [14]; (4) for associative gnosia – Columbia's b Test [15], (5) for memory – 5 mots de Dubois [16], (6) for executive functions – BREF (Batterie rapide d'evaluation frontale de Dubois 'The Frontal Assessment Battery') [17]. Total score = 18; cut-off = 15. Oral expression was still very severely impaired. She could repeat 10/18 isolated phonemes, and 9/19 isolated syllables. Word and nonwords repetition was not possible due to AOS. She started to repeat some disyllabic trained words although this did not appear on the formal evaluation. Oral naming was still impossible due to AOS and inability to initiate a phonation. Reading of words and nonwords was still impossible (Table 1, 2nd Column). The written expression had much better recovered at 9 months after stroke. Particularly, written naming performance improved from 60/144 at 3 months to 90/144(62%) at 9 months. There was no significant frequency effect (high-frequency words: 49/72; low-frequency words: 41/72, chi^2

TABLE 1: Language and neuropsychological performance.

Time after stroke	36 months	9 months	3 months
Period of therapy	18 months	pretherapy	pretherapy
Oral production			
Series	15/17	0*/10	0*/10
Description of a picture	nonfluent agrammatism	mute apraxia	mute apraxia
Pictures Naming	20/31	0*/31	0*/31
Verbal fluency (1')			
Letter « s »	3	0*	0*
Category « animals »	13	0*	0*
Oral Repetition			
Words	12/25	0*/25	0*/25
Nonwords	4/5	0*/5	0*/5
Sentences	0/3	0*/3	0*/3
Oral comprehension			
Words	9/9	8/9	9/9
Sentences	29/38	24/38	11/15**
Reading aloud			
Words	15/25	0*/25	0*/25
Nonwords	2/5	0*/5	0*/5
Sentences	0/3	0*/3	0*/3
Written Naming			
Words	NA	90/144	60/144
Writing to dictation (left hand)			
Name, last name, address	OK	OK	OK
Words	16/ 24**	19/28	7/18**
Written comprehension			
Words	4/5	4/5	5/5
Sentences	7/8	5/8	5/8
Praxia (Gestures)			
Buccofacial	11/13	5/7	not done
Symbolic gestures	4/5	3/5	1/4
Using objects gestures	9/10	7/10	0/4
No signification gestures (unimanual)	3/3	3/3	3/3
Calculation	1/5	0*/5	1/5
Multiple choice answer	8/8	7/8	not done
Others			
Memory Dubois 5 words	10/10	not done	not done
Executive functions (FAB)	11/18	9/18	0/12

0*: no production because of speech suppression due to apraxia of speech. **: simplified version used in this case.

is 1.89, p <.17), but a length effect was present (46/60 for 1 syllable words, 39/60 for 2 syllables words, 5/24 for 3 syllables words, chi^2=23, p < 0.001). In writing to dictation, she was able to write 64% of the presented items with neither regularity effect, nor significant frequency effect (Croisile's battery: 9/10 high-frequency words, 5/9 medium frequency words, and 4/9 low-frequency words, chi^2 = 4.7, p <.094). Concerning the error types in written production, she could write the first syllable, but could not always complete the word. Particularly, she helped herself with the vocalisation of some isolated syllables, but could not always vocalise or respect the order of the syllables in the word. There were mainly literal paragraphs (omission, substitution of letters) and nonphonologically plausible errors (examples: "canic" for "canary"; "abomas" for "abdomen") unless some random

words were correctly written (e.g., "oignon", "bapteme"). At the receptive and semantic levels, word comprehension was relatively preserved in the oral (8 correct word to image association /9) and the written (4/5) domain. T.W. partially preserved her ability to correctly classify in the semantic field 86% of the presented words in an intracategorical designation test. The score at the pyramid and palm tree test visual version had been 47/52 (lower limit) 3 months after stroke.

Her performances in the written and the oral domain at 9 months after stroke suggested preserved input (preserved writing to dictation) and semantic processing (satisfactory performance in oral and written comprehension). The results at our images designation test and the image pyramid and palm tree test also indicated that the general domain semantic system is preserved. The AOS was present in all

TABLE 2: Aphasia evolvement.

Time poststroke	initial	36 months
Types of aphasia	*Global*	*Broca's*
Speech	mute	non fluent
Comprehension	impaired	preserved
Repetition	impaired	effortful
Motor signs	right hemiplegia	right hemiparesis, buccofacial apraxia

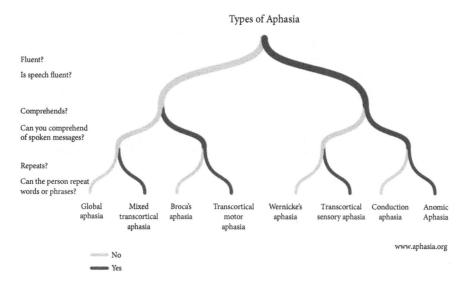

FIGURE 2: General types of aphasia (from https://www.aphasia.org).

oral outputs (naming, reading, repetition) for both words and nonwords in the oral domain sparing only isolated phonemes. Written expression was partially spared, but showed some nonphonological errors affecting words and nonwords, with a length effect but no consistent regularity and frequency. The whole pattern pointed to a locus of impairment mostly at the postlexical impairment, at the phonetic-phonological level in the oral domain, and a partially preserved writing ability with some milder graphemic buffer type of dysfunction. The difficulties in sentences comprehension were possibly syntactic.

T.W.'s initial global aphasia evolved at 9 months in a severe Broca's aphasia with severe postlexical oral impairment at the phonetic-phonological level leading to massive AOS. Interestingly, her writing was much better preserved despite moderate impairment at the graphemic buffer level. Some syntactic difficulties were also present. Main types of aphasia in general are presented in Figure 2. Aphasia evolvement in T.W. is presented in Table 2.

2.2. Speech Therapy. One year after the onset, given the dissociation between impossible oral and relatively preserved written expression, T.W. was instructed in the use of visual word imagery strategy by the language therapist (A.T.). The goals of the therapy were focused on (1) improving orthographic-visual skills to reinforce T.W.'s expertise to transform a set of letters into a visual word form; (2) memorising written form of the word based on a neurolinguistic

programming (NLP) technique to automate the visualisation strategy adding eventually upward eye movements [18]; (3) training of the visualisation (integration of the written word's picture, then visual mental rehearsal) so that T.W. could also improve written words production. The speech therapist observed the link between "visual orthographic imagery" of the word and its successful translation in articulatory movements. However, if the sound produced aloud was not congruent with the internal graphemic representation of the word, it immediately blocked its oral production. Thus, at the early stage, a "visualisation technique" was implemented to "reprogram" the articulation of phonemes. For each phoneme, a pictogram representing the correct articulatory movement was associated with the corresponding grapheme, and the set was memorised visually. This visualisation was cued using principles of NLP (increasing the capacity of imaging language representation by coinitiating eye movements towards up) for the 32 phonemes of the language [18]. Then T.W. focused her visualisation of mouth movements at the level of the syllables. Then T.W. was given as homework a sequence of pictograms corresponding to a certain number of basic words, as well as the written form of these words. She trained daily visually to memorise the succession of articulatory movements with this corresponding word (NLP visualisation technique [19], to develop progressively the oral form of the word and thus a "basic" oral lexicon). Support to construct the verbalisation of a word was through the simultaneous activation of the word visual orthographic image and the visible mental representations of the articulatory movements. Gradually, this visual stimulus enabled her to exploit initial lexical potential. T.W. was able to follow this new therapy program and could integrate it into her word finding strategies. To facilitate word visualisation, she developed eye movement techniques used by healthy subjects and aphasic persons in NLP approach. T.W. explained her personal method to find and articulate a word: *"I move my eyes in certain directions to facilitate certain aspects of language. First, I position my eyes downwards: in this way I know what I want to mean, but cannot yet articulate the words. Then, I lift my eyes towards up to see the written word, and I find it more "natural" to pronounce, particularly for simple words. For more difficult words, I block my mouth and stay silent until I have seen the written word. It is a way I have trained with the speech therapist"*.

The therapy lasted 18 months, twice a week for one hour sessions. After six months of this new technique, her spontaneous speech improved with a few comprehensible words, and after 18 months she could construct short sentences with a decreased number of phonetic and phonemic errors. She reported that using the visualisation technique of the written word gave her a more precise pronunciation. However, at the end of the therapy, she said that she used the visualisation technique less frequently and that the words were found easier also without visualisation techniques. The posttherapy language evaluation still revealed moderate-to-severe Broca's aphasia (nonfluent speech, but right comprehension) with AOS, phonetic and phonemic paraphasias, agraphia, mild oral-facial-lingual apraxia, dyscalculia and executive dysfunction – difficulty in inhibition and motor planning.

On posttherapy formal evaluation, she could name correctly 20 out of 31 items of the MT 86 battery in comparison to 0 at 9 months after stroke. Repetition and reading improved: 12 words out of 25 and 4 nonwords out of 5. She could also read aloud correctly 15 words out of 25 and 2 nonwords out of 5. Fluency for oral description of animals improved, but letter fluency remained impaired (see Table 1).

2.3. Experimental Design. At the end of therapy picture naming fMRI was recorded. Three fMRI experimental conditions were presented (see Table 3): (1) explicitly naming the picture activating the visual representation of the written word (cueing condition); (2) naming the picture and suppressing this cueing; (3) naming the picture by reading the written word below the picture (control condition). In total, 144 different pictures were presented in 3 separate experimental runs of 48 stimuli. Each run lasted 7 minutes and was composed of the three blocks of 16 pictures each: (i) one block in which T.W. explicitly used the cueing, (ii) one block of naming with suppressing cueing, and (iii) one control condition. Each picture lasted 6 seconds on the screen. Between the pictures, a fixation cross was displayed with a variable duration of 1.5-3 second. The position of the pictures was identical between conditions (centre of the screen) but with different colours on the border of the screen to help to recognise the task. The background colour around the black-white pictures was grey for each condition. Before the scan, a training session outside the scanner was performed to familiarise participants with the experimental design. The black and white line drawings were selected from the picture database of Cycowicz et al. [20]. The three lists of pictures (see Tables 3 and 4) were matched for frequency, name agreement, and visual complexity [21]. Moreover, the lists were matched by phonological neighbourhood density and syllabic structure, as these factors can have a strong effect on language production errors in aphasic patients [22, 23]. Grapheme-to-phoneme correspondence could play an important role on whether the words can be sounded out, a skill that is being encouraged by visualisation. So, we categorised the regularity of each word according to the following criteria: regular words: words with a one-to-one grapheme-phoneme correspondence or words with one-to-one grapheme-phoneme correspondence with a silent grapheme in a terminal position. All other words were defined as irregular. Kruskal Wallis test revealed that the word lists were matched for regularity. These items were not part of the therapy, although they may have been used in free communication training. The E-Prime 2 software (Psychology Software Tools, Inc.) was used for stimulus presentation.

MRI was carried out with Siemens 3T Prisma at the "Centre d'Imagerie BioMédicale" (CIBM, https://www.cibm.ch) of the University Hospital of Geneva. T1-weighted images were acquired with an MPRAGE sequence, voxel size: 0.5x0.5x1mm, number of sagittal slices: 176, TR/TE/TI=2300/2.27/900 ms, flip angle = 9°. Functional T2*weighted Echo Planar images with blood oxygenation level-dependent (BOLD) contrast were acquired with: voxel size: 2x2x3.5mm, 29 ascending axial slices, interslice spacing = 0.35mm, TR/TE=2000/30ms, Flip angle=85°. Diffusion Tensor Imaging (DTI) data was acquired using Echo Planar images with a voxel size of 1.6x1.6x1.6mm, 74 axial slices, TR/TE=3500/60ms, 64 noncollinear directions with b-value=1000 s/mm^2, 4 min duration.

2.4. Data Analysis. Data for the output in verbally identifying pictures was audiotaped and then scored by nomenclature accuracy and errors by a speech-language pathologist (C.G.M.) trained in clinical output analysis. She rated the first answer, except in cases where T.W. produced just a phoneme and then the correct answer (there were only 2 such productions). Since the errors were effectively complicated to decide between phonemic and phonetic, we clustered them in a single group, classifying them as segmental errors [24]. We defined the errors as follows:

(i) No response: no answer or just phoneme or unintelligible production.

(ii) Semantic error: the semantic link between production and the target word.

(iii) Segmental error: the phonological or phonetic transformation of the structure of the word, e.g., substitution, omission, addition, or transposition of phonemes/segments and also phonetic distortions [24–26].

(iv) Neologism: unrecognisable word, more than 50% transformation.

(v) Mixed: segmental + semantics.

TABLE 3: Experimental design, picture naming fMRI tasks.

(I) Cueing condition	(II) Suppressing the cueing	(III) Reading condition
abeille, aigle, aiguille, ampoule, ane, avion, balai, baleine, bras, bus, cactus, canard, chaise, chenille, ciseau, cle, coeur, coq, echelle, elephant, escargot, etoile, gant, girafe, hibou, jumelles, lampe, lion, maison, montagne, mouton, nez, ours, parapluie, peigne, piano, pinceau, pomme, prise, regle, renard, rhinoceros, sifflet, singe, tomate, tracteur, vache, voiture	araignee, arbre, arrosoir, autruche, bague, balle, banc, bougie, brosse, canape, carotte, cerise, chaussure, chemise, cheval, cheveux, chien, citron, cloche, commode, cravate, croissant, dauphin, douche, feu, fleche, fourchette, fourmi, fraise, lit, main, oeil, oiseau, oreille, panier, pasteque, pied, pipe, plume, poisson, requin, souris, table, tigre, tortue, trompette, violon, vis	ananas, banane, botte, boussole, bouteille, bouton, ceinture, cerf, cerveau, champignon, chat, chaussette, chauvesouris, cheminee, citrouille, corde, crabe, crayon, cuillere, cygne, ecureuil, enveloppe, louche, loup, montre, mouche, orteil, papillon, pingouin, poire, fleur, hache, jambe, kangourou, lapin, livre, louche, loup, montre, mouche, orteil, papillon, pingouin, poire, porte, pouce, poule, raisin, roue, scie, soleil, squelette, tournevis, velo, verre, zebre

ceinture

TABLE 4: Statistics of the word list in three conditions for the fMRI picture naming task.

Conditions	Frequency	Name agreement	Visual Complexity	Phonological neighborhood density	Syllable Structure	Regularity
			Mean			
I Cueing	43.97	95.77	2.97	8.60	1.37	0.58
II Suppressing	40.55	96.06	3.01	9.12	1.54	0.60
III Reading	27.21	95.83	2.88	9.83	1.43	0.72
			p value			
I vs II	843	841	833	775	103	837
I vs III	310	966	681	522	537	135
II vs III	248	882	480	721	312	197

fMRI images were analysed with SPM12 software (Welcome Trust Centre for Neuroimaging, Institute of Neurology, University College London). Unwarping, spatial realignment, slice timing, normalisation on the Montreal Neurological Institute (MNI) space with $2x2x2mm^3$ voxel size, and smoothing with a Gaussian kernel of 6-mm full-width-at-half-maximum (FWHM) were used for preprocessing [27]. The preprocessed volumes of T.W. and the control (healthy volunteer) were submitted to a fixed-effect analysis with movement parameters included as regressors of no interest. We studied the difference between fMRI picture naming tasks in both participants. A statistical threshold of $p<0.001$ at the voxel level, corrected for multiple comparisons with an extended cluster threshold size of 100 contiguous voxels ($p_{cluster} < 0.05$; family-wise error (FWE) corrected). Anatomical locations were checked with the neuromorphometrics probabilistic atlas provided in SPM12. Dynamic causal modelling (DCM) analysis was carried out with SPM12 using a mask from the interaction contrast between T.W. and control. We defined a region of interest (ROI) of 6 mm, centred inside the highest significantly activated clusters in T.W compared to the control. T.W.'s DCM model for picture naming was then studied firstly using orthographic visualisation priming (called strategy) and then without visualisation priming (called nonstrategy) in the second condition. We compared connection values between two ROIs in each condition.

3. Results

3.1. Picture Naming Performance. There was no significant difference of T.W.'s spoken correct responses across conditions (see in Table 5). The number of correct responses was between 33% and 45% in the three sessions. We did not find a difference between the different conditions in terms of errors. The vast majority of the errors was of segmental nature (phonetic-phonological type) in all conditions, confirming the evolution of aphasia. Some errors showed mixed pattern, e.g., for "violin" she said /gEtar/ (guitare = semantic paraphasie + "gEtar" instead of "guitar", so that was a segmental error). Simple syllable structure words were named 37/79, and complex structure words 23/65 (chi^2 statistic is 1.9, p value 0.165) and this difference was insignificant in all conditions.

3.2. fMRI Results. Naming visual pictures with an orthographic imagery prime in contrast with naming pictures without priming activated the left calcarine cortex (coordinates mm x y z: -14 -70 12, cluster size 609, $p_{FWE\ corr} = 0.000$) in T.W. brain. Naming visual pictures with an orthographic prime in contrast with reading activated the left and right superior and middle frontal gyrus (-24 60 -4; 34 54 -4, 40 52 2, cluster size 2787, $p_{FWE\ corr} = 0.000$) and left cuneus and left superior occipital gyrus (-12 – 76 20, -20 -78 16, -4 -86 28, cluster size 154, $p_{FWE\ corr} = 0.039$) in T.W. Picture naming without priming relative to reading activated the left medial frontal cortex and anterior cingulate gyrus in T.W. (-6 56 -10; -4 38 -6; 16 36 -4, cluster size 390, $p_{FWE\ corr} = 0.000$). T.W. brain activations during the picture naming with an orthographic visualisation prime were relative to naming without priming and relative to reading, as well as the superposition of both (see Figure 3). No significant occipital activations were found in T.W. for picture naming without priming contrasted with reading or the opposite. For the interaction contrast, there were significant activations in the left calcarine cortex and cuneus (-18 -68 12;-8 -80 24;-14 -78 16; cluster size 207, $p_{FWE\ corr} = 0.004$) and left superior and middle frontal cortex (-20 60 -4;-18 58 4;-32 -58 2; cluster size 202, $p_{FWE\ corr} = 0.004$) in comparison to the difference in orthographic visualisation priming versus without priming contrast between T.W. and the neurotypical control. Significant results of this interaction are presented in Figure 4. Based on the DCM model, which compared the priming (strategy) and without priming (no strategy) effects in T.W.'s second session, we found a priming effect on the strength of the functional connectivity between two ROIs—the left occipital and prefrontal. The strength of the connection between these two areas was higher during the priming in comparison without priming (see Figure 5).

4. Discussion

We reported an exceptional case of severe Broca's aphasia and AOS with a strong dissociation between severe mutism due to postlexical severe phonetic-phonological impairment and a partially preserved written ability, in a poststroke young female with largely affected Broca's, Wernicke's, motor, insular, subcortical areas, and interrupting the arcuate fasciculus.

Nine-month poststroke evaluation confirmed severe postlexical oral impairment at the phonetic-phonological level leading to massive AOS and functional writing despite moderate graphemic buffer dysfunction.

TABLE 5: Evaluation of T.W. naming production.

	Correct out of 48 items	No response	Semantic	Segmental	Neologism	Mixed
Naming with priming	n 17	n 6	n 5	n 15	n 3	n 2
Naming without priming	n 22	n 0	n 2	n 16	n 3	n 5
Reading	n 21	n 2	n 0	n 22	n 3	n 0

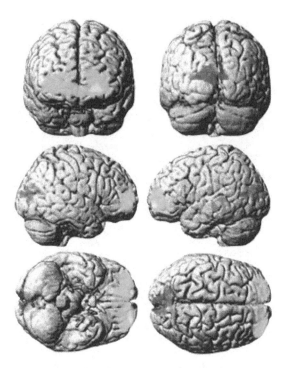

FIGURE 3: Brain activation during the picture naming with orthographic visualisation priming relative to naming without priming in red and relative to reading in green, as well as the superposition of both in yellow (p=0.01, cluster size≥100).

We could also demonstrate an improvement in the speech output in a severely chronic aphasic person (T.W.), using a speech therapy technique characterised by written words visualisation and mental training of articulatory movements.

By visualising written words during naming and word finding tasks, T.W. could regain oral expression of the word and correct the severe AOS. Functionally, we tried to mimic therapy sessions in an experiment where we asked the patient to use her visual strategy applying the visual priming explicitly. This priming condition, compared with control and without priming, resulted in the relative increase in brain activity in left visual and frontal areas.

Concerning the aphasiological case description, this is an intriguing case of dissociation between absent oral expression and preserved written expression. A similar case was described earlier after a lesion of the third frontal gyrus and the upper temporal gyrus [28]. The authors suggested that the rupture of the audio-phonological loop (with degradation of the verbal working, memory) made this dysfunction worse. However, in their case, Cambier et al. described no apraxia of speech, but an involuntary production of utterances. In the classical analyses of 500 aphasic patients, Basso et al. described 7 cases of selective impairment of speech. Three cases were with "pure anarthria," two patients with anarthria

in the context of Broca's aphasia, and two other aphasic patients with fluent aphasia except in writing [29]. Particularly, the two cases of Broca aphasia were characterised at the oral level by the absence of verbal production, clinical signs of "phonetic disintegration", very little speech outflow, and strenuous articulation and partially preserved (although not intact) writing abilities. This dissociation was longstanding in one patient (14 months). The lesion was not known, but both patients were young (< 35 yrs old), had less than 9 years of schooling, and suffered from right hemiplegia. One case also exhibited some problems in sentences (syntactic) comprehensions, as in our study. In their anatomic-clinical study, Kreisler et al. found that mutism depended on large front-putaminal lesions: "a finding consistent with the anatomy of severe Broca's and transcortical motor apraxia"; impaired repetition associated with insula-external capsule lesions, and paraphasia on external capsule lesions [30]. T.W.'s stroke involved frontal areas including Broca's, motor and insular cortex and basal ganglia. Moreover, T.W. had also a lesion of premotor cortex, which is known to cause AOS [31]. It has been confirmed that persistence of AOS after 12 months is associated with large left hemispheric stroke and strokes that involve Broca's area [32]. In our case, the dorsal parietal-frontal stream of the language (pre-

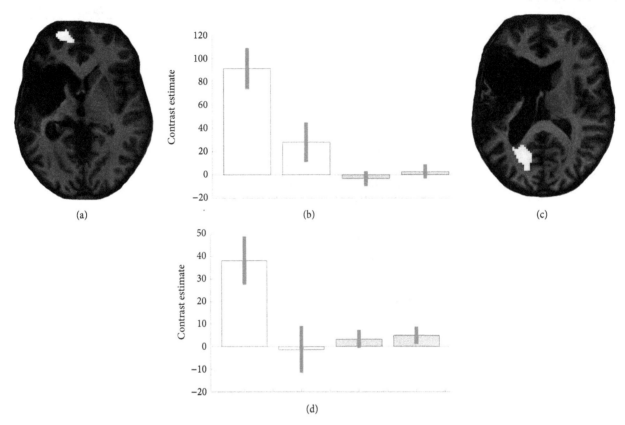

FIGURE 4: Interaction contrast (a, c) and 90% C.I. contrast estimates (b, d) between the patient (white bars) and the control (grey bars) during the picture naming with orthographic strategy (first and third bars) relative to naming without strategy (second and fourth bars). Cluster x y z coordinates (mm) in (a), (b): -18 -68 12, in (c), (d): -20 62 -4 (p=0.01, cluster size≥100).

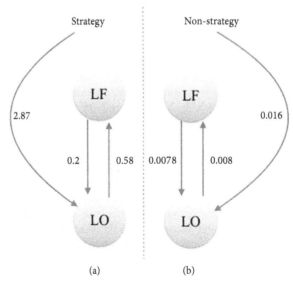

FIGURE 5: DCM model shows the strength (presented in numbers) and direction (arrows) of functional connectivity between two regions of interest: left frontal (LF) and left occipital (LO) during strategy in comparison to nonstrategy.

and postcentral gyri, left superior temporal and angular, the insula and Broca area) were affected. There was a complete disruption of the left arcuate fasciculus. Thus, we suggest that massive stroke involvement may explain the severe segmental (phonological-phonetic) impairment.

Nevertheless comprehension recovery was impressive. An initial reason for the retention of comprehension ability may be linked to the patient's young age. It has been reported that younger patients with equivalent lesions tend to have more Broca's aphasia pattern [33] and less comprehension deficit [34]. A second reason may be that the deficit was more syntactic than phonological or semantic, as shown by the good words and poor sentence comprehension. Thirdly, we suggest that the use of written imagery more easily compensated for the phonological impairment, not only in expression, but also in comprehension.

Concerning rehabilitation, to the best of our knowledge, our report is the first to describe in an aphasic patient the behavioural and brain changes associated with using visual imagery of the written words to name the objects in pictures and their appropriate verbalisation. The occipital cortex was previously reported to be involved in the ability to name correctly pictorial representations in people with aphasia [35]. Picture naming has also been shown to be mediated by a brain network independent of the classical arcuate fasciculus [9], which was destroyed in our poststroke participant. T.W.'s adoption of visual word imagery strategy was initially implemented to improve spelling through orthographic retraining [36].

Our findings were partly correlated to previous evidence that relying on visual speech perception for the treatment of nonfluent aphasia could improve speech production' possibly through activation of speech motor automatism through different channels [37]. In our study, there was no increase in occipital activations for reading as compared to picture naming without cueing, suggesting that visual form related activity was not higher for reading than for picture naming. In contrast, visual cortices activations were higher when T.W. used orthography visualisation for naming. Whether this pattern could be explained by previous evidence that orthographic processing in neurotypical adults is supported by the functional integration of visual processing, articulation and semantics remain to be elucidated with clinical group studies [38].

The superior frontal gyrus (SFG) has been involved in a wide range of functions such as cognitive control, execution, and motor control [39]. T.W.'s engagement of left prefrontal region and superior frontal gyrus could explain that for access to image orthography of the pictures she was using a phonological buffer. Because most of T.W.'s language network was damaged (the left arcuate fasciculus, Wernicke's and Broca's areas were impaired), T.W. necessarily used alternative pathways to support the interactions between an occipital prefrontal region and to improve articulation planning. Although it was not confirmed when compared to the control subject, an engagement of the right anterior structures in the case of imaging may have had a role in this left occipital-frontal activation. Adaptive plasticity of the right homologous area during speech production has been repeatedly shown

to contribute to recovery in certain circumstances [40]. Our results suggest that visual word imagery in naming is here associated with increased left occipital activation, which indirectly increases the left prefrontal network. Such activation pattern is proposed to be mediated by a nonclassical linguistic network which plays a role in speech output.

Recovery of speech output may depend on several factors, such as the amount of spared tissue in the left inferior frontal gyrus (LIFG) [41], damage to Broca's area, and treatment associated with the recruitment of areas in the left hemisphere [42]. The integrity of the left superior longitudinal fasciculus (SFL) [43] and the poststroke rehabilitation time [44] play an important role as well. Despite the complete necrosis of the LIFG and severely damaged left white matter tracts (especially SLF), T.W.'s speech output using an orthographic visualisation strategy has improved. The late stage at which the imaging strategy was introduced into rehabilitation suggests an indirect effect of this approach rather than a spontaneous recovery. Since there is no control case for T.W., one could argue that the visualisation technique used in the therapy is not necessarily the cause of the patient's verbal improvement. In fact, intensive training could also play an important role in the articulatory improvement of T.W. Indeed, speech therapist reported that after 1 month of the absence of therapy, e.g., during summer holidays, T.W. had more difficulties in pronouncing words. However, in this situation, T.W. had more difficulty to both visualise words and in motor movement. Access to visual support, in general, became less natural, and so communication. This required a "reexplanation" of the "strategies" allowing visual representation of articulatory movements, the spelling of words and verbal production.

No effect of syllabic complexity in word production was present, independently of the conditions. This absence of effect in postlexical impairment may be unexpected. However, it has been shown in another aphasic that it is possible to improve production of complex items with therapy [45]. It is possible that this absence of difference is related to the intensive therapy oriented towards orthographic imagery.

Based on fMRI findings, we postulate that T.W. was accessing word retrieval through the visual pathways and improved articulation planning using an adopted visual word imaging technique. More specifically, we postulate that the process of imagining the written words activated visual-spatial representations along the right sided dorsal route and modulated brain activity in the left occipital and left frontal regions.

Our study suffers several limitations. First, fMRI recording is challenging the aphasic participant, due to uncontrolled movements and AOS. To minimise movement effects, we immobilised T.W.'s head and applied unwarping during the postprocessing of the fMRI data. Also, we included the movement parameter of regressor of no interest in the statistical model for the patient and control. We also familiarised both participants with the task before image acquisition. Second, we did not carry out a full neuropsychological language evaluation and fMRI before the applied strategy, and therefore we cannot report any differences between the baseline and therapy-induced brain activation. Finally, we cannot exclude that the succession strategic and nonstrategic influenced the data. However, the mixing of conditions would have been too exhausting for T.W. The experiment lasted only 7 minutes, but fatigue may affect the accuracy of the 2nd and 3rd conditions. Moreover, it is possible that some of the prefrontal cortex activations are due to dealing with a novel task and this is less obvious, as the testing continues. Despite these limitations, T.W.'s data suggest that the visual imaging component of the orthographic strategy modulated intact left frontal region through occipital activation.

5. Conclusions

We suggest that visual imagery techniques in a rehabilitation setting may activate alternative nonlanguage networks and may improve articulation of the word in chronic aphasic individuals. This choice of rehabilitation methods can thus be logically based on the remaining capacities and, in this case, on a partially preserved capacity in written language.

Acknowledgments

The authors thank Dr. Lucas Spierer for his comments on an earlier version of the manuscript, Dr. Lea Jost and Maria Pestalozzi, from the Laboratory for Cognitive and Neurological Sciences, Fribourg University, for their outstanding work in preparation of stimuli, CIBM for technical support, and Ann Travis and Garry Joseph Dubickas for the English language revise. This project has received funding from a Lithuanian-Swiss cooperation program to reduce economic and social disparities within the enlarged European Union under project agreement No. CH-3- ŠMM-02/02.

References

[1] C. J. Price and J. Crinion, "The latest on functional imaging studies of aphasic stroke," *Current Opinion in Neurology*, vol. 18, no. 4, pp. 429–434, 2005.

[2] D. Saur, R. Lange, A. Baumgaertner et al., "Dynamics of language reorganization after stroke," *Brain*, vol. 129, no. 6, pp. 1371–1384, 2006.

[3] S. Abel, C. Weiller, W. Huber, K. Willmes, and K. Specht, "Therapy-induced brain reorganization patterns in aphasia," *Brain*, vol. 138, no. 4, pp. 1097–1112, 2015.

[4] S. Jarso, M. Li, A. Faria et al., "Distinct mechanisms and timing of language recovery after stroke," *Cognitive Neuropsychology*, vol. 30, no. 7-8, pp. 454–475, 2013.

[5] M. C. Brady, H. Kelly, J. Godwin, P. Enderby, and P. Campbell, "Speech and language therapy for aphasia following stroke," *Cochrane Database of Systematic Reviews*, vol. 16, no. 6, Article ID CD000425, 2016.

[6] A. E. Hillis, "Aphasia: Progress in the last quarter of a century," *Neurology*, vol. 69, no. 2, pp. 200–213, 2007.

[7] W. Heiss, "WSO leadership in stroke medicine award lecture Vienna, September 26, 2008: functional imaging correlates to disturbance and recovery of language function," *International Journal of Stroke*, vol. 4, no. 2, pp. 129–136, 2009.

[8] M. Richter, W. H. Miltner, and T. Straube, "Association between therapy outcome and right-hemispheric activation in chronic aphasia," *Brain*, vol. 131, no. 5, pp. 1391–1401, 2008.

[9] A. K. Pandey and K. M. Heilman, "Conduction aphasia with intact visual object naming," *Cognitive and Behavioral Neurology*, vol. 27, no. 2, pp. 96–101, 2014.

[10] M. P. Dean, "Use of orthography in spoken naming in aphasia: a case study," *Cognitive and Behavioral Neurology*, vol. 23, no. 4, pp. 262–268, 2010.

[11] P. M. Beeson and H. Egnor, "Combining treatment for written and spoken naming," *Journal of the International Neuropsychological Society*, vol. 12, no. 06, pp. 816–827, 2006.

[12] Y. Joanette, J.-L. Nespoulous, and A. Roch Lecours, *MT 86 - Protocole Montréal-Toulouse d'examen linguistique de l'aphasie*, vol. 86, Ortho Edition, 1998.

[13] L. E. Nicholas and R. H. Brookshire, "A system for quantifying the informativeness and efficiency of the connected speech of adults with aphasia," *Journal of Speech, Language, and Hearing Research*, vol. 36, no. 2, pp. 338–350, 1993.

[14] B. Croisile, "Une (petite) batterie d'évaluation de l'orthographe," *Glossa*, vol. 67, pp. 26–39, 1999.

[15] R. F. Street, "A Gestalt completion test," in *Contributions to Education*, Teachers College, Columbia University, 1931.

[16] B. Dubois, "L'épreuve des cinq mots. Fiche technique," *Neurologie-Psychiatrie-Geriatrie*, pp. 40–42, 2001.

[17] B. Dubois, A. Slachevsky, I. Litvan, and B. Pillon, "The FAB: a frontal assessment battery at bedside," *Neurology*, vol. 55, no. 11, pp. 1621–1626, 2000.

[18] E. H. Wertheim, C. Habib, and G. Cumming, "Test of the neurolinguistic programming hypothesis that eye-movements relate to processing imagery," *Perceptual and Motor Skills*, vol. 62, no. 2, pp. 523–529, 1986.

[19] K. O. Dooley and A. Farmer, "Comparison for aphasic and control subjects of eye movements hypothesized in neurolinguistic programming," *Perceptual and Motor Skills*, vol. 67, no. 1, pp. 233–234, 1988.

[20] Y. M. Cycowicz, D. Friedman, M. Rothstein, and J. G. Snodgrass, "Picture naming by young children: Norms for name agreement, familiarity, and visual complexity," *Journal of Experimental Child Psychology*, vol. 65, no. 2, pp. 171–237, 1997.

[21] F.-X. Alario, L. Ferrand, M. Laganaro, B. New, U. H. Frauenfelder, and J. Segui, "Predictors of picture naming speed," *Behavior Research Methods, Instruments, and Computers*, vol. 36, no. 1, pp. 140–155, 2004.

[22] E. L. Middleton and M. F. Schwartz, "Density pervades: An analysis of phonological neighbourhood density effects in aphasic speakers with different types of naming impairment," *Cognitive Neuropsychology*, vol. 27, no. 5, pp. 401–427, 2010.

[23] C. Romani and C. Galluzzi, "Effects of syllabic complexity in predicting accuracy of repetition and direction of errors in patients with articulatory and phonological difficulties," *Cognitive Neuropsychology*, vol. 22, no. 7, pp. 817–850, 2005.

[24] M. Laganaro, "Patterns of impairments in AOS and mechanisms of interaction between phonological and phonetic encoding," *Journal of Speech, Language, and Hearing Research*, vol. 55, no. 5, pp. S1535–S1543, 2012.

[25] K. Kurowski and S. E. Blumstein, "Phonetic basis of phonemic paraphasias in aphasia: Evidence for cascading activation," *Cortex*, vol. 75, pp. 193–203, 2016.

[26] M. McNeil, D. Robin, and R. Schmidt, "Apraxia of speech: definition and differential diagnosis," in *Clinical Management of*

Sensorimotor Speech Disorders, M. R. McNeil, Ed., vol. 2, Thieme Medical Publishers, New York, NY, USA, 2008.

[27] K. J. Friston and K. E. Stephan, "Free-energy and the brain," *Synthese*, vol. 159, no. 3, pp. 417–458, 2007.

[28] J. Cambier, C. Masson, and B. Robine, "Dissociated presevation of the written expression in a case of aphasia with recurrent utterances," *Revue Neurologique*, vol. 149, no. 8-9, pp. 455–461, 1993.

[29] A. Basso, A. Taborelli, and L. A. Vignolo, "Dissociated disorders of speaking and writing in aphasia," *Journal of Neurology, Neurosurgery & Psychiatry*, vol. 41, no. 6, pp. 556–563, 1978.

[30] A. Kreisler, O. Godefroy, C. Delmaire et al., "The anatomy of aphasia revisited," *Neurology*, vol. 54, no. 5, pp. 1117–1123, 2000.

[31] R. Itabashi, Y. Nishio, Y. Kataoka et al., "Damage to the left precentral gyrus is associated with apraxia of speech in acute stroke," *Stroke*, vol. 47, no. 1, pp. 31–36, 2016.

[32] L. A. Trupe, D. D. Varma, Y. Gomez et al., "Chronic apraxia of speech and Broca's area," *Stroke*, vol. 44, no. 3, pp. 740–744, 2013.

[33] J.-M. Annoni, F. Cot, J. Ryalls, and A. R. Lecours, "Profile of the aphasic population in a montreal geriatric hospital: A 6-year study," *Aphasiology*, vol. 7, no. 3, pp. 271–284, 1993.

[34] J. M. Ferro and M. Crespo, "Young adult stroke: Neuropsychological dysfunction and recovery," *Stroke*, vol. 19, no. 8, pp. 982–986, 1988.

[35] J. DeLeon, R. F. Gottesman, J. T. Kleinman et al., "Neural regions essential for distinct cognitive processes underlying picture naming," *Brain*, vol. 130, no. 5, pp. 1408–1422, 2007.

[36] P. M. Beeson, K. Higginson, and K. Rising, "Writing treatment for aphasia: a texting approach," *Journal of Speech, Language, and Hearing Research*, vol. 56, no. 3, pp. 945–955, 2013.

[37] J. Fridriksson, J. M. Baker, J. M. Whiteside et al., "Treating visual speech perception to improve speech production in nonfluent aphasia," *Stroke*, vol. 40, no. 3, pp. 853–858, 2009.

[38] C. J. Price, "A review and synthesis of the first 20 years of PET and fMRI studies of heard speech, spoken language and reading," *NeuroImage*, vol. 62, no. 2, pp. 816–847, 2012.

[39] W. Li, W. Qin, H. Liu et al., "Subregions of the human superior frontal gyrus and their connections," *NeuroImage*, vol. 78, pp. 46–58, 2013.

[40] G. Hartwigsen, D. Saur, C. J. Price, S. Ulmer, A. Baumgaertner, and H. R. Siebner, "Perturbation of the left inferior frontal gyrus triggers adaptive plasticity in the right homologous area during speech production," *Proceedings of the National Acadamy of Sciences of the United States of America*, vol. 110, no. 41, pp. 16402–16407, 2013.

[41] E. L. Meier, K. J. Kapse, and S. Kiran, "The relationship between frontotemporal effective connectivity during picture naming, behavior, and preserved cortical tissue in chronic aphasia," *Frontiers in Human Neuroscience*, vol. 10, no. 109, 2016.

[42] K. Marcotte, D. Adrover-Roig, B. Damien et al., "Therapy-induced neuroplasticity in chronic aphasia," *Neuropsychologia*, vol. 50, no. 8, pp. 1776–1786, 2012.

[43] Z. Han, Y. Ma, G. Gong, R. Huang, L. Song, and Y. Bi, "White matter pathway supporting phonological encoding in speech production: a multi-modal imaging study of brain damage patients," *Brain Structure & Function*, vol. 221, no. 1, pp. 577–589, 2016.

[44] F. Mattioli, C. Ambrosi, L. Mascaro et al., "Early aphasia rehabilitation is associated with functional reactivation of the left inferior frontal gyrus: a pilot study," *Stroke*, vol. 45, no. 2, pp. 545–552, 2014.

[45] E. Maas, J. Barlow, D. Robin, and L. Shapiro, "Treatment of sound errors in aphasia and apraxia of speech: Effects of phonological complexity," *Aphasiology*, vol. 16, no. 4-6, pp. 609–622, 2002.

10

Paving the Way for Speech: Voice-Training-Induced Plasticity in Chronic Aphasia and Apraxia of Speech—Three Single Cases

Monika Jungblut,[1] Walter Huber,[2] Christiane Mais,[1,3] and Ralph Schnitker[4]

[1] Interdisciplinary Institute for Music- and Speech-Therapy, Am Lipkamp 14, 47269 Duisburg, Germany
[2] Clinical Cognition Research, University Hospital Aachen University, RWTH Aachen,
  Pauwelsstraße 30, 52074 Aachen, Germany
[3] Aphasia Center North Rhine Westphalia, Laarmannstraße 21, 45359 Essen, Germany
[4] Interdisciplinary Centre for Clinical Research—Neurofunctional Imaging Lab, University Hospital Aachen,
  Pauwelsstraße 30, 52074 Aachen, Germany

Correspondence should be addressed to Monika Jungblut; jungblut@sipari.de

Academic Editor: Lin Xu

Difficulties with temporal coordination or sequencing of speech movements are frequently reported in aphasia patients with concomitant apraxia of speech (AOS). Our major objective was to investigate the effects of specific rhythmic-melodic voice training on brain activation of those patients. Three patients with severe chronic nonfluent aphasia and AOS were included in this study. Before and after therapy, patients underwent the same fMRI procedure as 30 healthy control subjects in our prestudy, which investigated the neural substrates of sung vowel changes in untrained rhythm sequences. A main finding was that post-minus pretreatment imaging data yielded significant perilesional activations in all patients for example, in the left superior temporal gyrus, whereas the reverse subtraction revealed either no significant activation or right hemisphere activation. Likewise, pre- and posttreatment assessments of patients' vocal rhythm production, language, and speech motor performance yielded significant improvements for all patients. Our results suggest that changes in brain activation due to the applied training might indicate specific processes of reorganization, for example, improved temporal sequencing of sublexical speech components. In this context, a training that focuses on rhythmic singing with differently demanding complexity levels as concerns motor and cognitive capabilities seems to support paving the way for speech.

1. Introduction

Functional imaging studies investigating therapy-induced recovery from aphasia after left-hemisphere stroke are rare (for review see [1]). This holds true even more for research with patients, who suffer from chronic nonfluent aphasia and concomitant apraxia of speech (AOS), a dysfunction of higher-order aspects of speech motor control characterized by deficits in programming or planning of articulatory gestures [2, 3].

Research results point out so far that neural correlates of functional recovery seem to involve both hemispheres. While in patients with small left-hemisphere lesions activation occurs to a greater extent in perilesional regions, in patients with large lesions involving the perisylvian language zone, there tends to be more activation of regions homologous to left-hemisphere language areas [4, 5]. Successful recovery seems to be correlated with perilesional activation; persistent right-hemisphere activation, however, seems to indicate slow and incomplete recovery [1, 6–11]. So far, only few studies demonstrated a direct impact of speech therapy on language recovery in chronic aphasia [12, 13].

The observation that even severely impaired aphasia patients are sometimes able to produce sung words more effectively than spoken words prompted many researchers and therapists to implement singing in the treatment of patients suffering from both motor speech disorders as well as aphasia [14–23]. Melodic intonation therapy (MIT), a form of speech therapy that was developed already in the 1970s, combines melodic intonation and rhythmic hand tapping with the objective to activate homologous language-capable regions in the right hemisphere [14, 22]. Neuroimaging research demonstrated conflicting results. The PET-study of Belin et al. included seven nonfluent aphasia patients, who received melodic intonation therapy (MIT) by comparing repetition of untrained MIT-loaded words to repetition of the same words spoken with a natural intonation [15]. Repetition of words using MIT strategies resulted in a significant increase of activation in left Broca's area as well as decrease in right-hemisphere regions. This result contradicts the essential objective of MIT to engage homologous right-hemisphere language regions. One criticism of this study is that activation changes were not measured by means of pre- and posttreatment image acquisition.

However, Schlaug et al. demonstrated treatment-associated fMRI changes in the right-hemisphere encompassing premotor, inferior frontal, and temporal lobes in a patient suffering from Broca's aphasia treated with MIT compared to a control patient [20]. Based on their post- and pretreatment results with diffusion tensor imaging, Schlaug et al. conclude that the right arcuate fasciculus can be remodeled by intense, long-term MIT [24].

As pointed out in detail in our previous studies, the greater bihemispheric organization for singing compared to speech might offer a chance for patients suffering from neurological speech and language disorders [25–27].

Singing combines pitch and intonation processing but also temporal processing and we are particularly interested in the latter. Temporal organization is an essential characteristic of language and speech processing and seems to be extremely vulnerable to left-hemisphere brain damage.

Lesion studies from the field of language as well as music demonstrate that patients with left-hemisphere lesions have problems with rhythm and time perception [28–31]. Many studies confirm deficits in aphasia patients with regard to temporal structuring of speech but also in AOS [3, 32, 69–71].

Stahl et al. investigated the importance of melody and rhythm for speech production in an experimental study with 17 nonfluent aphasia patients [33]. The authors conclude that rhythmic speech but not singing may support speech production. This applied particularly to patients with lesions including the basal ganglia.

Yet, timing deficits in these patient groups can be caused by very different reasons. While language production in aphasia patients may be nonfluent because of language-systematic reasons, for example, word retrieval deficits or agrammatic speech, temporal structuring in patients suffering from AOS is affected because of deficits in temporal coordination or sequencing of speech movements [34, 35]. Problems in accessing motor plans and programs result in temporal and prosodic distortions. Likewise, distortions of consonant and vowel segments are characteristic for AOS [36]. Extended segment and intersegment durations caused by disturbed anticipatory coarticulation result in slowed speech with visible and audible groping [37–39].

A number of treatment approaches from the field of speech therapy implemented strategies to control for rhythm or rate of speech production with patients suffering from AOS. Examples of such approaches are finger tapping [40], prolonged speaking [41], vibrotactile stimulation [42], metronomic pacing [3, 43, 44], or metrical pacing [45].

Taking the temporal organization of speech into account, we developed rhythmic-melodic voice training (SIPARI), a music therapy technique that is based on specific use of the voice [17, 25].

Over the past years, we performed several behavioral studies with patients suffering from chronic aphasia and AOS, which demonstrated that especially nonfluent patients significantly improved by this training [25, 26, 46, 47]. Since 2010, this treatment method is included in a Cochrane Review [48]. In a prestudy with 30 healthy control subjects, we investigated the neural substrates of chanted vowel changes in rhythm sequences by functional imaging in order to find explanations for the efficacy of this treatment [27]. Chanting is a rudimentary or simple form of singing, for example, on one pitch only.

According to our findings, rhythm structure is a decisive factor concerning lateralization as well as activation of specific, language-related areas during simple singing. With increasing demands on motor and cognitive capabilities additional activation of inferior frontal areas of the left hemisphere occurred, particularly in those areas, which are described in connection with temporal processing and sequencing [49–51]. These activations do not only comprise brain regions, whose lesions are causally connected with language disorders, but also regions of the left hemisphere (Broca's area, insular cortex, and inferior parietal cortex), whose lesions are reported to cause AOS [52, 53].

Our current study aims at investigating how the above-mentioned rhythmic-melodic voice training influences brain activation in patients with chronic nonfluent aphasia and concomitant AOS.

If it was possible to activate left-hemisphere language-related areas, as our imaging data with healthy subjects suggest, this might point to specific processes of reorganization, for example, improved temporal sequencing of sublexical speech components. Maybe, this explains at least in parts the efficacy of this treatment, which we already demonstrated in several behavioral studies mentioned above.

2. General Method

2.1. Patients. It is difficult to find relatively young and highly comparable patients. Therefore, only three patients with severe chronic nonfluent aphasia and concomitant AOS could be recruited from the Aphasia Center North Rhine Westphalia (Aphasiker-Zentrum NRW e.V.) for participation in this pilot study. Independently from the confirmation of the patients' therapists, three experienced speech therapists diagnosed the patients with AOS on the basis of direct observations involving inconsistently occurring phonemic and phonetic errors, initiation problems, prolonged segment durations, prolonged intersegment durations (sound/syllable/word segregation), disturbed prosody, visible groping, and effortful speech (see [36, 45]).

TABLE 1: Summary of the patients' characteristics. CCTs (obtained within 3 days after the cerebral accident); the left side of the brain is on the right.

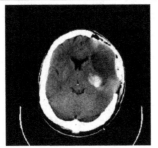 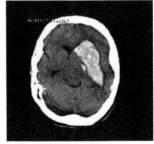 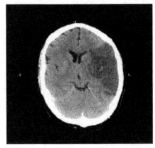

Patient	Mr. U.	Mrs. A.	Mr. H.
Sex	Male	Female	Male
Age	53	44	44
Months since incident	18	18	18
Diagnosis	Severe Broca's aphasia, moderate AOS	Severe global aphasia, severe AOS	Severe global aphasia, severe AOS
Aetiology	Left sylvian CVA with secondary hemorrhage	Extensive left frontotemporal hemorrhage, extension to caudate nucleus, basal ganglia, and internal capsule	Extensive left sylvian CVA with displacement of the midline

AOS: apraxia of speech; CVA: cerebral vascular accident.

All patients were right-handed as determined by means of the Edinburgh Handedness Scale [54], German speaking, and were included in the study 18 months after the incident. None of the patients had premorbid history of neurological or psychiatric problems. They had no perceptual hearing impairments and their auditory comprehension was sufficient to understand the instructions. Their capacity regarding concentration and attention was good and their general health condition was stable enough for continuous participation during the 6-month treatment period of this research study.

Apart from general school education, none of the patients had any special musical training. All patients gave written consent to abstain from speech therapy in this study. All patients gave written informed consent in line with the Declaration of Helsinki and the Institutional Review Board of the RWTH Aachen. This study was undertaken in compliance with national legislation.

2.1.1. Patient Mr. U. At the age of 53, Mr. U. suffered a left-hemisphere ischemic stroke involving in parts the area of the middle cerebral artery with secondary hemorrhage. The lesion encompassed frontotemporal regions. Clinical symptoms were spastic hemiparesis on the right and severe Broca's aphasia and moderate AOS. Up to the accident, Mr. U. was an industrial consultant in a leading position.

2.1.2. Patient Mrs. A. At the age of 44, Mrs. A. suffered an extensive left-hemisphere cerebral hemorrhage encompassing frontotemporal regions and the area of caudate nucleus with extension to the basal ganglia as well as left internal capsule. Clinical symptoms were spastic hemiparesis on the

right and severe global aphasia as well as severe AOS. Up to the accident, Mrs. A. was employed at an airline company.

2.1.3. Patient Mr. H. At the age of 44, Mr. H. suffered an extensive left-hemisphere ischemic stroke in the area of the middle cerebral artery with displacement of the midline. The lesion encompassed frontotemporoparietal regions. Clinical symptoms were spastic hemiparesis on the right and both severe global aphasia and AOS. Up to the accident, Mr. H. worked as a bookseller and publisher.

A summary of the patients' characteristics is given in Table 1.

2.2. Stimuli and Procedure. Before and after therapy patients underwent the same fMRI procedure as 30 healthy control subjects in our prestudy [27] in order to investigate if changes in brain activation occur due to the applied training.

Tasks of our fMRI paradigm comprised repetition of chanted vowel changes in rhythm sequences with differently demanding complexity levels for the following reasons: chanting is a rudimentary or simple form of singing, for example, on one pitch only and facilitates evaluating the influence of rhythm structure because melodic components are reduced. Rhythmic chanting (e.g., the vowel change /a/i/) requires exact temporal coordination and sequencing of speech movements. By focusing on sublexical processing with a single vowel change, we minimized the influence of semantic and lexical components of speech processing (for more details on the fMRI tasks see [27]). Stimuli consisted of quadruple measure groupings with duration of 4 sec. (8 vowels, alternately /a/i/) and differed as follows: (1) vowel changes with regular groupings, (2) vowel changes with regular groupings and rests, and (3) vowel changes with irregular groupings (see musical notations of Figures 1(a), 1(b), and 1(c)). Stimuli were sung by a female voice with the vowel change /a/i/ at a frequency of 220 Hz. Male patients were encouraged to transpose the heard stimuli down an octave. The length of each stimulus was electronically set to 4 sec. with a max. deviation of 0.05 sec. For each condition (1–3) four different grouping variations were available.

Patients had to listen and to immediately repeat the heard stimuli after the presentation had stopped. We used an event-related design with a total of 40 trials per condition and 40 randomly included null-events. The stimuli were presented in a pseudo-randomized order with a mean interstimulus interval of 9 sec. (jittered between 8 and 10 sec.). The presentation time took 4 sec. and the duration of the repetition period varied according to the estimated jitter time. The paradigm was implemented in Presentation (Neurobehavioral Systems) and synchronized to the scanner. Stimuli were presented binaurally through MR-compatible headphones with a sound absorption of 30 dBA (Resonance Technology). All conditions were performed with eyes closed.

Concerning movement artefacts, we point out that we compared three conditions utilizing the same response modality, that is, overt chanting. This allows generation of statistical maps that indicate activity more related to cognitive function than to movement [55]. Since our tasks are essentially demanding with regard to cognitive abilities (e.g., attention, short-term memory), which are often impaired in patients with frontal lobe damage, a sparse temporal scanning design was not used in this study. We wanted to avoid attention loss and consequently lower functional response caused by relatively long interscan intervals, which are required in sparse temporal schemes [56]. Moreover, stimuli were constantly sung at a frequency of 220 Hz, which is beyond the main frequency peaks of the scanner spectrum.

A remark in advance is that auditory stimulation was regarded as separately modeled condition in this design, which is not part of this paper. Auditory presentation and reproduction were time-shifted; patients did not sing along but after the presentation had stopped. Hence, the expected auditory activations in the auditory areas caused by the auditory stimulus presentation will not be present in the reported results (see [27]).

2.3. Musical Analyses.

2.3. Musical Analyses. Recorded data of pre- and postrhythmic chanting of all patients were analyzed by 2 professional musicians (singer and percussionist) post hoc. They transcribed by ear and scored each stimulus repetition with either "correct" (score 1) or "incorrect" (score 0) regarding correct rhythm repetition. Tone repetitions (a total of 8 tones per stimulus) had to be timed correctly with a max. deviation of ±0.2 sec. each. Only unanimous assessments that rhythm production had been performed without error were scored 1. Comparison of pre- and posttreatment performance of the patients for each of the three tasks was statistically assessed by McNemar's test using exact binomial probability calculations (see Table 3).

2.4. Assessment of Language and Speech Motor Performance. Additionally, two experienced speech therapists of the Aphasia Center North Rhine Westphalia (Aphasiker-Zentrum NRW e.V.) who were blinded to the experiment performed two well-established diagnostic procedures for the German language as control tests at baseline and at the end of the 6-month treatment period in order to assess potential changes in language and speech motor capabilities.

2.4.1. Aachener Aphasie Test. One instrument used for assessment of the efficacy of the treatment was the Aachener Aphasie Test (AAT) [57]. The AAT is a standardized procedure for evaluating type and severity of aphasia, developed and validated in the German language, subsequently translated into several European languages including English [58], and also validated and standardized in Dutch and Italian. The AAT may also be applied repeatedly in order to assess the efficacy of speech therapy interventions. The presence and type of aphasia were established using the ALLOC classification procedure, a nonparametric discriminant analysis computer program [57] using the normative data of the AAT. The AAT consists of six description levels for spontaneous speech (communicative verbal behavior, articulation and prosody, automatized language, semantic structure, phonemic structure, and syntactic structure) and five subtests (token test, repetition, written language, naming, and comprehension) for the assessment of specific language impairments. For an assessment of the degree of language impairment related to the entire group of aphasia patients, the AAT assesses percentile scores from the score values of the five subtests, that is, token test, repetition, written language, naming, and comprehension. The percentile score found for one test value indicates the percentage of patients of the exercise sample ($n = 376$) who have achieved the same or a lower score [57].

Although our primary focus was on expressive verbal behavior and motor speech performance, written language and comprehension were also assessed because reliable data regarding the speech profile can only be achieved if the AAT is administered in its complete version.

Apart from that, a more general transfer to other language modalities like written language and comprehension could not be excluded.

2.4.2. Hierarchical Word List. Although not standardized, the hierarchical word list (HWL) is the first German diagnostic procedure, which allows systematic assessment of the symptoms caused by AOS [59]. The procedure contains a word/nonword repetition test (48 words and 48 matched nonwords) with word length varying between one and four syllables. Half of the items are phonologically simple (single consonants in syllable onsets or codas) and half are complex (consonant clusters in onsets or codas). All repeated words or nonwords (max. 96 items) are assessed in a quantitative analysis as regards *number* of assessable items, *phonetic structure, phonemic structure,* and *speech fluency.*

Qualitative analysis evaluates *speech effort, groping, syllabic speech,* and *deviant word accent* on a scale from 0 (without abnormality) to 3 (very pronounced) on an overall visual analogue scale. Each of these symptoms is precisely delineated in the HWL manual [59].

3. Data Analysis and General Procedure

3.1. Image Acquisition. Functional images were obtained with a whole-body 3 T Siemens Trio MRI-system. Participants were fixated in the head coil using Velcro straps and foam paddings to stabilize head position and minimize motion artefacts. After orienting the axial slices in the anterior-posterior commissure (AC-PC) plane functional images were acquired using a T2*-weighted echo planar imaging (EPI) sequence with a repetition time (TR) of 2200 ms, an echo time (TE) of 30 ms, and a flip angle (FA) of 90 degrees. 640 volumes consisting of 41 contiguous transversal slices with a thickness of 3.4 mm were measured. A 64 × 64 matrix with a field of view (FOV) of 220 mm was used, yielding an effective voxel size of 3.44 × 3.44 × 3.74 mm.

3.2. Image Analysis. Functional images were preprocessed and analyzed using SPM8 (Wellcome Department of Cognitive Neurology London, UK). During preprocessing, images were realigned and unwarped in order to correct for motion and movement-related changes in magnetic susceptibility. Translation and rotation correction did not exceed 1.8 mm and 1.9°, respectively, for any of the participants. The anatomical T1 images of the patients were coregistered to the mean functional image using a rigid-body transformation implemented in SPM8 so that activation maps could be displayed on the structural images. As this study included patients with extended lesions, which may cause problems with the normalizing algorithm, images were not normalized into MNI space. Finally, all functional images were smoothed using a Gaussian filter of 8 × 8 × 8 mm to increase signal-to-noise ratio in the images [60].

3.3. Statistical Analysis. In the first-level statistical analyses, each preprocessed functional volume was entered into a subject specific, fixed-effect analysis using the general linear model approach for time-series data suggested by Friston and coworkers [60, 61] and implemented in SPM8. All stimulus onset times were modeled as single events.

Afterwards, stimulus functions were convolved with a canonical hemodynamic response function.

The data were high-pass filtered using a set of discrete cosine basis functions with a cut-off period of 128s in order to exclude low frequency confounds. For each of the 3 conditions of interest the contrasts of interest were generated. Statistical parametric maps (SPMs) were evaluated and voxels were considered significant if their corresponding linear contrast t values were significant at a voxelwise threshold of $P = 0.05$ (FDR-corrected). Only regions comprising at least 5 voxels will be reported.

3.4. General Procedure. For all patients therapy was started 18 months after the onset. None of the patients had ever received rhythmic-melodic voice training SIPARI before.

Each patient received 50 individual therapy sessions (60 minutes, twice a week) over a period of 25 weeks. During this period, no speech therapy took place. In order to control for comparable treatment conditions patients received exactly the same treatment program. We emphasize that none of the stimuli of the fMRI paradigm was trained during the treatment period of 6 months.

3.4.1. Treatment Method. Therapy was conducted by the first author. The applied rhythmic-melodic voice training (SIPARI) comprises six components: singing, intonation, prosody, breathing (German: Atmung), rhythm, and improvisation. The efficacy of this treatment could be demonstrated in several behavioral studies with patients suffering from chronic aphasia and AOS [25, 26, 46, 47]. In 2010 a pseudorandomized controlled study with chronic nonfluent aphasia patients (mean duration of aphasia: 11,5 years), which examined the effects of the SIPARI method, was included in a Cochrane Review [48].

The main part of this treatment is based on specific use of the voice. Focusing initially on melodic speech components, which are mainly processed in the right hemisphere, a stepwise change to temporal-rhythmic speech components is carried out with the objective to stimulate phonological and segmental capabilities of the left hemisphere. To this end, an essential core of the treatment constitutes rhythmic singing with differently demanding complexity levels as concerns motor and cognitive capabilities. Since this treatment has been developed especially for severely impaired patients, an essential part of the verbal material comprises sublexical tasks (i.e., single vowels, vowel changes, consonant-vowel changes, etc.) in order to enable those patients to practice motor and cognitive function like planning, programming, and sequencing, that is, basics of language processing. The objective is a general transfer from the level of sublexical speech components to the level of words and phrases.

In terms of linguistics, SIPARI intervenes at the interface of phonological and phonetic encoding where access to the mental syllabary is supposed to take place [62, 63]. By embedding segmental and syllabic speech elements in rhythmic sequences with differently demanding complexity levels, specific grouping strategies are trained [64]. Apart from the fact that grouping or chunking (i.e., bundling events together into larger units) serves to enhance maintenance of information in working memory [65, 66], temporal-rhythmic chunking promotes speech motor processes by training intersyllabic programming, which is supposed to play an important role in phonetic planning [67]. In contrast to other treatment approaches mentioned in the introduction, which use pacing techniques or synchronous singing to an external timekeeper, SIPARI focuses on encouraging self-initiated planning and sequencing performance. Therefore, we give special emphasis on vocal training in connection with cognitive function, for example, executive control and working memory. This implies training of auditory short-term maintenance of melodic and rhythmic information in order to enable patients in a second step to coordinate the maintained information with verbal material.

TABLE 2: Anatomical location, cluster sizes (k, number of voxels), and t values of areas of significant activation.

Condition 1

	Anatomical location	Side	Cluster size k	t value
Mr. U	Subtraction post-minus pre-therapy			
	Insula	L	119	4.64
	Inferior frontal gyrus	L	28	4.01
	Superior temporal gyrus	L	20	3.92
	Nucleus caudatus	L	99	4.89
Mrs. A	Subtraction post-minus pre-therapy			
	Superior temporal gyrus	R	2737	5.4
	Middle temporal gyrus	R		
	Superior temporal gyrus	L	341	5.16
	Middle temporal gyrus	L		
	Insula	L		
	Precentral gyrus	R	15	3.56
Mr. H	Subtraction post-minus pre-therapy			
	Superior temporal gyrus	L	42	5.37
	Superior temporal gyrus	R	7	4.81

Condition 2

	Anatomical location	Side	Cluster size k	t value
Mr. U	Subtraction pre-minus post-therapy			
	Precentral gyrus	R	19	4.49
	Subtraction post-minus pre-therapy			
	Precentral gyrus	L	9	3.69
	Superior temporal gyrus	L	11	3.62
Mrs. A	Subtraction post-minus pre-therapy			
	Superior temporal gyrus	L	143	4.89
	Inferior frontal gyrus	L		
	Middle temporal gyrus	R	11	3.34
	Inferior frontal gyrus	R	14	3.31
	Cingulate gyrus	R	31	3.78
Mr. H	Subtraction pre-minus post-therapy			
	Superior temporal gyrus	R	16	3.59
	Middle temporal gyrus	R		
	Subtraction post-minus pre-therapy			
	Superior temporal gyrus	L	12	4.48
	Superior temporal gyrus	R	28	5.07
	Precentral gyrus	R	15	4.60

Condition 3

	Anatomical location	Side	Cluster size k	t value
	Subtraction post-minus pre-therapy			
	Middle temporal gyrus	L	71	5.34
	Superior temporal gyrus	L	24	4.07

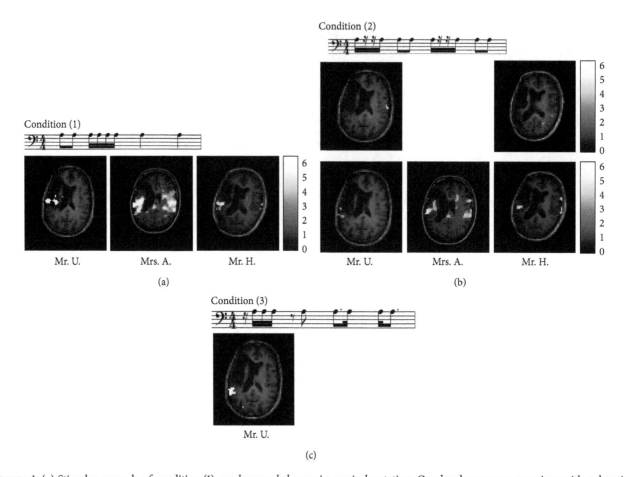

FIGURE 1: (a) Stimulus example of condition (1) *regular vowel changes* in musical notation. Quadruple measure groupings with a duration of 4 sec. (1 beat per sec.; 8 vowels alternately /a/i/) sung at a frequency of 220 Hz (A3), fMRI post-minus pretreatment results; (b) stimulus example of condition (2) *regular vowel changes* with rests in musical notation. Quadruple measure groupings with a duration of 4 sec. (1 beat per sec.; 8 vowels alternately /a/i/) sung at a frequency of 220 Hz (A3), fMRI results, upper row: pre-minus posttreatment and lower row: post-minus pretreatment; (c) stimulus example of condition (3) *irregular vowel changes* in musical notation. Quadruple measure groupings with a duration of 4 sec. (1 beat per sec.; 8 vowels alternately /a/i/) sung at a frequency of 220 Hz (A3) fMRI post-minus pretreatment results of Mr. U.

Treatment objectives are to improve motor, linguistic, and cognitive functions and thus to support speech motor processes and also language-systematic processes, that is, to encourage planning, programming, and sequencing.

An appendix containing the treatment interventions can be provided. We did not include a description of the method because detailed information on the method as well as selection of exercises has been already published elsewhere [17, 25, 46, 68].

4. Results

4.1. fMRI Data. To determine how neural activity differed before and after therapy, both subtractions (i.e., pre-minus post-therapy and post-minus pre-therapy) were performed for all conditions. The anatomical localizations were determined by two experienced experts (neuroanatomist and neuroradiologist) from the University Hospital Aachen.

4.1.1. Subtractions for Condition (1) Vowel Changes with Regular Groupings. Subtraction pre-minus post-therapy yielded no significant activation for any patient.

(1) *Mr. U.* Subtraction post-minus pre-therapy yielded significant activation in the left hemisphere, comprising the basal ganglia (caudate nucleus), insula, and inferior frontal regions. Left superior temporal gyrus was also activated significantly.

Comparison with the anatomical image showed that Mr. U. has a tissue bridge in the infarcted area.

(2) *Mrs. A.* Subtraction post-minus pre-therapy demonstrated significant activations in both hemispheres, including superior and middle temporal gyrus. Further activation was also found in the left insula. Precentral gyrus was activated in the right hemisphere.

(3) *Mr. H.* Subtraction post-minus pre-therapy yielded bilateral activation of the superior temporal gyrus, however, more pronounced in the left hemisphere.

TABLE 3: McNemar's test comparison of pre- and posttreatment rhythmic chanting (40 tasks per each condition) condition (1) regular vowel changes; condition (2) regular vowel changes with rests; condition (3) irregular vowel changes.

	Mr. U		Mrs. A		Mr. H	
Condition 1	14	22	16	20	17	20
	0	4	1	3	2	1
$P=$	Two-tailed	**<0.001**	Two-tailed	**<0.001**	Two-tailed	**<0.001**
Condition 2	7	17	28	8	10	18
	4	12	1	3	5	7
$P=$	Two-tailed	**<0.01**	Two-tailed	Not sign.	Two-tailed	0.01
Condition 3	27	10	37	0	33	4
	1	2	1	2	3	0
$P=$	Two-tailed	<0.012	Two-tailed	Not sign.	Two-tailed	Not sign.
	No—no	No—yes				
	Yes—no	Yes—yes				

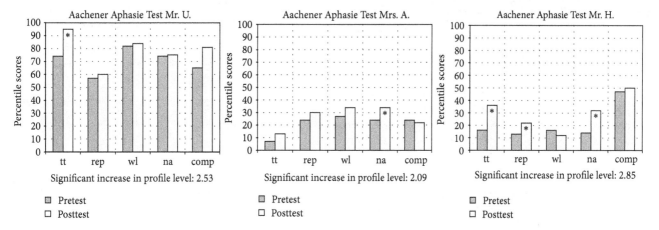

FIGURE 2: Results of the Aachener Aphasie Test (AAT) (in percentile scores) and changes in profile level (in t-scores); * indicates significant improvement tt = token test, rep = repetition, wl = written language, na = naming, and comp = comprehension.

4.1.2. Subtractions for Condition (2) Vowel Changes with Regular Groupings and Rests

(1) *Mr. U.* While subtraction pre-minus post-therapy demonstrated significant activation in the right precentral gyrus, the reverse subtraction yielded a shift of significant activation to the left precentral gyrus and superior temporal gyrus.

(2) *Mrs. A.* Subtraction pre-minus post-therapy yielded no significant activation. The reverse subtraction, however, showed significant activation of the left superior temporal gyrus and bilateral inferior frontal gyrus. Middle temporal gyrus and cingulate gyrus were activated in the right hemisphere.

(3) *Mr. H.* Pre-minus post-therapy subtraction showed activation in the right middle and superior temporal gyrus. The reverse subtraction demonstrated significant bilateral activation in the superior temporal gyrus and precentral gyrus activation in the right hemisphere.

4.1.3. Subtractions for Condition (3) Vowel Changes with Irregular Groupings.
For Mrs. A and Mr. H., neither subtraction pre-minus post-therapy nor the reverse subtraction showed any results.

Mr. U. While no significant activation could be found in subtraction pre-minus post-therapy, the reverse subtraction yielded significant activation in the left hemisphere comprising the superior and middle temporal gyrus.

With regard to anatomical locations, cluster sizes, and *t* values see Table 2.

4.2. Behavioral Analysis

4.2.1. Musical Analyses. Recorded data of pre- and post-rhythmic chanting of all patients were analyzed by 2 professional musicians (singer and percussionist) post hoc. Only unanimous assessments that rhythm production had been performed without error were scored 1. Overall interrater agreement resulted in 6 = 0.99, *P* < 0.002. Comparison of pre- and posttreatment performance of the patients for each

TABLE 4: Spontaneous speech.

		cvb	ap	al	sem s	ps	syn s
Mr. U.	Pre	2	2	3	3	2	2
	Post	3*	3*	4*	4*	3*	2
Mrs. A.	Pre	1	1	2	2	2	1
	Post	2*	2*	2	2	2	1
Mr. H.	Pre	1	1	1	0	0	0
	Post	2*	2*	2*	1*	2**	1

*substantial; **significant.
Aachener Aphasie Test, evaluation of spontaneous speech; min = 0, max = 5 points.
cvb: communicative verbal behavior; ap: articulation and prosody; al: automatized language.
sem s: semantic structure; ps: phonemic structure; syn s: syntactic structure.

of the three tasks was statistically assessed by McNemar's test using exact binomial probability calculations (see Table 3). All patients improved statistically significant ($P < 0.001$) in condition (1) *vowel changes with regular groupings*. Analyses of condition (2) *vowel changes with regular groupings and rests* yielded statistically significant improvements for Mr. U. ($P < 0.01$) and Mr. H. ($P = 0.01$). Mr. U. achieved a statistically significant improvement ($P < 0.012$) in condition (3) *vowel changes with irregular groupings*.

4.2.2. Aachener Aphasie Test (AAT). Clinically significant improvements could be assessed in the subtests token test, repetition, and naming. Further significant improvements were achieved regarding changes in profile level and spontaneous speech.

4.2.3. Hierarchical Word List (HWL). Quantitative analysis revealed improvements concerning *number* of assessable items (Mr. H.), *phonetic structure* (Mr. U. and Mr. H.), *phonemic structure* (Mr. U. and Mr. H.), and speech *fluency* (Mrs. A. and Mr. H.).

Qualitative analysis yielded for Mr. U. less speech effort and less syllabic speech (improvement of 1.5 points each out of an overall scale of 3 points) and for Mrs. A. and Mr. H. less speech effort and less groping (improvement of 1 point each).

5. Discussion

Difficulties with temporal coordination or sequencing of speech movements are frequently reported in patients suffering from aphasia and AOS [3, 32, 69–71]. Our own experiences are in accordance with these findings and prompted us to develop rhythmic-melodic voice training SIPARI [17, 25], which was applied in this study (see Sections 1 and 3.4.1).

The major objective of this pilot study was to investigate how this training influences brain activation in three patients with severe chronic nonfluent aphasia and AOS (1 Broca's, 2 global aphasia patients). Before and after therapy each patient underwent the same fMRI procedure as 30 control subjects in our prestudy [27].

To determine how neural activity differed before and after therapy, both subtractions (i.e., pre-minus post-therapy and post-minus pre-therapy) were performed for all three conditions (see Section 4.1 and Figures 1(a), 1(b), and 1(c)).

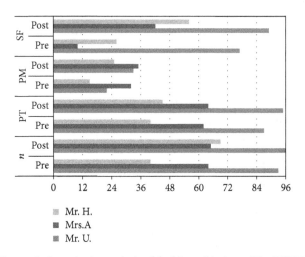

FIGURE 3: Quantitative analysis of the hierarchical word list (HWL), n = number of assessable items (max. 96 items); PT = phonetic structure; PM = phonemic structure; and SF = speech fluency.

In addition, pre- and posttreatment results of patients' vocal production as well as their language and speech motor performance were examined by cognitive methods.

5.1. Rhythm Production and Brain Activation. All patients improved most in *condition (1) vowel changes with regular groupings.*

Musical analyses of the recorded data revealed that before therapy none of the patients had any strategy to manage the demands of this condition. It should be mentioned that this condition comprises either no vowel change within one beat or the same tone durations and regular changes within one beat. From beat to beat tone durations change in even-numbered ratios (see musical notation of condition (1) Figure 1(a)). A conceivable strategy to keep the respective stimulus in short-term memory in order to reproduce it afterwards could be, for example, to group vowel changes on the basis of tones with equal durations [64, 72, 73]. We suggest that due to therapy patients could use an adequate strategy in the post-therapy assessments more effectively. First, musical analyses corroborate this assumption. Secondly, subtraction post-minus pre-therapy resulted in brain activation comprising areas, which are described not only in connection with temporal processing and sequencing [49–51] but also with language and speech processing, for example, inferior frontal gyrus, insula, basal ganglia (caudate nucleus), and particularly superior temporal gyrus [1, 74–76].

However, while significant activations of the Broca's aphasia patient (Mr. U.) were found exclusively in the left hemisphere, in both global aphasia patients (Mrs. A. and Mr. H.) significant activations were measured in perilesional and also in homologous areas in the right hemisphere (see Figure 1(a)). Moreover, comparison of all three conditions points to increases or changes of activation that differ depending on task demand; for example, for all patients, activation was most pronounced in this post-minus pre-therapy comparison. Task-dependent activation changes are in line with our prestudy with healthy subjects [27]. However, these findings are all the more remarkable as our study also included chronic global aphasia patients with large lesions. Since Mr. H. also improved in basically all measures regarding his language performance a possible explanation could be that in contrast to the other two patients at least parts of his arcuate fasciculus are still intact. However, we cannot verify this assumption because diffusion tensor imaging data are not available.

Further research is needed, especially if we compare our results with other studies, which investigated the therapeutic effect of singing on language rehabilitation. For instance, Schlaug et al. demonstrated treatment-associated fMRI changes in the right-hemisphere encompassing premotor, inferior frontal, and temporal lobes in a patient suffering from Broca's aphasia treated with melodic intonation therapy (MIT) [20]. Based on their post- and pretreatment results with diffusion tensor imaging, Schlaug et al. even conclude that the right arcuate fasciculus can be remodeled by intense, long-term MIT [24].

Musical analyses of *condition (2) vowel changes with regular groupings and rests* demonstrated that Mr. U. and Mr. H coped better with this task already at the beginning of the treatment (see Table 3). Comparison of image analyses revealed for Mr. U. a shift of activation from right precentral gyrus in the pre-minus posttreatment subtraction to left precentral gyrus and superior temporal gyrus activation in the reverse subtraction (see Figure 1(b)). The same way, data of Mr. H. demonstrate that activation changed from right middle and superior temporal gyrus activation in the pre-minus posttreatment subtraction to bilateral superior temporal gyrus activation in the reverse subtraction. Additional activation could be measured in the right precentral gyrus. What is special about this condition is that implementation of rests brings about higher demands on timing because legato and staccato vocalization changes from beat to beat (see musical notation of condition (2) Figure 1(b)). This way of vocalization requires precise execution of articulatory movements because staccato and legato vocalizations change from beat to beat. Particularly, the initial phase of vocal preparation becomes the focus of attention, which is reported to be dominated by the left hemisphere [77]. Since findings of our prestudy with healthy subjects also corroborate this assumption [27], this may explain the shift from right to left superior temporal and precentral gyrus (Mr. U.) representing improved auditory-motor interaction in a task, which requires exact executed vocalization. This

may also hold true for Mr. H., who additionally activated left superior temporal gyrus but had to compensate with regard to motor preparation by activating right precentral gyrus due to his lesion in the left homologue. Musical evaluations confirmed more correct entries and improved legato and staccato differentiation in the post-therapy analyses. While Mrs. A. was not able to manage this task before therapy, musical evaluation as well as post-minus pre-therapy subtraction point to improved planning with significant activations in the left superior temporal gyrus. Bilateral inferior frontal gyrus activation but also activation of right cingulate gyrus suggest that this task was demanding for Mrs. A. Based on the results of our prestudy [27], we assume that these activations are related not only to sustaining attention in order to maintain temporal information in memory [78] but also to coordination of response generation and respective action planning [79].

The only patient, who developed a strategy to manage *condition (3) vowel changes with irregular groupings* posttherapy, was Mr. U. His post-minus pre-therapy subtraction data yielded significant left-hemisphere activation in the superior and middle temporal gyrus (see Figure 1(c)). Since irregularity of this condition caused by implementation of syncopations, dottings, and rests further increases the demands on auditory-motor interaction, activity seems to be focused on this area, which is reported to be interfacing with motor planning systems for sublexical aspects of speech [75, 76]. One may object that posterior superior temporal gyrus activation in basically all of our post-minus pre-contrasts, with an asymmetry towards the left, might only indirectly reflect any improvements but merely auditory processing. This may hold true if we had limited our analysis to the fMRI data only. However, language and speech motor outcomes were additionally tested by blinded assessors.

5.2. Improvements of Language and Speech Motor Capabilities. Post- and pretest comparisons revealed clinically significant improvements for all patients in the Aachener Aphasie Test (AAT) concerning the subtests Token Test (Mr. U. and Mr. H.), repetition (Mr. H.), and naming (Mrs. A. and Mr. H.). Furthermore, all patients achieved a clinically significant increase in profile, thus testifying to the fact that an improvement in the overall range of all five subtests occurred (see Figure 2). These improvements are remarkable as they concern expressive language capabilities (in particular naming) of two severely impaired global aphasia patients (Mrs. A., Mr. H.). Particularly in connection with further improvements in the Token Test (Mr. U., Mr. H.), which represents a measure to evaluate the severity of the aphasic disorder, these results imply that more comprehensive activation of language-systematic processes must have been initiated. Likewise, this assumption is corroborated by substantial improvements in spontaneous speech for all patients (see Table 4). Our findings are in line with our previous therapy studies [25, 26, 46, 47]. We suggest that specifically focusing on improving cognitive function (e.g., auditory short-term and working memory performance), which is one of the main objectives of the applied treatment, is an essential reason for these improvements (see Section 3.4.1 and [17]).

Moreover, assessments of speech motor capabilities of the patients revealed improvements concerning *number* of assessable items (Mr. H.), *phonetic structure* (Mr. U. and Mr. H.), *phonemic structure* (Mr. U. and Mr. H.), and speech *fluency* (Mrs. A. and Mr. H.) (see Figure 3).

All patients produced the items with significantly less speech effort in the posttest, two of them, namely, the global aphasia patients with severe AOS (Mrs. A. and Mr. H.), also with less groping.

The improvements concerning *phonetic structure* and *phonemic structure* are remarkable insofar as they indicate that not only retrieval of motor plans for phones but also sequential organization of movements for a series of phones improved, exactly those processes that are particularly impaired in patients with AOS [34, 80]. Likewise, one frequently cited temporal characteristic of apraxic speech is a reduction in overall speech rate [34]. Since qualitative analysis yielded that all patients improved in *speech fluency*, it would appear that also patients with AOS benefit from a treatment, which combines motor and cognitive training.

6. Conclusion

In this therapy study including three patients with chronic nonfluent aphasia and AOS, we demonstrated the effects of rhythmic-melodic voice training (SIPARI) by functional imaging. While post-minus pretreatment imaging data of the Broca's aphasia patient (Mr. U.) yielded significant left-hemisphere activation in perilesional regions, activation patterns of both global aphasia patients (Mrs. A. and Mr. H.) comprised perilesional regions as well as homologous areas in the right hemisphere. A neural correlate of a system, which is supposed to interface with motor planning systems for sublexical aspects of speech [75, 76], was consistently located in the left superior temporal gyrus. This auditory-motor circuit provides the essential neural mechanisms for phonological short-term memory [81, 82]. Functional reintegration of this region is mentioned in the literature in connection with language improvement [1, 10, 83–85].

Although patients of our study are already in the chronic stage and have large lesions, they improved significantly with regard to language but also speech motor capabilities. They recruited parts of the neural network that we previously found in healthy subjects using the same fMRI paradigm, for example, inferior frontal gyrus, insula, and basal ganglia [27]. In addition, our findings indicate that also in severely impaired patients activations vary with task demand. These results are new and significant in particular for directed therapy interventions. Therefore, further research will elucidate potential influences in greater detail, for example, the relationship between rhythm structure, grouping strategy, and phonological working memory.

Based on our results, we assume that, for example, an improvement of short-term storage of sublexical phonolog-

ical material and, as a result of this, improved temporal sequencing possibly represent one essential prerequisite for improvements of speech motor but also language capabilities. Planning, programming, and sequencing include motor as well as cognitive capabilities. In this context, the singing voice may serve as a gateway be it that linguistic as well as musical components are applied systematically.

Acknowledgment

This work was supported in part by the Gebrüder Werner Stiftung.

References

[1] B. Crosson, K. McGregor, K. S. Gopinath et al., "Functional MRI of language in aphasia: a review of the literature and the methodological challenges," *Neuropsychology Review*, vol. 17, no. 2, pp. 157–177, 2007.

[2] R. D. Kent and J. C. Rosenbek, "Prosodic disturbance and neurologic lesion," *Brain and Language*, vol. 15, no. 2, pp. 259–291, 1982.

[3] J. L. Wambaugh and A. L. Martinez, "Effects of rate and rhythm control treatment on consonant production accuracy in apraxia of speech," *Aphasiology*, vol. 14, no. 8, pp. 851–871, 2000.

[4] W.-D. Heiss and A. Thiel, "A proposed regional hierarchy in recovery of post-stroke aphasia," *Brain and Language*, vol. 98, no. 1, pp. 118–123, 2006.

[5] A. E. Hillis, "Aphasia: progress in the last quarter of a century," *Neurology*, vol. 69, no. 2, pp. 200–213, 2007.

[6] E. G. Chrysikou and R. H. Hamilton, "Noninvasive brain stimulation in the treatment of aphasia: exploring interhemispheric relationships and their implications for neurorehabilitation," *Restorative, Neurology, and Neuroscience*, vol. 29, no. 6, pp. 375–394, 2011.

[7] M. A. Naeser, P. I. Martin, E. H. Baker et al., "Overt propositional speech in chronic nonfluent aphasia studied with the dynamic susceptibility contrast fMRI method," *NeuroImage*, vol. 22, no. 1, pp. 29–41, 2004.

[8] M. A. Naeser, P. I. Martin, E. Treglia et al., "Research with rTMS in the treatment of aphasia," *Restorative Neurology and Neuroscience*, vol. 28, no. 4, pp. 511–529, 2010.

[9] C. J. Price and J. Crinion, "The latest on functional imaging studies of aphasic stroke," *Current Opinion in Neurology*, vol. 18, no. 4, pp. 429–434, 2005.

[10] D. Saur, R. Lange, A. Baumgaertner et al., "Dynamics of language reorganization after stroke," *Brain*, vol. 129, no. 6, pp. 1371–1384, 2006.

[11] R. Zahn, M. Schwarz, and W. Huber, "Functional activation studies of word processing in the recovery from aphasia," *Journal of Physiology Paris*, vol. 99, no. 4-6, pp. 370–385, 2006.

[12] M. Meinzer and C. Breitenstein, "Functional imaging studies of treatment-induced recovery in chronic aphasia," *Aphasiology*, vol. 22, no. 12, pp. 1251–1268, 2008.

[13] M. Meinzer, D. Djundja, G. Barthel, T. Elbert, and B. Rockstroh, "Long-term stability of improved language functions

in chronic aphasia after constraint-induced aphasia therapy (CIAT)," *Stroke*, vol. 36, no. 7, pp. 1462–1466, 2005.

[14] M. L. Albert, R. W. Sparks, and N. A. Helm, "Melodic intonation therapy for aphasia," *Archives of Neurology*, vol. 29, no. 2, pp. 130–131, 1973.

[15] P. Belin, P. van Eckhout, M. Zilbovicius et al., "Recovery from nonfluent aphasia after melodic intonation therapy: a PET study," *Neurology*, vol. 47, no. 6, pp. 1504–1511, 1996.

[16] N. S. Cohen and J. Ford, "The effect of musical cues on the nonpurposive speech of persons with aphasia," *Journal of Music Therapy*, vol. 32, pp. 46–57, 1995.

[17] M. Jungblut, "SIPARI: a music therapy intervention for patients suffering with chronic, nonfluent aphasia," *Music and Medicine*, vol. 1, no. 2, pp. 102–105, 2009.

[18] R. L. Keith and A. E. Aronson, "Singing as therapy for apraxia of speech and aphasia: report of a case," *Brain and Language*, vol. 2, no. 4, pp. 483–488, 1975.

[19] M. A. Pilon, K. W. McIntosh, and M. H. Thaut, "Auditory versus visual speech timing cues as external rate control to enhance verbal intelligibility in mixed spastic-ataxic dysarthric speakers: a pilot study," *Brain Injury*, vol. 12, no. 9, pp. 793–803, 1998.

[20] G. Schlaug, S. Maechina, and A. Norton, "From singing to speaking: why singing may lead to recovery of expressive language function in patients with broca's aphasia," *Music Perception*, vol. 25, no. 4, pp. 315–323, 2008.

[21] R. W. Sparks and J. W. Deck, "Melodic intonation therapy," in *Language Intervention Strategies in Aphasic Adults*, R. Chapey, Ed., pp. 368–379, Williams and Wilkins, Baltimore, Md, USA, 3rd edition, 1994.

[22] R. Sparks, N. Helm, and M. Albert, "Aphasia rehabilitation resulting from melodic intonation therapy," *Cortex*, vol. 10, no. 4, pp. 303–316, 1974.

[23] P. van Eeckhout, C. Honrado, P. Bhatt, and J. C. Deblais, "De la TMR et de sa pratique," *Rééducation Orthophonique*, vol. 21, pp. 305–316, 1983.

[24] G. Schlaug, S. Marchina, and A. Norton, "Evidence for plasticity in white-matter tracts of patients with chronic broca's aphasia undergoing intense intonation-based speech therapy," *Annals of the New York Academy of Sciences*, vol. 1169, pp. 385–394, 2009.

[25] M. Jungblut, "Music therapy for people with chronic aphasia: a controlled study," in *Music Therapy and Neurological Rehabilitation: Performing Health*, D. Aldridge, Ed., pp. 189–211, Jessica Kingsley, London, UK, 2005.

[26] M. Jungblut, M. Suchanek, and H. Gerhard, "Long-term recovery from chronic global aphasia: a case report," *Music and Medicine*, vol. 1, no. 1, pp. 61–69, 2009.

[27] M. Jungblut, W. Huber, M. Pustelniak, and R. Schnitker, "The impact of rhythm complexity on brain activation during simple singing: an event-related fMRI study," *Restorative Neurology and Neuroscience*, vol. 30, no. 1, pp. 39–53, 2012.

[28] R. Efron, "Temporal perception, aphasia and Déjà VU," *Brain*, vol. 86, no. 3, pp. 403–424, 1963.

[29] C. Liégeois-Chauvel, J. B. De Graaf, V. Laguitton, and P. Chauvel, "Specialization of left auditory cortex for speech perception in man depends on temporal coding," *Cerebral Cortex*, vol. 9, no. 5, pp. 484–496, 1999.

[30] D. A. Robin, D. Tranel, and H. Damasio, "Auditory perception of temporal and spectral events in patients with focal left and right cerebral lesions," *Brain and Language*, vol. 39, no. 4, pp. 539–555, 1990.

[31] P. Tallal, S. Miller, and R. H. Fitch, "Neurobiological basis of speech: a case of preeminence of temporal processing," *The Irish Journal of Psychology*, vol. 16, no. 3, pp. 195–219, 1995.

[32] S. R. Baum and J. P. Boyczuk, "Speech timing subsequent to brain damage: effects of utterance length and complexity," *Brain and Language*, vol. 67, no. 1, pp. 30–45, 1999.

[33] B. Stahl, S. A. Kotz, I. Henseler, R. Turner, and S. Geyer, "Rhythm in disguise: why singing may not hold the key to recovery from aphasia," *Brain*, vol. 134, no. 10, pp. 3083–3093, 2011.

[34] K. J. Ballard, J. P. Granier, and D. A. Robin, "Understanding the nature of apraxia of speech: theory, analysis, and treatment," *Aphasiology*, vol. 14, no. 10, pp. 969–995, 2000.

[35] H. S. Kirshner, "Apraxia of speech," in *Handbook of Neurological Speech and Language Disorders*, H. S. Kirshner, Ed., pp. 41–57, Marcel Dekker, New York, NY, USA, 1995.

[36] M. R. McNeil, S. R. Pratt, and T. R. D. Fossett, "The differential diagnosis of apraxia of speech," in *Speech Motor Control in Normal and Disordered Speech*, B. Maassen, R. D. Kent, H. F. M. Peters, P. H. M. van Lieshout, and W. Hulstijn, Eds., pp. 389–413, Oxford University Press, Oxford, UK, 2004.

[37] M. R. McNeil, D. A. Robin, and R. A. Schmidt, "Apraxia of speech: definition, differentiation, and treatment," in *Clinical Management of Sensorimotor Speech Disorders*, M. R. McNeil, Ed., pp. 311–344, Thieme, New York, NY, USA, 1997.

[38] H. Southwood, P. A. Dagenais, S. M. Sutphin, and J. M. Garcia, "Coarticulation in apraxia of speech: a perceptual, acoustic and electropalatographic study," *Clinical Linguistics and Phonetics*, vol. 11, pp. 179–203, 1997.

[39] W. Ziegler and D. Von Cramon, "Anticipatory coarticulation in a patient with apraxia of speech," *Brain and Language*, vol. 26, no. 1, pp. 117–130, 1985.

[40] N. N. Simmons, "Finger counting as an intersystemic reorganizer in apraxia of speech," in *Clinical Aphasiology Conference Proceedings*, R. H. Brookshire, Ed., pp. 174–179, BRK, Minneapolis, MN, USA, 1978.

[41] H. Southwood, "The use of prolonged speech in the treatment of apraxia of speech," in *Clinical Aphasiology Conference Proceedings*, R. H. Brookshire, Ed., pp. 277–287, BRK, Minneapolis, MN, USA, 1978.

[42] R. T. Rubow, J. Rosenbek, and M. D. Collins Longstreth, "Vibrotactile stimulation for intersystemic reorganization in the treatment of apraxia of speech," *Archives of Physical Medicine and Rehabilitation*, vol. 63, no. 4, pp. 150–153, 1982.

[43] J. P. Dworkin and G. G. Abkarian, "Treatment of phonation in a patient with apraxia and dysarthria secondary to severe closed head injury," *Journal of Medical Speech-Language Pathology*, vol. 2, pp. 105–115, 1996.

[44] J. P. Dworkin, G. G. Abkarian, and D. F. Johns, "Apraxia of speech: the effectiveness of a treatment regimen," *Journal of Speech and Hearing Disorders*, vol. 53, no. 3, pp. 280–294, 1988.

[45] B. Brendel and W. Ziegler, "Effectiveness of metrical pacing in the treatment of apraxia of speech," *Aphasiology*, vol. 22, no. 1, pp. 77–102, 2008.

[46] M. Jungblut and D. Aldridge, "The musictherapy intervention SIPARI with chronic aphasics: research findings," *Neurologie und Rehabilitation*, vol. 10, no. 2, pp. 69–78, 2004 (German).

[47] M. Jungblut, H. Gerhard, and D. Aldridge, "Recovery from chronic global aphasia by a specific music therapy treatment: report of a case," *Neurologie und Rehabilitation*, vol. 12, no. 6, pp. 339–347, 2006 (German).

[48] J. Bradt, W. L. Magee, C. Dileo, B. Wheeler, and E. McGilloway, "Music therapy for acquired brain injury," *Cochrane Database of Systematic Reviews*, no. 4, 2007.

[49] D.-E. Bamiou, F. E. Musiek, and L. M. Luxon, "The insula (Island of Reil) and its role in auditory processing: literature review," *Brain Research Reviews*, vol. 42, no. 2, pp. 143–154, 2003.

[50] D.-E. Bamiou, F. E. Musiek, I. Stow et al., "Auditory temporal processing deficits in patients with insular stroke," *Neurology*, vol. 67, no. 4, pp. 614–619, 2006.

[51] D. J. Levitin, "The neural correlates of temporal structure in music," *Music and Medicine*, vol. 1, no. 1, pp. 9–13, 2009.

[52] N. F. Dronkers, "A new brain region for coordinating speech articulation," *Nature*, vol. 384, no. 6605, pp. 159–161, 1996.

[53] J. Ogar, H. Slama, N. Dronkers, S. Amici, and M. L. Gorno-Tempini, "Apraxia of speech: an overview," *Neurocase*, vol. 11, no. 6, pp. 427–432, 2005.

[54] R. C. Oldfield, "The assessment and analysis of handedness: The Edinburgh Inventory," *Neuropsychologia*, vol. 9, no. 1, pp. 97–113, 1971.

[55] D. M. Barch, F. W. Sabb, C. S. Carter, T. S. Braver, D. C. Noll, and J. D. Cohen, "Overt verbal responding during fMRI scanning: empirical investigations of problems and potential solutions," *NeuroImage*, vol. 10, no. 6, pp. 642–657, 1999.

[56] N. J. Shah, S. Steinhoff, S. Mirzazade et al., "The effect of sequence repeat time on auditory cortex stimulation during phonetic discrimination," *NeuroImage*, vol. 12, no. 1, pp. 100–108, 2000.

[57] W. Huber, K. Poeck, D. Weniger, and K. Willmes, *Aachener Aphasie Test (AAT). Protokollheft und Handanweisung*, Hogrefe, Göttingen, Germany, 1983.

[58] N. Miller, R. De Bleser, and K. Willmes, *The English Version of the Aachener Aphasia Test (EAAT)*, Hogrefe, Göttingen, Germany, 2000.

[59] M. Liepold, W. Ziegler, and B. Brendel, *Hierarchische Wortlisten. Ein Nachsprechtest für die Sprechapraxiediagnostik*, Borgmann, Dortmund, Germany, 2003.

[60] K. J. Friston, C. D. Frith, R. Turner, and R. S. J. Frackowiak, "Characterizing evoked hemodynamics with fMRI," *NeuroImage*, vol. 2, no. 2, pp. 157–165, 1995.

[61] K. L. Friston, J. T. Ashburner, S. J. Kiebel, T. E. Nichols, and W. E. Penny, Eds., *Statistical Parametric Mapping: The Analysis of Functional Brain Images*, Academic press, San Diego, Calif, USA, 1st edition, 2007.

[62] W. J. M. Levelt, A. Roelofs, and A. S. Meyer, "A theory of lexical access in speech production," *Behavioral and Brain Sciences*, vol. 22, no. 1, pp. 1–75, 1999.

[63] W. Ziegler, "Psycholinguistic and motor theories of apraxia of speech," *Seminars in Speech and Language*, vol. 23, no. 4, pp. 231–243, 2002.

[64] N. P. M. A. Todd, "The auditory "primal sketch": a multiscale model of rhythmic grouping," *Journal of New Music Research*, vol. 23, no. 1, pp. 25–70, 1994.

[65] A. M. Glenberg and M. Jona, "Temporal coding in rhythm tasks revealed by modality effects," *Memory and Cognition*, vol. 19, no. 5, pp. 514–522, 1991.

[66] M. C. Payne and T. G. Holzman, "Rhythm as a factor in memory," in *Rhythm in Psychological, Linguistic and Musical Processes*, J. R. Evans and M. Clynes, Eds., pp. 41–54, Charles C Thomas, Springfield, Ill, USA, 1986.

[67] K. Deger and W. Ziegler, "Speech motor programming in apraxia of speech," *Journal of Phonetics*, vol. 30, no. 3, pp. 321–335, 2002.

[68] N. Lauer and B. Birner-Janusch, *Sprechapraxie im Kindes- und Erwachsenenalter*, Georg Thieme, New York, NY, USA, 2007.

[69] M. Danly and B. Shapiro, "Speech prosody in Broca's aphasia," *Brain and Language*, vol. 16, no. 2, pp. 171–190, 1982.

[70] A. Schirmer, "Timing speech: a review of lesion and neuroimaging findings," *Cognitive Brain Research*, vol. 21, no. 2, pp. 269–287, 2004.

[71] E. Maas, D. A. Robin, D. L. Wright, and K. J. Ballard, "Motor programming in apraxia of speech," *Brain and Language*, vol. 106, no. 2, pp. 107–118, 2008.

[72] E. F. Clarke, "Rhythm and timing in music," in *The Psychology of Music*, D. Deutsch, Ed., pp. 473–500, Academic Press, San Diego, Calif, USA, 2nd edition, 1999.

[73] D. J. Povel and P. Essens, "Perception of temporal patterns," *Music Perception*, vol. 2, no. 4, pp. 411–440, 1985.

[74] K. Cornelissen, M. Laine, A. Tarkiainen, T. Järvensivu, N. Martin, and R. Salmelin, "Adult brain plasticity elicited by anomia treatment," *Journal of Cognitive Neuroscience*, vol. 15, no. 3, pp. 444–461, 2003.

[75] G. Hickok and D. Poeppel, "Dorsal and ventral streams: a framework for understanding aspects of the functional anatomy of language," *Cognition*, vol. 92, no. 1-2, pp. 67–99, 2004.

[76] G. Hickok and D. Poeppel, "The cortical organization of speech processing," *Nature Reviews Neuroscience*, vol. 8, no. 5, pp. 393–402, 2007.

[77] U. Jürgens, "Neural pathways underlying vocal control," *Neuroscience & Biobehavioral Reviews*, vol. 26, no. 2, pp. 235–258, 2002.

[78] A. M. Ferrandez, L. Hugueville, S. Lehéricy, J. B. Poline, C. Marsault, and V. Pouthas, "Basal ganglia and supplementary motor area subtend duration perception: an fMRI study," *NeuroImage*, vol. 19, no. 4, pp. 1532–1544, 2003.

[79] F. Macar, H. Lejeune, M. Bonnet et al., "Activation of the supplementary motor area and of attentional networks during temporal processing," *Experimental Brain Research*, vol. 142, no. 4, pp. 475–485, 2002.

[80] A. van der Merwe, "A theoretical framework for the characterization of pathological speech sensorimotor control," in *Clinical Management of Sensorimotor Speech Disorders*, M. R. McNeil, Ed., pp. 1–25, Thieme, New York, NY, USA, 1997.

[81] B. R. Buchsbaum, R. K. Olsen, P. Koch, and K. F. Berman, "Human dorsal and ventral auditory streams subserve rehearsal-based and echoic processes during verbal working memory," *Neuron*, vol. 48, no. 4, pp. 687–697, 2005.

[82] G. Hickok, B. Buchsbaum, C. Humphries, and T. Muftuler, "Auditory-motor interaction revealed by fMRI: speech, music, and working memory in area Spt," *Journal of Cognitive Neuroscience*, vol. 15, no. 5, pp. 673–682, 2003.

[83] J. I. Breier, J. Juranek, L. M. Maher, S. Schmadeke, D. Men, and A. C. Papanicolaou, "Behavioral and neurophysiologic response to therapy for chronic aphasia," *Archives of Physical Medicine and Rehabilitation*, vol. 90, no. 12, pp. 2026–2033, 2009.

[84] D. Cardebat, J.-F. Démonet, X. De Boissezon et al., "Behavioral and neurofunctional changes over time in healthy and aphasic subjects: a PET language activation study," *Stroke*, vol. 34, no. 12, pp. 2900–2906, 2003.

[85] H. Karbe, A. Thiel, G. Weber-Luxenburger, K. Herholz, J. Kessler, and W.-D. Heiss, "Brain plasticity in poststroke aphasia: what is the contribution of the right hemisphere?" *Brain and Language*, vol. 64, no. 2, pp. 215–230, 1998.

11

Can Combination Therapy of Conventional and Oriental Medicine Improve Poststroke Aphasia? Comparative, Observational, Pragmatic Study

WooSang Jung,[1] SeungWon Kwon,[1] SeongUk Park,[2] and SangKwan Moon[1]

[1] Department of Cardiovascular and Neurologic Diseases, Kyung Hee University Oriental Medicine Hospital, 1 Hoegi-dong, Dongdaemun-gu, Seoul 130-702, Republic of Korea
[2] Department of Cardiovascular and Neurologic Diseases, Kyung Hee University Hospital at Gangdong, Republic of Korea

Correspondence should be addressed to SeungWon Kwon, kkokkottung@hanmail.net

Academic Editor: Il-Moo Chang

The aim of the present study was to determine the effectiveness of oriental medicine therapy on poststroke aphasia. The outcome was measured as the delta value of the Aphasic Quotient score. Patients completed test at two timepoints: baseline and discharge time. Patients who received conventional therapy and language therapy were grouped in the Only Language Therapy group. Patients who received conventional therapy, language therapy, and an Oriental medicine regimen were grouped in the Combined oriental Medicine Therapy group. We compared the delta value of the Aphasic Quotient score between two groups. The Combined Oriental Medicine group exhibited a greater improvement than the Only Language Therapy group in the total Aphasic Quotient score and most subsection scores. In particular, there were statistically significant differences in total Aphasic Quotient score and subsections such as spontaneous speech, content delivery, comprehension, auditory verbal comprehension, and command performance. Among severe aphasic patients, the improvement of the Combined oriental Medicine group was better than that of the Only Language Therapy group. Through this study, we suggest combination therapy with the administration of oriental medicine and language therapy can be helpful in the treatment of post-stroke aphasic patients.

1. Introduction

Approximately 38% of stroke patients suffer from aphasia. Among them, 50% have aphasia with long-term disabilities after 6 months [1]. Recovery from aphasia is commonly achieved within 6 months after the onset of stroke. However, post-stroke aphasia can become a permanent deficit after 6 months. Therefore, post-stroke aphasia must be treated effectively within the first 6 months after the stroke. Some studies suggest that the duration of an effective aphasia treatment regimen should be 2–6 months [2–7].

Donepezil [8], bromocriptine,amphetamine, and piracetam [9, 10] are generally suggested for the treatment of aphasia. However, these drugs are not always prescribed because there is a lack of evidence concerning their overall effect on aphasia. Compared with conventional therapy strategies for the treatment of aphasia, Oriental medicine doctors have used several different modalities to treat this disease. Some case reports suggested that herbal complexes such as *jihwangeumja* [11–13], *cheongshinhaeeo-tang* [14], *seonghyangjeongkisan* [13], *cheongshindodam-tang* [13], and others [15] are effective in the treatment of aphasia. Other reports describe the use of "*scalp acupucnture*" a form of acupuncture, to heal aphasia [16, 17]. However, these reports were based on case studies. Furthermore, these studies did not include a control group.

The aim of the present study was to determine the effectiveness of oriental medicine (consisting of herbal medicine, acupuncture, and moxibustion) on post-stroke aphasia by comparing the Aphasia Quotient (AQ) scores between a combined Oriental medicine therapy group and a non-Oriental medicine therapy group. Present study was performed as a pragmatic method understanding character of Oriental medicine, reflecting individuation of patients' general condition and symptoms.

2. Methods

2.1. Participants. The Kyung Hee University Oriental Medicine Hospital Institutional Review Board approved the present study (KOMC IRB 2009-14), which was conducted as a comparative, observational, and pragmatic study. Over a 31-month period spanning from March 2009 to September 2011, 77 Korean Asian patients in total (mean ± SD age 53.7 ± 14.4 years) with a clinical diagnosis of post-stroke aphasia of different severities (mild to severe) were enrolled in the study. Participants who were treated with language therapy after 6 months from the onset of stroke were also excluded from the study.

2.2. Study Design (Figure 1). After admission to Kyung Hee Medical Center (Department of Cardiovascular and Neurologic Diseases of the Oriental Medicine Hospital, and Department of Neurology, Neurosurgery, and Rehabilitation of the Western Medicine Hospital), the participants received language therapy until they were discharged. The frequency and intensity of language therapy were adjusted individually according to the severity and the type of the participants' aphasia. Participants completed the K-WAB (Korean version of the Western Aphasia Battery) AQ test (Table 7) at 2 time-points: an initial ("baseline") test was administered at the time of recruitment of the participants, and a second test was administered after the last language therapy session (discharge time). Discharge time was decided according to the Korean health policy which limit the admission duration of one hospital to 6–8 weeks. The AQ test was performed by four language therapists. All participants were evaluated by language therapist in charge twice. These language therapists did not know that they were participating in the present study. Calculation of the AQ test scores included the total AQ score and the AQ subsection score. The type of stroke was determined by the results of the initial AQ test. Medical records of each participant's age, medical history, and associated symptoms were recorded. The patients were diagnosed with stroke when neurological deficits were accompanied by abnormal findings in computed tomography (CT) or magnetic resonance imaging (MRI) of the brain.

The participants were assigned to one of the two treatment groups. The Combined Oriental Medicine Therapy (COT) group admitted to the Oriental Medicine Hospital of Kyung Hee Medical Center and received conventional therapy that included taking antiplatelet agent, control risk factor (e.g. hypertension, diabetes mellitus, dyslipidemia and cardiac disease), rehabilitation exercise, working exercise for stroke, language therapy for aphasia, and an oriental medicine regimen that included herbal medicine, acupuncture, and moxibustion. oriental medicine therapy administered to patients in the COT group was adjusted individually according to the severity and type of aphasia, general condition, and associated symptoms. Details of the Oriental medicine therapies (herbal medicine type and contents, using frequency, acupuncture, method, and moxibustion method) were recorded in Table 1. Herbal medicine adjusted in each patient was selected by patient's condition, characters, and oriental diagnosis (pattern recognition).

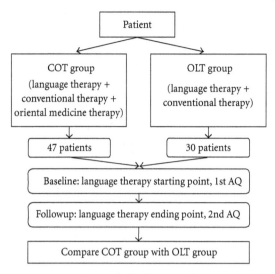

FIGURE 1: Study protocol.

Acupuncture and moxibustion were conducted equally in all COT group patients. The Only Language Therapy (OLT) group was admitted to the Western Medicine Hospital of Kyung Hee Medical Center and received conventional therapy for stroke and language therapy for aphasia. In Kyung Hee Medical Center, there are two hospitals, Western Medicine Hospital which treat patients with conventional therapy and Oriental Medicine Hospital which treat patients with conventional therapy and oriental medicine therapy. Each patient who is admited Kyung Hee Medical Center can choose one of the two hospitals according to their preference. Therefore, inclusion in each group was not randomized, but based on the participants' choice.

2.3. Measurements. The AQ test was used to estimate the effectiveness of the oriental medicine combination therapy for aphasia. The primary outcome of this study was measured as the delta value of the total AQ score (difference between the initial total AQ score and the final total AQ score, "final total AQ score—initial total AQ score"). The secondary outcome was the delta value of each subsection score of the AQ test, such as spontaneous speech, comprehension, repetition, and naming. The third outcome was the change of aphasia severity distribution. Patients were classified into two severity groups according to the AQ scores as follows: non-severe aphasia: AQ 36.3 ~ 92.2, severe aphasia: AQ 0–36.2. We compared the scores of AQ test and the distribution of severity (severe, and non-severe) of the COT group with the OLT group.

2.4. Statistical Analysis. All data and results were analyzed using SPSS 12.0 for Windows. Fisher's exact test was used to compare categorical variables, including gender, handedness, type of stroke, type of aphasia, risk factors, frequency of related symptoms, and distribution of aphasia severity between the two groups. The Mann-Whitney U test was used to compare continuous variables such as age, education, treatment periods from onset, duration of treatment, and differences in AQ scores between the 2 groups.

TABLE 1: Oriental medicine therapies referred to COT group.

Therapy	Contents	Proportion (%)
Herbal medicine (g/day)	*Cheongshinhaeeo-tang*	Arisaematis Rhizoma, Pinelliae Rhizoma 8 Saposhnikovia Radix, Poria, Paeoniae Radix Alba, Rehmanniae Radix, Acori Graminei Rhizoma, Linderae Radix, Polygalae Radix, Aurantii Immaturus, Citri Pericarpium, Ligustici Rhizoma, Coptidis Rhizoma, Angelicae Gigantis Radix, Liriopes Radix, Glycyrrhizae Radix, and Notopterygii Rhizoma 4	21 (44.7)
	Jasoohaeeo-tang	Glycyrrhizae Radix, Notopterygii Rhizoma 6, Cinnamomi Ramulus, Gazellae Cornu 8, Saposhnikovia Radix, Pulvis Aconiti Tuberis Purificatum, Zizyphi Spinosae Semen, Gastrodiae Rhizoma 4	3 (6.4)
	Hyungbangjihwang-tang	Poria, Alismatis Rhizoma, Corni Fructus, Rehmanniae Radix Preparata 16 Notopterygii Rhizoma, Angelicae Pubescentis Radix, Schizonepeta Spica, Saposhnikovia Radix, and Plantaginis Semen 8	6 (12.8)
	Yeoldahanso-tang	Puerariae Radix 32 Ligustici Sinense Radix, Scutellariae Radix 16 Platycodi Radix, Raphani Semen, Angelicae Dahuricae Radix, and Cimicifugae Rhizoma 8	8 (17)
	Seonghyangjeonggi-san	Pogostemi Herba 12 Platycodi Radix, Arecae Pericarpium, Perillae Folium 8 Citri Pericarpium, Magnoliae Cortex, Aucklandiae Radix, Pinelliae Rhizoma, Poria, Angelicae Dahuricae Radix, Atractylodis Rhizoma Alba, Arisaematis Rhizoma, and Glycyrrhizae Radix 4	3 (6.4)
	Bojoongikgi-tang	Astragali Radix 12 Glycyrrhizae Radix, Atractylodis Rhizoma Alba, Ginseng Radix 8 Angelicae Gigantis Radix, Citri Pericarpium 4 Cimicifuga Rhizoma, and Bupleuri Radix 2	6 (12.8)
Acupuncture (1 time/day)	LI4, LI11, GB20, LR3 (both sides), LI10, ST36, ST37, TE3, GB34, GB39, GB41, TE5 (affected side), HT7, PC6 (nonaffected side), GV15, GV20, and GV23	47 (100)
Electroacupuncture (1 time/day)	LI4, LI10, LI11, ST36, ST37, GB39, GB41, and TE5 (affected side)	47 (100)
Moxibustion (1 time/day)	CV4 and CV12	47 (100)

COT group: group that received language therapy with oriental medicine therapy.

TABLE 2: Patient characteristics in the 2 groups.

	COT group ($n = 47$)	OLT group ($n = 30$)	P-value
Gender, male (%)	31 (66)	14 (46.7)	0.104
Age, yr (SD, median)	54.5 (12.1, 54)	52.5 (17.6, 55.5)	0.790
Education, yr (SD, median)	10.8 (5.1, 12)	11.2 (3.8, 12)	0.918
Handedness, right (%)	46 (97.9)	30 (100)	1.000
Treatment period from onset, day (SD, median)	48 (45.4, 29)	41 (28.7, 39)	0.954
Duration of treatment, weeks (SD, median)	6.6 (7.1, 4.9)	7.8 (5.7, 6.4)	0.104
Hypertension (%)	31 (65.96)	20 (66.67)	1.000
Diabetes mellitus (%)	12 (25.53)	3 (10)	0.140
Dyslipidemia (%)	8 (17.02)	3 (10)	0.513
Heart disease (%)	7 (14.89)	4 (13.33)	1.000
AQ scores (SD, median)	28.1 (25.6, 19.2)	26.7 (26.2, 19)	0.875
Total score	5.5 (5.1, 3)	5.7 (5.4, 5)	0.757
Spontaneous speech	3.3 (2.8, 2)	3.4 (3, 3)	0.987
Content delivery	2.2 (2.4, 1)	2.5 (2.8, 1.5)	0.928
Fluency	3.6 (2.9, 3.2)	3.6 (2.7, 3.1)	0.979
Comprehension	32.1 (17.9, 33)	29.6 (18.9, 32)	0.645
Yes-no	21.1 (20.9, 11)	21.9 (20.4, 18.5)	0.892
Auditory verbal comprehension	19.8 (23.4, 10)	19.7 (21.4, 12)	0.834
Command performance	3.3 (3.6, 1.2)	2.4 (3.4, 0.6)	0.179
Repetition	1.9 (2.6, 0.5)	1.6 (2.6, 0.2)	0.405
Naming	12.9 (17.9, 4)	11.4 (18.1, 0.5)	0.457
Naming things	1.2 (2.8, 0)	1.2 (2.5, 0)	0.510
Control word association	2.5 (3.6, 0)	2 (3.3, 0)	0.472
Sentence completion	1.9 (3.3, 0)	1.7 (3.3, 0)	0.670
Sentence answers			

COT group: group that received language therapy with oriental medicine therapy.
OLT group: group that received language therapy only.
AQ: aphasia Quotient.
P value was obtained by the Mann-Whitney U test (age, education, treatment period from onset, duration of treatment, and AQ scores) and Fisher's exact test (gender and handedness).
SD: standard deviation.

The Wilcoxon-signed rank test was performed to compare changes of AQ scores in each group. The McNemar test was performed to compare changes of the distribution of severity of aphasia.

3. Results

3.1. Baseline Assessment. Among the 77 participants, 47 were included in the COT group and 30 in the OLT group. However, the baseline characteristics of the two groups exhibited no significant differences with regard to gender, age, education, handedness, treatment period from onset, and duration of language therapy. There was no significant difference in stroke risk factors such as hypertension, diabetes mellitus, dyslipidemia, and heart disease (Table 2).

The total AQ score was 28.1 ± 25.6 in the COT group and 26.7 ± 26.2 in the OLT group. There were small differences in the total score between the 2 groups, which were not statistically significant. The subsection scores such as spontaneous speech, comprehension, repetition, and naming (naming things, control word association, sentence completion, and answers) demonstrated no statistically significant differences either (Table 2).

3.2. Type of Stroke. In the COT group, there were 30 infarction patients and 17 hemorrhage patients. In the OLT group, there were 14 infarction patients and 16 hemorrhage patients. The proportion of cerebral infarction subtypes based on the TOAST (Trials of Org 10172 in Acute Stroke Treatment) classification was not significantly different between the two groups (Table 3), nor was the proportion of cerebral hemorrhage subtypes (Table 3).

3.3. Type of Aphasia, and Related Symptoms. Twenty-five patients in the COT group and 16 patients in the OLT group had global aphasia at baseline. There was no significant difference between the two groups. The proportions of other types of aphasia were not significantly different between the 2 groups either (Table 4). There were 12 patients in the COT group and 5 patients in the OLT group who had dysphagia, which can affect aphasia. However, there was no significant difference between the two groups ($P = 0.412$). Deafness and dysphonia were not found in these participants.

3.4. AQ Score before and after Treatment in the OLT Group. Before language therapy, the total AQ score was 26.7 ± 26.2 in the OLT group. After 7.8 ± 5.7 weeks of conventional therapy

TABLE 3: Type of stroke.

	COT group ($n = 47$)	OLT group ($n = 30$)	P value
Infarction : hemorrhage	30 : 17	14 : 16	
Infarction			
LAA (%)	26 (55.32)	10 (33.33)	0.670
CE (%)	2 (4.26)	1 (3.33)	1.000
SAO (%)	0 (0)	1 (3.33)	0.390
Other causes (%)	1 (2.13)	1 (3.33)	1.000
Undetermined causes (%)	1 (2.13)	0 (0)	1.000
Hemorrhage			
ICH (%)	13 (27.66)	13 (43.33)	0.217
IVH (%)	1 (2.13)	0 (0)	1.000
SDH (%)	0 (0)	2 (6.67)	0.149
SAH (%)	3 (6.39)	1 (3.33)	1.000

COT group: group that received language therapy with oriental medicine therapy.
OLT group: group that received language therapy only.
LAA: large artery atherosclerosis. CE: cardioembolism.
SAO: small artery occlusion. ICH: intracerebral hemorrhage.
IVH: intraventricular hemorrhage. SDH: subdural hemorrhage.
SAH: subarachnoid hemorrhage.
P value was obtained by Fisher's exact test.

TABLE 4: Type of aphasia at time of admission.

	COT group ($n = 47$)	OLT group ($n = 30$)	P value
Motor (%)	7 (14.89)	6 (20)	0.756
Sensory (%)	3 (6.38)	3 (10)	0.673
Global (%)	25 (53.19)	16 (53.33)	1.000
Conduction (%)	1 (2.13)	0 (0)	1.000
Transcortical (%)	7 (14.89)	2 (6.67)	0.469
Anomic (%)	4 (8.51)	3 (10)	1.000

COT group: group that received language therapy with oriental medicine therapy.
OLT group: group that received language therapy only.
P value was evaluated by Fisher's exact test.

with language therapy, the total AQ score increased to 39 ± 31.1, which was a statistically significant change according to the Wilcoxon-signed rank test ($P = 0.001$). All subsections demonstrated improvements in the score and the differences were statistically significant in all subsection scores (Table 5).

3.5. AQ Score before and after Treatment in the COT Group. Before language therapy, the total AQ score was 28.1 ± 25.6 in the OLT group. After 6.6 ± 7.1 weeks of oriental medicine therapy combined with language therapy, the total AQ score increased to 45.3 ± 27.4, which was a statistically significant change according to the Wilcoxon signed rank test ($P < 0.001$). All subsections demonstrated improvements in the score and the differences were statistically significant (Table 5).

3.6. Comparison of the AQ Score Improvements between the COT and OLT Groups: Total Score and Subsection Scores. The COT group (+17.2 ± 11.6) demonstrated greater improvements in the total AQ score than the OLT group did (+12.3 ± 13.6). This result was statistically significant ($P = 0.021$). The subsections demonstrating better results in the COT group were those for spontaneous speech, content

delivery, comprehension, auditory verbal comprehension, command performance, repetition, naming, and naming things. Among them, spontaneous speech, content delivery, comprehension, auditory verbal comprehension, and command performance were statistically significant. The yes-no section exhibited better results in the OLT group with a delta value (value after − value before) of 9 in the OLT group, and 6 in the COT group. However, these differences were not statistically significant (Table 5).

3.7. Comparison of the AQ Score Improvements between the COT and OLT Groups: Distribution of Severity. Before language therapy, 66% of patients in the COT group and 76.7% of patients in the OLT group demonstrated severe aphasia. After language therapy, 38.3% of the COT group and 56.7% of the OLT group demonstrated severe aphasia. After language therapy, 41.9% of patients in the COT group and 26.1% of patients in OLT group with severe aphasia were converted into non-severe aphasia. The aphasia subsided in one patient in the COT group. In this change of severe aphasia distribution, the COT group reveals statistically significance. The OLT group also shows statistically significance. Before and after treatment, there

TABLE 5: AQ scores before and after language treatment in the OLT and COT group.

AQ	OLT group (SD, median)			COT group (SD, median)			P value*
	Before	After	Delta value	Before	After	Delta value	
Total score	26.7 (26.2, 19)	39# (31.1, 31.6)	12.3 (13.6, 7.2)	28.1 (25.6, 19.2)	45.3# (27.4, 41.3)	17.2 (11.6, 16.9)	0.021
Spontaneous speech	5.7 (5.4, 5)	8.2# (6.4, 6.8)	2.5 (3.4, 1.5)	5.5 (5.1, 3)	9# (5.4, 8.5)	3.5 (2.9, 3)	0.049
Content delivery	3.4 (3, 3)	4.6# (3.5, 4)	1.2 (2.1, 1)	3.3 (2.8, 2)	5.2# (2.7, 5)	1.9 (1.7, 2)	0.024
Fluency	2.5 (2.8, 1.5)	3.7# (3.3, 2.3)	1.2 (1.9, 1)	2.2 (2.4, 1)	3.9# (4.4, 6.2)	1.8 (1.7, 1)	0.097
Comprehension	3.6 (2.7, 3.1)	4.8# (3, 4.4)	1.3 (1.4, 0.9)	3.6 (2.9, 3.2)	6.2# (4.4, 6.2)	2.7 (4.3, 1.9)	0.009
Yes-no	29.6 (18.9, 32)	35.7# (19.3, 37.5)	7.9 (10.4, 9)	32.1 (17.9, 33)	43# (15.6, 48)	11 (13.1, 6)	0.574
Auditory verbal comprehension	21.9 (20.4, 18.5)	29.8# (21.3, 26.5)	8 (9.3, 4)	21.1 (20.1, 11)	36.2# (19.8, 36)	15.1 (13.7, 12)	0.019
Command performance	19.7 (21.4, 12)	28.2# (26, 21.5)	8.7 (15.6, 1.5)	19.8 (23.4, 10)	34.1# (26, 32)	14.2 (15.5, 8)	0.031
Repetition	2.4 (3.4, 0.6)	3.6# (3.7, 2.6)	1.3 (1.8, 0.5)	3.3 (3.6, 1.2)	5.5# (5.3, 5.2)	2.1 (3.9, 1.3)	0.100
Naming	1.6 (2.6, 0.2)	2.8# (3.2, 1.2)	1.2 (1.5, 0.8)	1.9 (2.6, 0.5)	3.4# (3, 2.1)	1.5 (1.7, 1.2)	0.274
Naming things	11.4 (18.1, 0.5)	19.3# (21.1, 9.5)	8 (11, 4.5)	12.9 (17.9, 4)	21.1# (19.2, 14)	8.2 (10.8, 6)	0.626
Control word association	1.2 (2.5, 0)	3.1# (4.6, 0)	1.9 (2.9, 0)	1.2 (2.8, 0)	2.7# (4.2, 0)	1.5 (3.4, 0)	0.427
Sentence completion	2 (3.3, 0)	2.9# (3.8, 1)	0.9 (1.8, 0)	2.5 (3.6, 0)	4# (3.7, 4)	1.5 (2.5, 0)	0.391
Sentence answer	1.7 (3.3, 0)	2# (4.1, 0)	1 (2.3, 0)	1.9 (3.3, 0)	3.3# (3.8, 2)	1.5 (2.7, 0)	0.215

COT group: group that received language therapy with oriental medicine therapy.
OLT group: group that received language therapy only.
*P value was obtained by the Mann-Whitney U test for comparing delta values between the OLT and the COT group.
#P value means "<0.05." It was obtained by the Wilcoxon-signed rank test for evaluating significance of change in each group.

TABLE 6: Comparison of the AQ Score improvements between the COT and OLT groups: distribution of severity.

Group	Aphasia severity	COT group ($n = 47$)	OLT group ($n = 30$)	P value
Before treatment (%)	Severe	31 (66)	23 (76.7)	0.445
	Nonsevere	16 (34)	7 (23.3)	
After treatment (%)	Severe	18 (38.3)	17 (56.7)	0.159
	Non-severe	29 (61.7)	13 (43.3)	

COT group: group that received language therapy with oriental medicine therapy.
OLT group: group that received language therapy only.
P value was obtained by Fisher's exact test for evaluating significance of distribution of severe aphasia in each point (before treatment and after treatment).

was no statistically significant difference between the COT and the OLT group in distribution of severe aphasia (Table 6, Figure 2). Therefore, severe aphasia patients who belonged to the COT group revealed better improvements rather than patients who belonged to the OLT group.

4. Discussion

The results of the present study suggest that the administration of language therapy in combination with oriental medicine therapy is effective for the treatment of post-stroke aphasia. Among patients with severe aphasia at onset, those in the COT group exhibited better improvements than those in the OLT group, suggesting that the co-administration of oriental medicine therapy with language therapy revealed more effective tendency in the treatment of patients with severe aphasia.

The efficacy of language therapy for aphasia has received much attention in recent years. Wertz et al. reported a 6% improvement in patients receiving language therapy compared to those that did not receive conventional language therapy [18]. In a recent meta-analysis, patients who received

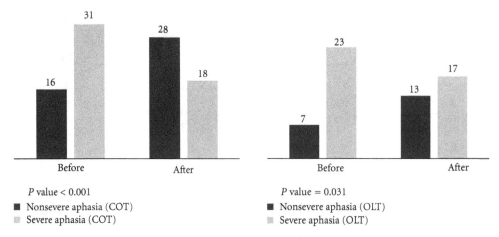

FIGURE 2: Change of distribution of aphasia severity. COT: group that received language therapy with oriental medicine therapy, OLT: group that received language therapy only, non-Severe: Aphasia Quotient 36.3–92.2, Severe: Aphasia Quotient 0–36.2, P value was obtained by the McNemar test for evaluating significance of change of distribution of severe aphasia in each group.

TABLE 7: AQ (Aphasia Quotient) test subsection.

Spontaneous speech
   Content delivery
   Fluency
Comprehension
   Yes-no
   Auditory verbal comprehension
   Command performance
Repetition
Naming
   Naming things
   Control word association
   Sentence completion
   Sentence answer

Total AQ score = spontaneous speech + comprehension + repetition + naming.

intense language therapy exhibited a greater improvement than patients who did not receive language therapy [19, 20]. The American BI-ISIG (Brain Injury Interdisciplinary-Specific Interest Group) classified language therapy as a practice standard and an essential item for post-stroke aphasic patients [21]. Therefore, most patients who suffer from post-stroke aphasia usually receive language therapy during their rehabilitation.

In addition to language therapy, the treatment of patients with aphasia may include pharmacological intervention. Bromocriptine, amphetamines, and piracetam are sometimes used for post-stroke aphasia treatment [9, 10]. The efficacy of these medications has been demonstrated in previous studies. However, it is still controversial whether the improvement of aphasia in patients treated with bromocriptine and amphetamines is caused by an improvement of the aphasia itself or an improvement in their attention. Furthermore, the routine prescription of amphetamines should be avoided because of its potential negative effects on the central nervous system and addiction [22]. Piracetam has been associated with exacerbation of intracerebral hemorrhage and effects on the central nervous system [23].

Therefore, pharmacological interventions have not been used routinely in aphasic patients. In this respect, safe and effective treatments that can be administered in association with language therapy are needed for the treatment of patients with aphasia.

According to previous studies, oriental medicine is an effective therapy for the treatment of the effects of stroke [24–26]. However, the aim of these studies was to evaluate the effects of oriental medicine on the general sequelae of stroke, in particular, motor function disorders. Studies focusing on aphasia were not comparative, but rather case reports or case series [11–17]. The present study was therefore designed to evaluate the effect of the co-administration of oriental medicine with language therapy using a comparative method.

In addition, the present study assessed the individualized nature of oriental medicine. When Oriental medicine doctors use oriental medicine therapy to treat stroke patients, they adjust the treatment regimen according to each patient's individual needs, general condition, and constitution such as oriental diagnosis. Patients admitted to Oriental medicine hospitals may receive different types of treatment. Therefore, in this study, we used a pragmatic method to investigate the effects of oriental medicine therapy itself on post-stroke aphasia recovery. For example, oriental medicine doctors prescribed *Hyungbangjihwang-tang*, when patients were diagnosed with *Yin deficiency*.

The present study has following limits. First, because of the study design (non-randomized case-control study), the numbers of participants in each group were not the same. However, there were no significant differences between the two groups in terms of baseline characteristics, type of stroke, type of aphasia, stroke risk factors, and related symptoms. Second, the duration of followup was not the same for all patients. However, there were no significant differences between the 2 groups regarding the duration of language therapy.

The present data suggest that co-administration of oriental medicine with language therapy can be an effective method for the treatment of post-stroke aphasia. The factors that can affect the improvement of aphasia are first, individual factors such as age, sex, education, and handedness; second, neurological factors such as the severity of aphasia at onset [3], treatment period [3], and cause and sites of brain damage; third, treatment-related factors, including the intensity and duration of language therapy, and the methods used. There were no significant differences in these factors between the two groups in the present study. The exclusion of differences in the factors that affect aphasia recovery between the groups enabled the acquisition of more accurate results. In addition, we believe that this study reflects clinical circumstances more accurately than previous studies. We used a pragmatic method to investigate the effects of oriental medicine therapy itself on post-stroke aphasia recovery. We believe that this method better reflects the individualized character of oriental medicine. Furthermore, we used an objective tool such as the K-WAB to estimate the effect of oriental medicine therapy on post-stroke aphasia. K-WAB is a standardized test for the evaluation of aphasia. The above points demonstrate the reliability and objectivity of the present results.

A possible mechanism which can explain the result obtained is as follows: oriental medicine therapy affects neural plasticity related to the recovery of language functions such as diaschisis, redundancy, and vicariation [27]. "Diaschisis" means language function that is indirectly damaged has declined for a short period since onset and these functions will be recovered as time passes. "Redundancy" indicates that a language area that is not involved can lead to the recovery of aphasia. Lastly, "vicariation" refers to a brain area that is not in charge of everyday language, but assumes an important role in the recovery from aphasia. Vicariation is assumed a major mechanism of Large artery atherosclerosis (LAA) type stroke patients' aphasia recovery. Vicariation has been considered ineffective because most patients with severe aphasia and extensive brain damage have a tendency to recover slowly. Howevere, we think that a major mechanism of oriental medicine on the recovery of post-stroke aphasia is thought to be vicariation. In this study, 55.3% of COT group patients exhibited an LAA-type ischemic stroke, which was of a higher proportion than in the OLT group. However, the improvement of the COT group was better than that of the OLT group. Furthermore, the COT group exhibited a greater improvement than the OLT group among severely aphasic patients at onset (Figure 2). Therefore, we consider the effect of conventional therapy to be mostly mediated by diaschisis and redundancy and only slightly by vicariation. However, the co-administration of oriental medicine therapy may increase the influence of vicariation. As a result, the COT group exhibited a greater improvement among severely aphasic patients, indicating that oriental therapy can act as a catalyst of vicariation and that it can be effective when it is administered in combination with language therapy.

However, this effect is not limited to the language function area. According to previous studies, oriental medicine can also affect the improvement of motor functions in stroke patients [24]. The results of previous studies showed that oriental medicine can have an effect on neural plasticity related to the recovery of motor function. Together with the present results, these studies suggest that oriental medicine can affect brain neural plasticity in relation to both language and motor functions, and the improvement of aphasia may be the result of the activation of whole-brain neural plasticity. Future studies should assess the recovery of language disorders together with other stroke symptoms to validate this hypothesis.

5. Conclusion

The present study assessed the effect of co-administration of oriental medicine therapy with language therapy on post-stroke aphasia 6 months before stroke onset. This study was conducted as a comparative, observational, and pragmatic study. The results of this study are as follows.

(1) The COT group exhibited a greater improvement than the OLT group in the total AQ score and most subsection scores. In particular, there were statistically significant differences in total AQ score and subsections such as spontaneous speech, content delivery, comprehension, auditory verbal comprehension, and command performance.

(2) Among severe aphasic patients, the improvement of the COT group was better than that of the OLT group There was statistically significant differences in distribution of severe aphasia of the COT group. However, there were no statistically significance in the OLT group.

Therefore, we suggest that combination therapy with the administration of oriental medicine therapies and language therapy can be helpful in the treatment of post-stroke aphasic patients 6 months before stroke onset.

References

[1] P. M. Pedersen, H. S. Jørgensen, H. Nakayama, H. O. Raaschou, and T. S. Olsen, "Aphasia in acute stroke: Incidence, determinants, and recovery," *Annals of Neurology*, vol. 38, no. 4, pp. 659–666, 1995.

[2] K. Hojo, S. Watanabe, H. Tasaki et al., "Recovery in aphasia (Part 1)," *No To Shinkei*, vol. 37, no. 8, pp. 791–797, 1985.

[3] C. M. Shewan and A. Kertesz, "Effects of speech and language treatment on recovery from aphasia," *Brain and Language*, vol. 23, no. 2, pp. 272–299, 1984.

[4] W. Lendrem and N. B. Lincoln, "Spontaneous recovery of language in patients with aphasia between 4 and 34 weeks after stroke," *Journal of Neurology Neurosurgery and Psychiatry*, vol. 48, no. 8, pp. 743–748, 1985.

[5] A. C. Laska, A. Hellblom, V. Murray, T. Kahan, and M. Von Arbin, "Aphasia in acute stroke and relation to outcome," *Journal of Internal Medicine*, vol. 249, no. 5, pp. 413–422, 2001.

[6] C. M. Godfrey and E. Douglass, "The recovery process in aphasia," *Canadian Medical Association Journal*, vol. 80, no. 8, pp. 618–624, 1959.

[7] N. B. Lincoln, E. McGuirk, G. P. Mulley et al., "Effectiveness of speech therapy for aphasic stroke patients. A randomised controlled trial," *The Lancet*, vol. 1, no. 8388, pp. 1197–1200, 1984.

[8] M. L. Berthier, C. Green, C. Higueras, I. Fernández, J. Hinojosa, and M. C. Martín, "A randomized, placebo-controlled study of donepezil in poststroke aphasia," *Neurology*, vol. 67, no. 9, pp. 1687–1689, 2006.

[9] M. L. Berthier, "Poststroke aphasia: epidemiology, pathophysiology and treatment," *Drugs and Aging*, vol. 22, no. 2, pp. 163–182, 2005.

[10] N. Marjorie, *Recovery after Stroke*, Cambridge University Press, 2005.

[11] W. S. Jung, Y. J. Lee, Y. J. Jeong et al., "A case report on broca aphasia," *Korean Journal of Oriental Internal Medicine*, vol. 25, pp. 401–409, 2004.

[12] J. Yeo, I. S. Jang, G. Yoo et al., "Korean medical treatment and language therapy in patient with fluent aphasia after stroke: case report," *Journal of Oriental Neuropsychiatry*, vol. 17, pp. 137–143, 2006.

[13] L. Hsing, J. Yeo, G. Yoo et al., "A case of subcortical aphasic stroke treated with speech-language therapy and Korean medical therapy," *Korean Journal of Oriental Internal Medicine*, vol. 26, pp. 733–740, 2005.

[14] T. K. Yang and J. M. Park, "Two cases of combination therapy of acupuncture, herbal medication and language therapy for aphasic stroke patients," *Journal of Korean Oriental Medicine*, vol. 23, pp. 196–202, 2002.

[15] D. M. Kim, H. K. Kim, S. Y. Ha et al., "A case report of communication disorder associated with post-stroke," *Journal of Meridian & Acupoint*, vol. 24, pp. 47–54, 2007.

[16] Y. J. Han, J. E. Lee, H. H. Bae et al., "The effects of the bang's scalp acupuncture on poststroke aphasia," *Korean Journal of Oriental Physiology & Pathology*, vol. 17, pp. 1560–1563, 2003.

[17] J. M. Yun, S. W. Park, M. G. Lee et al., "Clinical study of scalp acupuncture effects on patients with broca aphasia," *Korean Journal of Oriental Internal Medicine*, vol. 25, pp. 167–176, 2004.

[18] R. T. Wertz, D. G. Weiss, and J. L. Aten, "Comparison of clinic, home, and deferred language treatment for aphasia: a Veterans Administration Cooperative study," *Archives of Neurology*, vol. 43, no. 7, pp. 653–658, 1986.

[19] S. K. Bhogal, R. W. Teasell, N. C. Foley, and M. R. Speechley, "Rehabilitation of aphasia: more is better," *Topics in Stroke Rehabilitation*, vol. 10, no. 2, pp. 66–76, 2003.

[20] S. K. Bhogal, R. Teasell, and M. Speechley, "Intensity of aphasia therapy, impact on recovery," *Stroke*, vol. 34, no. 4, pp. 987–993, 2003.

[21] K. D. Cicerone, C. Dahlberg, J. F. Malec et al., "Evidence-based cognitive rehabilitation: updated review of the literature from 1998 through 2002," *Archives of Physical Medicine and Rehabilitation*, vol. 86, no. 8, pp. 1681–1692, 2005.

[22] C. H. Hong and B. H. Oh, "Inappropriate prescribing in the elderly patients," *Journal of the Korean Medical Association*, vol. 52, no. 1, pp. 91–99, 2009.

[23] B. Winblad, "Piracetam: a review of pharmacological properties and clinical uses," *CNS Drug Reviews*, vol. 11, no. 2, pp. 169–182, 2005.

[24] Y. J. Kim, M. Y. Kim, S. Y. Lee et al., "The study about characteristics affecting functional recovery of stroke patients treated in oriental medical center," *Korean Journal of Oriental Internal Medicine*, vol. 30, pp. 719–731, 2009.

[25] T. S. Cho, I. S. Son, I. B. Park et al., "Effects of scalp acupuncture on short-term NIHSS and MBI in stroke patients," *Journal of Korean Oriental Medicine*, vol. 24, pp. 65–73, 2003.

[26] T. S. Cho, I. S. Son, C. H. Kim et al., "Effects of added tong's acupuncture on NIH stroke scale and MBI in stroke patients," *The Journal of Korean Acupuncture & Moxibustion Society*, vol. 19, pp. 35–45, 2002.

[27] M. Musso, C. Weiller, S. Kiebel, S. P. Müller, P. Bülau, and M. Rijntjes, "Training-induced brain plasticity in aphasia," *Brain*, vol. 122, no. 9, pp. 1781–1790, 1999.

12

Right Hemisphere Remapping of Naming Functions Depends on Lesion Size and Location in Poststroke Aphasia

Laura M. Skipper-Kallal,[1] **Elizabeth H. Lacey,**[1,2] **Shihui Xing,**[1,3] **and Peter E. Turkeltaub**[1,2]

[1]*Department of Neurology, Georgetown University Medical Center, Washington, DC, USA*
[2]*Research Division, MedStar National Rehabilitation Hospital, Washington, DC, USA*
[3]*Department of Neurology, First Affiliated Hospital of Sun Yat-Sen University, Guangzhou, China*

Correspondence should be addressed to Peter E. Turkeltaub; turkeltp@georgetown.edu

Academic Editor: Cynthia K. Thompson

The study of language network plasticity following left hemisphere stroke is foundational to the understanding of aphasia recovery and neural plasticity in general. Damage in different language nodes may influence whether local plasticity is possible and whether right hemisphere recruitment is beneficial. However, the relationships of both lesion size and location to patterns of remapping are poorly understood. In the context of a picture naming fMRI task, we tested whether lesion size and location relate to activity in surviving left hemisphere language nodes, as well as homotopic activity in the right hemisphere during covert name retrieval and overt name production. We found that lesion size was positively associated with greater right hemisphere activity during both phases of naming, a pattern that has frequently been suggested but has not previously been clearly demonstrated. During overt naming, lesions in the inferior frontal gyrus led to deactivation of contralateral frontal areas, while lesions in motor cortex led to increased right motor cortex activity. Furthermore, increased right motor activity related to better naming performance only when left motor cortex was lesioned, suggesting compensatory takeover of speech or language function by the homotopic node. These findings demonstrate that reorganization of language function, and the degree to which reorganization facilitates aphasia recovery, is dependent on the size and site of the lesion.

1. Introduction

One-third of stroke survivors suffer from loss of language ability [1, 2]. Recovery rates vary greatly, for reasons that are poorly understood [3]. The relationships between lesion site, activity pattern changes, and recovered language functions remain unclear.

1.1. Reorganization of Language Function after Stroke. In neuroimaging studies, patterns of increased activation during language tasks in chronic aphasia have been broadly consistent across studies. In a meta-analysis of neuroimaging studies, collapsing across a wide range of language tasks, we found that people with aphasia consistently overactivated perilesional regions in the left hemisphere, as well as right hemisphere regions that were homotopic to the left hemisphere language network [4]. In particular, people with

lesions in the left inferior frontal gyrus (IFG) were more likely to recruit right IFG than those without lesions in that area. However, the behavioral and biological drivers of these changes, as well as the degree to which they promote, inhibit, or are even relevant to recovery, remain open questions.

The increased activation in the preserved left hemisphere in people with aphasia has generally been associated with overall better performance [5–8]. However, the relationship between lesion size, location, and ability to use these preserved regions has not been carefully examined. For example, particularly severe participants may have larger lesions or lesions in highly critical areas. If this is the case, then the relationship between left hemisphere activity and language performance may be indirect, in that both are actually dependent on the severity and size of the stroke itself, as well as the availability of left hemisphere tissue adjacent to the critical areas.

Within the right hemisphere, the relationship between plasticity and language performance is even less clear. A number of lines of evidence suggest that engagement of the right hemisphere serves overall to support aphasia recovery (for review, see [9]), suggesting a compensatory role for the right hemisphere homologues to language nodes. However, transcranial magnetic stimulation (TMS) studies show that inhibiting the right IFG pars triangularis (PTr) improves fluency, naming, and other language measures in people with left hemisphere stroke [10–15]. This suggests that the right IFG, specifically right PTr, may be limiting recovery in people with left hemisphere lesions. Furthermore, neuroimaging studies show that early engagement of the right hemisphere during the acute phase promotes recovery but that disengagement of the right hemisphere in later stages is related to ongoing successful recovery [16–19]. Increased activation in the right hemisphere during the chronic stage of aphasia is associated with naming errors [20] and overall worse performance, especially in picture-word naming and rhyme judgment [16, 21].

Unfortunately, the same concerns arise when examining the function of the right hemisphere as were raised for the left, specifically, confounding with lesion size and location. The usefulness of a shift from right to left hemisphere activation during the chronic stages likely depends on the availability of remaining healthy left hemisphere tissue [5]. Additionally, right hemisphere recruitment identified in neuroimaging studies may not be a consequence of plasticity at all. In neurologically healthy control subjects, right hemisphere activation has been shown to increase as a function of task difficulty [22, 23]. Furthermore, right hemisphere activity appears to be greater in participants with larger overall left hemisphere lesions [24], although this finding is only for some language tasks (picture naming, but not semantic judgment). Right hemisphere activity in people with aphasia, therefore, may actually be driven by the unique difficulty of the language tasks for people with aphasia. Right hemisphere activity may also reflect overactivation of any preserved tissue, of which there is less for people with large lesions, rather than actually remapping of function. However, the relationship between activity in the right hemisphere in people with aphasia, the rate of recovery, and actual plasticity remains unclear.

Beyond the general anatomical patterns of reorganization and their association with good or bad outcomes, the mechanisms underlying reorganization remain unclear. Such mechanisms may include behaviorally driven reorganization, as in the plasticity induced by speech-language therapy [18], or direct biological effects of the stroke itself. With regard to direct biological mechanisms underlying plasticity in language networks, relatively few specific hypotheses have been put forth. While some investigators, including ourselves, have previously described different patterns of reorganization (e.g., compensatory "takeover" by a new area), these descriptions do not generally hypothesize a specific biological basis for these changes. The great virtue of specific biological hypotheses is that they generate specific testable predictions, especially with regard to the timing of plasticity, the relationship of specific lesion features such as size and location to the pattern of reorganization, and the relationship of brain changes to behavioral outcomes.

One such biological hypothesis which has gained a great deal of traction in recent years is the interhemispheric inhibition model, which is commonly invoked to explain recruitment of homotopic right hemisphere processors, negative relationships between right hemisphere activity and language performance, and the beneficial effects of right PTr inhibition [25]. This hypothesis states that, in healthy people, there is transcallosal cross-hemispheric inhibition between language areas, similar to what has been demonstrated in motor areas [26, 27]. A stroke in the left hemisphere theoretically disrupts the interhemispheric inhibitory balance, leading to overactivation of right hemispheric language areas homotopic to the lesion. In the context of the interhemispheric inhibition theory, the overactivated right hemisphere is thought to maladaptively inhibit perilesional left hemisphere areas, resulting in worse outcomes [14].

In particular, the interhemispheric inhibition model makes at least three specific testable claims. First, larger lesions in the left hemisphere should be associated with more activity in the right hemisphere. Second, left hemisphere lesions should be associated with increased activity specifically in homotopic regions in the right hemisphere. Finally, increased right hemisphere activity in homotopic areas should be related to worse language abilities, even at the chronic stage. Some of the prior evidence regarding the latter two claims is outlined above. The predicted relationship between lesion size and right hemisphere recruitment is frequently mentioned in reviews on aphasia recovery either in the context of interhemispheric inhibition or based on the logical argument that if no left hemisphere tissue remains, the right hemisphere must be recruited for any recovery to occur [7, 28, 29]. However, the empirical evidence supporting this relationship is lacking and based primarily on small case series using methods that do not control for the accuracy of task performance [30].

1.2. Cognitive Models of Naming. Lexical-retrieval processes involve accessing concept knowledge and mapping phonological representations, stored in long-term memory [31] and these two stages are supported by distinct cortical regions. Phonological retrieval is ascribed to a ventral stream of processing, in which phonological representations in the posterior superior temporal lobe map onto semantic and conceptual information in the angular gyrus and anterior temporal lobes [32].

Postlexical output is the production stage, in which phonological representations are mapped to motor representations and speech occurs. Some dual-stream models assign this stage to the dorsal stream, in that the phonological representations in the superior temporal gyrus (STG) are mapped to motor sequence representations in the temporoparietal junction and posterior inferior frontal lobes [32].

1.3. Design of This Experiment. We tested these three predictions of the interhemispheric inhibition model in a cross-sectional study of people with chronic aphasia following left hemisphere stroke. The experiment used an fMRI task to isolate covert (phonological retrieval) and overt (postlexical output) phases of picture naming; we first examined the general patterns of activity in our aphasia group compared to matched controls and the relationship between activity and overall lesion size. We then used the activity in the control group to define the normal brain network for naming in older people without language impairment or brain injury and tested how lesions at key nodes in this network affected activity throughout the rest of the brain, in particular within the remaining bilateral language sites. The goal of the study was to examine whether plastic changes in chronic aphasia would be related to the size and site of the lesion, with particular interest in right hemisphere plasticity occurring in regions that were homotopic to the left hemisphere lesions. We further tested whether any changes in activity associated with lesion site were related to naming performance, in order to assess whether these regions are successfully adapting to support language function or are inhibiting successful recovery.

2. Materials and Methods

2.1. Participants. Forty-nine chronic left hemisphere stroke survivors with a history of aphasia were recruited. Ten participants were then excluded based on fMRI task performance (<10% accuracy) resulting in a final sample of 39 participants in the aphasia group.

All participants in the aphasia group were native English speakers and testing occurred at least six months after their stroke (mean chronicity = 52.9 months). Participants were screened based on ability to follow testing instructions and had no history of other significant neurological illnesses. The distribution of lesions and individual demographic information for the aphasia group can be found in the Supplementary Material available online at https://doi.org/10.1155/2017/8740353.

Thirty-seven healthy control subjects, with no neurologic or psychiatric disorders, were also tested. Participants in the control group were matched to the aphasia group on age ($t(67.5) = -0.42, P > 0.60$), sex ($\chi^2(1) = 0.79, P > 0.30$), education ($t(73.0) = 0.85, P > 0.30$), and handedness ($\chi^2(3) = 3.1, P > 0.30$). Group means can be found in Table 1.

The study was approved by the Georgetown University Institutional Review Board, and written informed consent was obtained from all study participants prior to enrollment in the study.

2.2. Experimental Design. Visual stimuli consisted of 54 line drawings, with 92–100% name agreement based on norming in an independent sample of 55 older controls, representing one-, two-, and three-syllable words. To reduce individual differences in in-scanner performance, participants were presented with one of two 32-item sets during scanning based on the severity of their deficits. Fourteen participants whose naming and repetition deficits were severe in pre-MRI testing were given 32 one- and two-syllable items, while all other participants, including controls, were given 32 two- and three-syllable items during scanning. The one-syllable words

TABLE 1: Demographic information for the aphasia group and control group. Standard deviations are shown in parentheses. There were no differences between the groups on age, sex, education, or handedness.

	Aphasia group	Control group
Age (years)	59.8 (10.1)	58.7 (13.2)
Sex (male/female)	26/13	20/17
Education (years)	16.4 (2.8)	16.9 (2.6)
Handedness (right/left/ambidextrous/unknown)	33/4/0/4	33/3/1/0
Time since stroke (months)	52.9 (51.4)	—
WAB naming/word finding	7.1 (2.5)	—
WAB auditory-verbal comprehension	8.3 (1.5)	—
WAB repetition	7.0 (2.5)	—
WAB spontaneous speech	15.1 (4.9)	—

also had overall higher frequency than the three-syllable words.

The fMRI task followed a slow jittered event related design. The trials were presented in a pseudo-randomized order. The task was a delayed naming task, which allows for the independent analysis of name retrieval and name production [33]. First, a single line drawing appeared centered on the screen, surrounded by a red border. This image remained on the screen for 7500–9000 ms, during which time the participant named the object in the image silently (covert naming). Then, the border around the image changed from red to green and remained on screen for 5500 ms. During this time, the participant was asked to produce the name of the object aloud (overt naming). Finally, the line drawing and the surrounding box disappeared and the participant fixated on a crosshair for 14000 ms. A slow event related design was chosen to allow for wash out of the hemodynamic response, which may be slower in stroke survivors [34]. Images were presented using E-Prime software (Psychology Software Tools Inc., Pittsburg, PA), and responses were recorded using a MRI safe microphone (Opto-acoustics, FOMRI-III). Before the scan, participants practiced the task on images not included in the fMRI task. If a participant produced the correct name at any point during the overt naming period, the item was counted as correct. Only trials in which the correct response was produced during the overt phase were included in the analysis. If a participant made an incorrect or no response during the overt naming phase of the trial, the entire trial (both covert and overt phases) was removed from further analysis.

Naming ability was tested using a 60-item version of the Philadelphia Naming Test (PNT) [35], made up of items independent of those used in the scanning task. Testing took place within one week of the MRI scan. We counted the total number of items on the PNT that were named correctly on the first attempt.

2.3. Scanning Parameters and Preprocessing. MRI data were collected on a 3.0 T Siemens Trio Scanner at the Georgetown University Medical Center. A high resolution T1-weighted MPRAGE was collected with the following parameters: repetition time = 1900 ms, echo time = 2.56 ms, flip angle = 9°, 160 contiguous 1 mm slices, field of view = 250 × 250 mm, matrix size = 246 × 256, and voxel size = 1 × 1 × 1 mm. Functional T2*-weighted images were acquired using a gradient-echo echo-planar pulse sequence, with the following parameters: repetition time = 2000 ms, echo time = 30 ms, flip angle = 90°, 38 contiguous 3.2 mm slices, field of view = 250 × 250 mm, and voxel size = 3.2 × 3.2 × 3.2 mm. The functional scan consisted of 32 trials, including an opening and closing screen, totaling approximately 15 minutes.

Lesion masks were created by manually tracing stroke damage on the T1-weighted images, in native space, in MRIcron [36], following a preestablished set of guidelines for determining lesion borders. Ventricular expansion was not included in the lesion. All lesion masks were checked by two board certified neurologists (Shihui Xing and Peter E. Turkeltaub) after the tracing and again after the lesion masks were warped to the template.

fMRI data were preprocessed and analyzed using FSL 5.0.6 [37]. Preprocessing included application of a high pass temporal filter, standard correction for head motion using MCFLIRT, interleaved slice timing correction, intensity normalization across volumes, and spatial smoothing to 5 mm FWHM. Registration and normalization were carried out to the MNI standardized brain provided by FSL. For each condition in each trial, a canonical double-gamma hemodynamic response function was constructed for the duration of the event. Motion parameters were then included as covariates in the model.

2.4. fMRI Analysis. First, we examined where participants in the aphasia group over- and underactivated relative to controls during covert and overt naming. In between-group contrasts, only areas that were significantly active ($z > 2.3$) in the aphasia group were included in the aphasia > control contrast, and vice versa. All whole-brain analyses were examined at cluster corrected $P < 0.01$, after a grey matter mask was applied.

2.4.1. Effects of Lesion Volume on Activity. We tested whether right hemisphere activity in people with aphasia is driven by the extent of overall damage in the left hemisphere. To do this, we quantified the size of the lesion, warped to template, for each individual. Lesion size was measured in mm³ after warping to a standardized template and then entered as a voxelwise continuous predictor variable in a group analysis. Clusters identified as significant in this analysis are areas where activation, for either covert or overt naming, differed as a function of lesion size.

2.4.2. Regions of Interest Used to Examine Remapping. In order to examine how lesions within the normal language network affect naming ability, we identified regions of interest (ROIs) using the within-group contrasts from the control group. The peak voxel in each active cluster was identified,

excluding primary visual cortex, for both the covert > fixation and overt > fixation contrasts. Then, 5 mm spheres were drawn around the peak voxel.

For each of the left hemisphere ROIs, aphasia group participants were grouped based on lesion status at the ROI. As these were very small ROIs, not large clusters, the distributions of percent lesions in the ROIs were highly bimodal, so an all or nothing approach was used: If a participant had a lesion that overlapped with the ROI in even one voxel, the participant was counted in the "lesion" group for that ROI. Then we tested whether lesions at each left hemisphere site led to worse naming performance on the PNT. Whole-brain analyses were then carried out, contrasting activity in these two groups (lesion versus intact at ROI site) of people with aphasia, while controlling for overall lesion volume.

Finally, we examined more closely the relationships between damage in sites normally active in controls and activity in the remaining nodes in the network. Regressions were carried out which tested whether lesion status in a left hemisphere ROI predicted activity levels in each of the other left and right hemisphere ROIs, controlling for lesion volume. ROIs in which activity was modulated by lesion status at another site were then further tested to see whether activity in that area related to naming ability.

3. Results

3.1. Whole-Brain Activity during Covert and Overt Naming. In the covert > fixation contrast (Table 2, Figures 1(a)-1(b)), the aphasia group showed greater activity than the control group mostly in bilateral basal ganglia, bilateral cerebellum, but also the right ventral central sulcus and right IFG. The aphasia group underactivated the left frontal pole, cingulate cortex, and bilateral clusters in the superior frontal gyrus compared to controls. In within-group contrasts, both groups showed significant activation in the visual cortex. The control group showed bilateral activation in the inferior parietal sulcus (IPS), while the aphasia group only showed significant activation in the right IPS. Likewise, the control group showed activation in the bilateral insula and pars opercularis (POp), as well as left PTr, while the aphasia group only activated the right PTr.

During overt naming (Table 3, Figures 1(c)-1(d)), the aphasia group overactivated dorsal regions bilaterally, in particular bilateral central sulcus, as well as right insula, right angular gyrus, and right Heschl's gyrus. The aphasia group underactivated, relative to controls, the left IFG, insula, superior temporal gyrus (STG), and cerebellum. In the within-group contrasts, both the aphasia group and control group activated the right superior temporal sulcus (STS), STG, temporal pole, and central sulcus. Only the control group activated these regions in the left hemisphere, while only the aphasia group showed activity in the right IFG.

3.2. Effect of Lesion Size on Activity. Next, we looked for regions, within the aphasia group, where activity during covert and overt naming was predicted by large lesions (Table 4, Figure 2). During covert naming, larger lesion size predicted widespread right hemisphere activity, especially

TABLE 2: MNI coordinates of activity in the covert naming > fixation contrast.

Group contrast	Peak z-value	x	y	z	Label
Aphasia > control	4.8	−22	16	8	Left basal ganglia
Aphasia > control	4.8	−20	−62	−28	Left lateral cerebellum
Aphasia > control	4.5	10	−40	−12	Right medial cerebellum
Aphasia > control	4.4	20	14	−2	Right basal ganglia
Aphasia > control	4.1	14	−62	−22	Right lateral cerebellum
Aphasia > control	4	−10	−28	0	Left thalamus
Aphasia > control	4.0	42	16	2	Right insula
Aphasia > control	4.0	65	10	0	Right ventral POp
Aphasia > control	3.9	62	−8	8	Right inferior central sulcus
Control > aphasia	3.9	−52	−40	60	Left IPS
Control > aphasia	3.7	−26	64	−2	Left frontal pole
Control > aphasia	3.7	26	54	26	Right superior frontal gyrus
Control > aphasia	3.5	−2	48	42	Left anterior cingulate cortex
Control > aphasia	3.1	−28	44	32	Left superior frontal gyrus
Aphasia group	8.1	36	90	0	Right visual cortex
Aphasia group	7.6	8	−84	−18	Right medial cerebellum
Aphasia group	6.8	10	0	6	Right thalamus
Aphasia group	6.6	−4	16	42	Left cingulate cortex
Aphasia group	6.2	50	20	−6	Right PTr
Aphasia group	6.2	−30	−92	4	Left visual cortex
Aphasia group	6.0	4	−34	−4	Right brainstem
Aphasia group	5.9	0	−22	6	Medial thalamus
Aphasia group	5.6	48	8	22	Right central sulcus
Aphasia group	5.2	30	−56	50	Right IPS
Aphasia group	5.2	−44	30	14	Left POp
Aphasia group	5.1	−16	6	6	Left thalamus
Aphasia group	5.1	50	18	−16	Right anterior STS
Aphasia group	5.0	18	−32	−8	Right posterior hippocampus
Control group	8.9	32	−92	12	Left visual cortex
Control group	7.2	0	28	36	Medial cingulate cortex
Control group	6.9	30	−66	54	Right dorsal IPS
Control group	6.6	−30	−60	48	Left dorsal IPS
Control group	6.6	38	22	−6	Right insula
Control group	6.5	−36	20	−4	Left insula
Control group	6.4	−50	28	24	Left dorsal POp
Control group	6.3	4	−36	−4	Right brainstem
Control group	6.3	54	16	−16	Right anterior STS
Control group	6.1	−48	12	24	Left ventral POp
Control group	6.0	48	10	24	Right central sulcus
Control group	6.0	54	38	12	Right POrb
Control group	5.9	−46	32	12	Left PTr
Control group	5.8	−32	56	14	Left frontal pole
Control group	5.7	28	−70	34	Right ventral IPS
Control group	5.5	−36	−50	44	Left ventral IPS

in the central sulcus, POp, and PTr, but also in bilateral visual cortex, cingulate, IPS, and basal ganglia. During overt naming, larger lesion size predicted activation in bilateral central sulcus, cingulate, and cerebellum, but activity was heavily right lateralized, especially in right PTr, posterior STS, and posterior STG.

We also looked for regions where activity was greater in participants with smaller lesions. There were no areas where

TABLE 3: MNI coordinates of activity in the overt naming > fixation contrast.

Group contrast	Peak z-value	x	y	z	Label
Aphasia > control	4.7	−28	−22	48	Left dorsal central sulcus
Aphasia > control	4.6	44	−66	0	Right visual cortex
Aphasia > control	4.6	24	0	66	Right dorsal central sulcus
Aphasia > control	4.0	−12	−26	64	Left middle cingulate cortex
Aphasia > control	4.0	−38	−10	48	Left central gyrus
Aphasia > control	3.9	40	−6	52	Right central gyrus
Aphasia > control	3.9	−14	10	42	Left anterior cingulate cortex
Aphasia > control	3.9	28	16	2	Right insula
Aphasia > control	3.8	40	−30	18	Right Heschl's gyrus
Aphasia > control	3.4	48	−34	24	Right angular gyrus
Aphasia > control	3.2	−32	−38	46	Left ventral IPS
Control > aphasia	5.2	−62	−4	−4	Left temporal pole
Control > aphasia	5.1	−62	−2	24	Left middle central sulcus
Control > aphasia	4.6	−10	−18	6	Left thalamus
Control > aphasia	4.5	−66	−40	4	Left posterior STS
Control > aphasia	4.1	−40	−14	−12	Left posterior insula
Control > aphasia	4.1	−4	−24	0	Left brainstem
Control > aphasia	4.0	−46	−30	6	Left posterior STG
Control > aphasia	3.9	−44	18	−6	Left PTr
Control > aphasia	3.9	−68	−30	8	Left middle STG
Control > aphasia	3.6	−16	−30	−16	Left hippocampus
Control > aphasia	3.4	−40	−82	−22	Left cerebellum
Aphasia group	7.7	54	4	36	Right central gyrus
Aphasia group	7.4	28	−80	−20	Right visual cortex
Aphasia group	7.4	6	6	52	Right cingulate cortex
Aphasia group	6.4	66	−22	−2	Right middle STG
Aphasia group	6.1	48	−34	2	Right posterior STS
Aphasia group	5.9	−46	−16	36	Left central sulcus
Aphasia group	5.6	12	−16	0	Right thalamus
Aphasia group	5.4	44	10	−6	Right PTr
Aphasia group	5.4	36	20	2	Right anterior insula
Aphasia group	5.4	56	−32	8	Right posterior STG
Aphasia group	5.3	−26	−94	12	Left visual cortex
Aphasia group	5.3	64	−40	22	Right angular gyrus
Aphasia group	5.1	40	−12	14	Right posterior insula
Aphasia group	5.0	−8	8	40	Left middle cingulate cortex
Aphasia group	5.0	38	−30	18	Right Heschl's gyrus
Aphasia group	4.9	32	−14	−10	Right middle hippocampus
Aphasia group	4.5	22	10	0	Right basal ganglia
Aphasia group	3.3	2	−54	−26	Right medial cerebellum
Aphasia group	3.3	−34	−20	48	Left central gyrus
Aphasia group	3.2	10	−28	−24	Right brainstem
Control group	8.5	−10	−104	−2	Left visual cortex
Control group	7.8	−50	−12	26	Left central sulcus
Control group	6.5	−16	−28	−12	Left middle hippocampus
Control group	6.5	22	−28	−10	Right middle hippocampus
Control group	6.4	68	−28	2	Right posterior STS
Control group	6.2	14	−18	2	Right basal ganglia

TABLE 3: Continued.

Group contrast	Peak z-value	x	y	z	Label
Control group	6.2	−64	−42	6	Left posterior STS
Control group	6.1	−2	2	58	Left middle cingulate cortex
Control group	6.0	−66	−2	−6	Left temporal pole
Control group	5.8	58	14	−16	Right temporal pole
Control group	5.6	−40	−30	8	Left Heschl's gyrus
Control group	5.3	66	−6	10	Right MTG
Control group	5.0	14	−24	−12	Right brainstem
Control group	4.1	−32	24	2	Left anterior insula
Control group	3.8	−46	8	22	Left dorsal POp
Control group	3.6	−36	4	2	Left middle insula

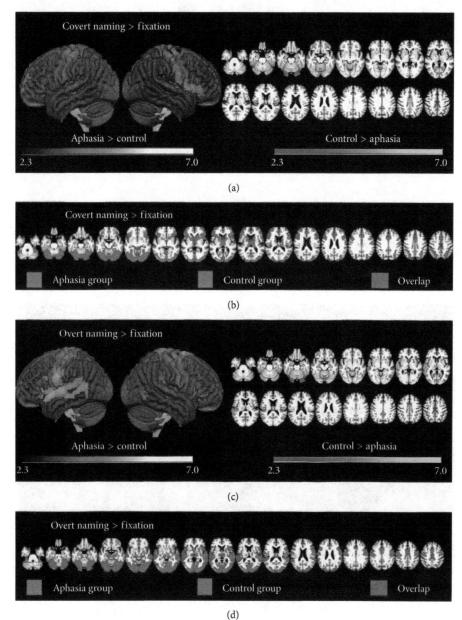

FIGURE 1: (a) Between-group contrasts showing activity during covert naming. (b) Within-group contrasts showing activity for both the aphasia and control groups during covert naming. (c) Between-group contrasts showing activity during overt naming. (d) Within-group contrasts showing activity for both the aphasia and control groups during overt naming.

TABLE 4: MNI coordinates of activity associated with large lesions, for both the covert naming and overt naming contrasts.

Task	Peak z-value	x	y	z	Label
Covert > fixation	5.5	4	−82	−16	Right visual cortex
Covert > fixation	5.4	34	−64	−24	Right cerebellum
Covert > fixation	5.3	−40	−88	−14	Left visual cortex
Covert > fixation	5.3	6	−32	−8	Right brainstem
Covert > fixation	5.1	12	0	2	Right basal ganglia
Covert > fixation	4.9	−26	−76	40	Left ventral IPS
Covert > fixation	4.8	30	−56	50	Right IPS
Covert > fixation	4.7	4	6	56	Right cingulate cortex
Covert > fixation	4.3	66	0	10	Left central gyrus
Covert > fixation	4.1	−18	8	4	Left basal ganglia
Covert > fixation	3.8	−24	−64	56	Left dorsal IPS
Overt > fixation	6.6	32	−58	−24	Right cerebellum
Overt > fixation	6.1	−26	−64	−28	Left cerebellum
Overt > fixation	5.4	4	4	52	Right cingulate cortex
Overt > fixation	5.4	68	−18	0	Right middle STS
Overt > fixation	5.3	66	2	10	Right PTr
Overt > fixation	5.1	52	−38	−6	Right MTG
Overt > fixation	4.3	−46	−16	36	Left central sulcus
Overt > fixation	4.3	22	8	0	Right basal ganglia
Overt > fixation	4.0	38	−12	14	Right posterior insula
Overt > fixation	3.9	−14	−34	54	Left cingulate cortex
Overt > fixation	3.8	−20	−20	0	Left external capsule
Overt > fixation	3.4	32	−14	−12	Right hippocampus

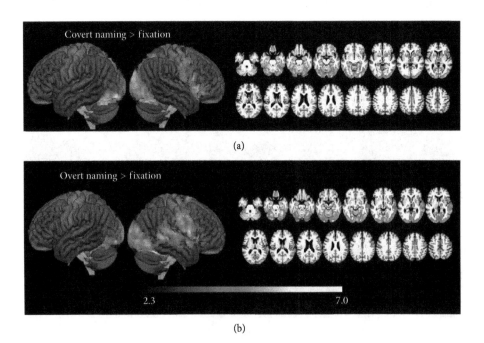

FIGURE 2: Regions where large left hemisphere lesions were related to greater activity during (a) covert naming and (b) overt naming.

activity was significantly predicted by smaller lesions at our threshold.

3.3. Lesions at ROIs and Behavior.

Regions of interest were drawn based on peaks from the control group maps (Table 5). For covert naming, ROIs included the left and right IPS, left and right insula, and a left dorsal POp peak. Another peak in the left cingulate met requirements for an ROI, but only one participant in the aphasia group had a lesion in this area, so it was removed from further analysis. For overt naming, ROIs were selected in both the left and right motor cortex and STS.

We then tested whether lesion statuses in the left ROIs were related to naming performance in the scanner, using linear regression. Lesions in the left insula were related to worse naming, $t(37) = -2.4$, $P < 0.05$, but this effect did not hold when lesion size was introduced as a control variable, $P > 0.30$. Lesions in the left insula, dorsal POp, motor cortex, and STS had no relationship with naming performance in the scanner.

3.4. Effect of Lesion Location on Remapping and Whole-Brain Analysis.

We then carried out whole-volume analysis using the aphasia group, testing whether lesion status at each left hemisphere ROI resulted in different patterns of activity in the rest of the brain, with lesion volume added as a nuisance variable. For covert naming, at a cluster corrected $P < 0.01$, there was no difference between people with left IPS lesions versus those without lesions at the IPS site.

People with left insula lesions showed less activity in the right middle and inferior frontal gyri, with peaks in the right middle frontal gyrus and right dorsal PTr. Participants with left POp lesions also showed less activation in nearly overlapping regions, including right dorsal POp (Figure 3, Table 6). The similarity of these results is likely due to the significant overlap between participants with left insula lesions and participants with left POp lesions.

We then took the cortical peak in this right hemisphere cluster, located in dorsal PTr, and extracted the activation levels for covert naming relative to baseline. The activation level in each participant with aphasia was transformed into a z-score centered on the control group mean. We carried out two tests, to examine whether activity in this area was related to PNT score, in the group with left POp lesions ($N = 16$) and in the group with intact left POp ($N = 23$), again controlling lesion size. There was no significant relationship between activity in the right peak activation and naming in either group (both P's > 0.25). The same analyses were also done, dividing participants based on lesion status at left insula (intact $N = 21$, lesion $N = 18$), but again no relationship was found for either group (both P's > 0.80).

No group differences in activity in the whole-volume analysis were identified based on lesion status at the two left hemisphere overt naming ROIs, left motor cortex and left STS, at this threshold.

3.5. Effect of Lesion Status in One ROI on Activity in Other ROIs.

Finally, we tested whether lesion status in each left hemisphere ROI affected activity levels in all other, left and right hemisphere, ROIs derived from the healthy control sample, controlling for lesion size.

For covert naming, only one relationship was marginally significant. Participants with left insula lesions had marginally greater activity in the left POp, but this effect was unreliable at $P = 0.07$.

For overt naming, lesions in the left motor cortex were related to significantly greater activity in the right motor cortex, $t(36) = 2.91$, $P < 0.01$, while lesions in the left STS were associated with lower activity in right motor cortex, $t(36) = -2.24$, $P < 0.05$ (Figure 4).

We then tested whether right motor cortex over- or underactivation predicted naming performance in people with and without left motor lesions. As with the IFG analysis above, we calculated z-scores for activity in participants with aphasia, centered on the control group mean. For participants in the aphasia group with intact left motor cortex ($N = 15$), there was no relationship between right motor activity and naming, $t(12) = -0.28$, $P = 0.75$. However, for participants with left motor lesions ($N = 24$), right motor activity was positively associated with naming, $t(21) = 3.67$, $P = 0.001$.

4. General Discussion

This study addressed the relationship between stroke distribution and naming activity in chronic left hemisphere stroke survivors. Specifically, we examined whether overall size of the lesion, and damage of different nodes in the normal naming network, results in different patterns of brain activity. The analysis approach allowed us to test several current hypotheses regarding poststroke plasticity in language networks. Overall, the results support the prevalent notion that larger strokes result in greater usage of right hemisphere areas and further demonstrate that damage to different left hemisphere language nodes results in different patterns of activity in surviving nodes. The specific results, however, present challenges for the interhemispheric inhibition model and suggest that other mechanisms of behavioral and biological plasticity might better account for the data.

4.1. Residual Left Hemisphere Language Activity and Perilesional Recruitment.

A striking finding from the overall group analysis was a failure of people with aphasia to activate normal left hemisphere brain areas associated with speech production, including the ventral sensorimotor cortex and the superior temporal cortex [38], during overt naming. These areas were robustly activated by the control group but not the group with aphasia, a difference confirmed in the direct between-group comparison. This finding cannot be related to direct lesion damage to these areas, as lesioned voxels were excluded from the analysis on a person-by-person basis. Rather, this pattern suggests a failure to activate spared left hemisphere speech production areas due to lesions elsewhere in the network. This explanation was not clearly supported by the ROI analysis, however, in which lesions in left hemisphere overt naming nodes did not relate to decreased activity in other spared left hemisphere nodes. Of note, because the ROIs were based on peak locations of activity in the control group, they were all located in the grey matter. It is possible the decreased activity observed in normal left hemisphere speech areas was primarily driven by

TABLE 5: Regions of interest drawn from the contrasts in the control group.

Contrast	Control group peak	x	y	z	Label	Subjects in aphasia group with lesions at ROI (out of 39 in total)
Covert > fixation	6.61	−30	−60	48	Left IPS	11
Covert > fixation	6.48	−36	20	−4	Left insula	18
Covert > fixation	6.38	−50	28	24	Left dorsal POp	16
Covert > fixation	6.91	30	−66	54	Right IPS	—
Covert > fixation	6.56	38	22	−8	Right insula	—
Overt > fixation	7.77	−50	−12	26	Left motor cortex/central sulcus	24
Overt > fixation	6.18	−64	−42	6	Left posterior STS	20
Overt > fixation	7.12	52	−10	26	Right motor Cortex/central sulcus	—
Overt > fixation	6.4	68	−28	2	Right posterior STS	—

TABLE 6: Areas where decreased activity was related to lesions in the left frontal lobe ROIs.

Lesion status ROI	Peak z-value	x	y	z	Label
Insula	−3.8	30	10	18	Right subcortical IFG
Insula	−3.6	46	22	32	Right superior frontal gyrus
Insula	−3.6	44	30	14	Right dorsal POp
Opercularis	−3.8	42	26	16	Right dorsal POp
Opercularis	−3.7	30	10	18	Right subcortical IFG
Opercularis	−3.2	48	26	30	Right superior frontal gyrus

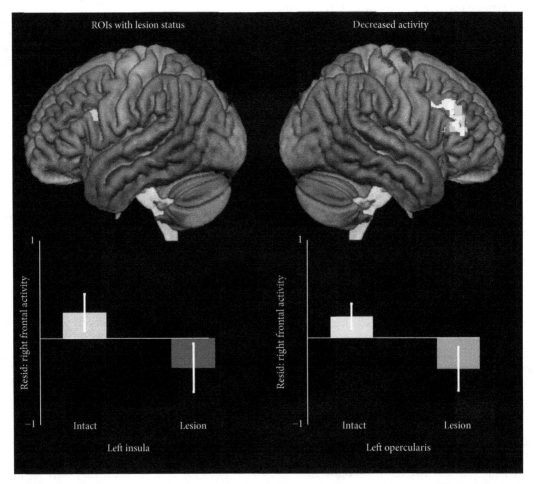

FIGURE 3: Lesions in the left insula and left opercularis were associated with less activity in the right middle frontal gyrus and right pars triangularis. Bar graphs show activity level in the right ROIs relative to the control sample, controlling for lesion volume.

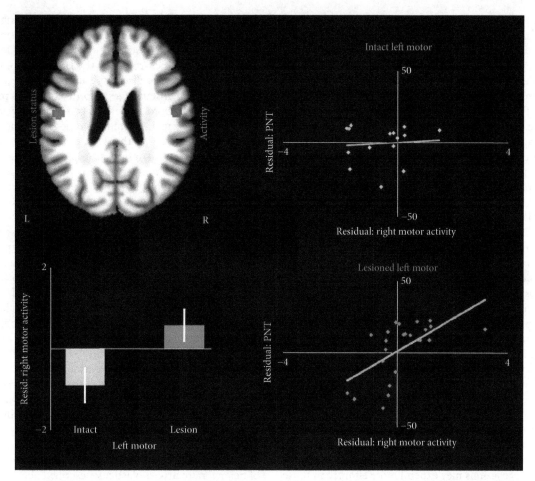

FIGURE 4: Lesions in the left motor cortex were associated with greater activity in the right motor cortex. The bar graph shows activity level in the right motor ROI relative to controls, controlling for lesion volume. Scatter plots show the relationship between activity and performance on the PNT, controlling for lesion volume, in the intact left motor group and in the group with lesions in left motor cortex.

disconnection from other network nodes due to white matter damage, which was not examined here. Regardless, the failure to activate normal left hemisphere areas involved in naming begs the question of whether and where compensation might be occurring in spared brain areas.

One prominent idea regarding poststroke language network plasticity proposes that left hemisphere perilesional areas surrounding the stroke that were previously involved in other functions are recruited into the language network to compensate for loss of language nodes [8]. In our voxelwise analysis, we found only weak evidence for these effects, with small areas of increased activity relative to controls in left dorsal frontal cortex during overt naming. We note that the analysis may not have been sensitive to these effects due to variability in stroke distributions. In the more sensitive ROI analysis, we found that lesions in the left insula were associated with marginally higher covert naming activity levels in the left dorsal POp, but this effect was weak and difficult to interpret given how few of our participants had one of these nodes lesioned and the other intact. Overall, this study provides little evidence either for or against perilesional compensation.

4.2. Lesion Size and Right Hemisphere Recruitment.
Another prominent mode of proposed reorganization after stroke is the recruitment of homotopic areas in the right hemisphere. It has frequently been suggested that overall lesion size in the left hemisphere may relate to right hemisphere recruitment [7, 28, 29]. This proposed relationship is sometimes based on the interhemispheric inhibition model, even though a relationship between lesion size and contralesional recruitment is not supported by animal models, in which small sensorimotor lesions result in an increase in synaptogenesis and astrocytic volume contralateral to the stroke, while large lesions result in decreases in both of these measures, likely due to denervation-induced atrophy [37]. Alternatively, the proposed relationship between lesion size and right hemisphere engagement is sometimes based on the logical argument that people with relatively small lesions have sufficient viable left hemisphere tissue to support language and may not require right hemisphere compensation, whereas people with large lesions have little viable left hemisphere tissue and must rely on the right hemisphere to a greater extent. Although a positive relationship between lesion size and right hemisphere recruitment is frequently discussed

in the literature, there is surprisingly little direct empirical evidence of this relationship. One prior study examined the laterality indices of eight people with aphasia and found that large lesions were associated with greater right than left hemisphere activation during picture naming but not during a semantic decision task [17]. Here, we present strong support for this effect in both covert and overt naming in a large sample. Participants with larger lesions showed greater activity in right hemisphere areas homotopic to the normal left hemisphere language network. Notably, for overt naming, the specific pattern of activity related to lesion size in the right hemisphere (Figure 2(b)) closely mirrored the pattern of decreased activity relative to controls in the left hemisphere (Figure 1(c)).

The mechanisms underlying the increased activation of the right hemisphere in people with large lesions are unclear. This effect may not reflect plasticity at all but rather the increased effort required for language tasks by people with larger lesions. It is not unusual for more difficult tasks to elicit greater activity throughout the brain, including homotopic right hemisphere areas for language tasks [23]. Participants with large lesions likely exert greater effort in retrieving and producing the names of items and thus show overactivation during the task. Notably, activity in the bilateral visual cortex was also related to lesion size during both covert and overt naming here, suggesting that greater activity in general may be related to greater effort and longer looking times. Like other recent studies, we restricted our analysis to correct trials only in part to minimize these effort effects. However, even when producing a correct naming response, it is likely the people with large lesions may expend more effort than those with small lesions.

Similarly, it has recently been proposed that some right hemisphere overactivation observed in aphasia could be explained by recruitment of domain general attentional systems [39, 40] rather than language system reorganization per se. As above, the right hemisphere activity may similarly relate to the overall greater difficulty of language tasks for people with aphasia, although, under this hypothesis, the right hemisphere activity does not contribute to computations specific to language at all. Although this may explain part of the effect, we think it is unlikely to explain all right hemisphere overactivation in aphasia, given evidence here and elsewhere that activation of some right hemisphere nodes relates to the location of damage in the left and that the tasks that activate specific right hemisphere nodes are the same as those that activate the homotopic left hemisphere nodes in healthy controls [4].

Alternatively, explicit or implicit strategies used to compensate for deficits may result in recruitment of brain networks not used by healthy controls for language tasks, including the right hemisphere. As in the proposed overreliance on domain general systems, activity related to use of these strategies during scanning would not reflect any true plasticity in the language network. However, ultimately, reliance on domain general resources or alternate strategies in the long term could reinforce new neuronal connections and result in permanent neuroplastic changes in the network. In this case, differential activity could be observed even if the person does not actively use any alternate strategies during scanning. Melodic intonation therapy provides a clear example of an explicit compensatory strategy that can induce long lasting changes in network structure [41]. However, compensatory strategies need not be directly related to specific therapeutic experiences. For instance, a person who fails to retrieve the phonology of a word may attempt to visualize its spelling without any therapeutic training to do so. Changes in brain organization related to these type of strategic shifts may or may not relate to lesion size and location. For example, compensatory strategies involving pragmatic aspects of language or alternate forms of communication might be most used by people with large lesions and severe aphasia, potentially resulting in a relationship between lesion size and remodeling in brain areas involved in these functions. In the example of melodic intonation therapy, people with large frontal lesions causing nonfluent aphasias are most likely to receive this type of treatment [42], so this bias in exposure to intonation-based treatment could result in a relationship between left frontal strokes and right hemisphere changes that are behaviorally, rather than neurobiologically, driven. Spontaneous strategies such as mental visualization of word spellings could similarly relate to lesion location, assuming specific stroke distributions give rise to a pattern of deficits and preserved abilities that make these strategies advantageous. Importantly, however, reorganization related to strategic shifts should not necessarily occur in areas that are homotopic to the lesion.

4.3. Remapping in Homotopic Nodes. In contrast to the types of behaviorally driven plasticity described above, some neuroplasticity after stroke may occur as a direct biological result of the stroke itself. The interhemispheric inhibition model is the most prominent theory of biologically driven plasticity in the intact hemisphere after stroke. One prediction of this model is that remapping into the right hemisphere in aphasia should be homotopic to the lesion and not only driven by an overall lack of remaining left hemisphere tissue. A second predication is that as right hemisphere regions inhibit the remaining left hemisphere tissue, activity in the right should be associated with worse performance.

Contrary to this hypothesis, we found that lesions in the left POp and insula led to robustly decreased covert naming activity in the right PTr and in the MFG just dorsal to the POp, even when controlling for lesion volume. Furthermore, activity in this right frontal region was not related to naming ability. This finding also stands in contrast to a recent meta-analysis showing, across many studies using various language tasks, people with left IFG lesions were more likely to activate the right IFG [4]. There are several possible explanations for this discrepancy. First, the right hemisphere activity here is not perfectly homotopic with the lesioned nodes, although the difference in location, compared to the dorsal POp node, is very small. Second, we did not account for the proportion of the region affected by stroke. Greater right IFG activity might be more likely in people with a greater proportion of the left IFG damaged, while we treated all participants with lesions at the left insula (or POp) site as one group. However, a recent study using a semantic task found no relationship between proportion of intact left IFG and right IFG activity [43], and as noted above, the animal literature shows that larger lesions can be associated with atrophy of contralateral cortex, rather than enhanced plasticity [44], corresponding with our findings here. Second, our study controlled for total lesion volume, which is rarely done in fMRI studies of aphasia, particularly in case studies or case series with few participants. It is likely that increased right IFG activity in prior studies is related to large lesions that include the left IFG and not specifically to lesions in the left IFG themselves. In support of this explanation, Figure 2 demonstrates that increased total lesion volume is associated with increased right IFG activity, among other areas. Finally, our study excluded participants with severe anomia, who could not correctly name at least 10% of the trials in the scanner. Other studies involving more severe patients, especially those that do not isolate activity related exclusively to correct trials, might reasonably produce a different result in the IFG. Therefore, questions for future study include whether homotopic remapping in the inferior frontal lobes is more likely in people with more severe aphasia and is related primarily to erroneous responses, as has previously been suggested in a small case series [20].

We did find evidence for homotopic remapping in motor cortex, in that left motor cortex lesions led to significantly greater right motor cortex activation during overt naming, controlling for total lesion volume. However, in contrast to the predictions of the interhemispheric inhibition model, overactivation of right motor cortex was associated with better naming performance in people with left motor lesions. These results join a growing body of literature suggesting that the right hemisphere may play a largely compensatory role, even in chronic stages of aphasia. Evidence for this begins in neuropsychological case studies, which have identified people who had recovered at least partially from aphasia following left hemisphere stroke and then redeveloped aphasia after a later right hemisphere disruption, whether due to intracarotid amobarbital injection or a second stroke [45–48]. These studies suggest that the right hemisphere can, to some degree, take over the language functions that the left hemisphere can no longer perform. A recent structural study found that greater grey matter volume in the right temporoparietal cortex related to better language production outcomes in chronic aphasia [49]. Other neuroimaging studies have shown positive relationships between right hemisphere activation and various language outcomes, supporting right hemisphere compensation [50–52]. Based on performance decrements after inhibitory TMS, other studies have also suggested that right hemisphere areas may be involved to some degree in phonology and naming in healthy people [53, 54]. Damage to left hemisphere language nodes may thus result in increased reliance on these right hemisphere language processors [55]. However, this explanation cannot account for the effects observed here, since the activity in right motor cortex related to naming performance only in people with left motor cortex lesions. This pattern strongly suggests a true compensatory relationship in which the right hemisphere node "takes over" for the corresponding lesioned left hemisphere area and demonstrates that specific biological mechanisms of plasticity beyond the interhemispheric inhibition model must be considered.

4.4. Alternate Biological Mechanisms of Right Hemisphere Recruitment. If not interhemispheric inhibition, what biological mechanism might explain recruitment of a homotopic node in the right hemisphere? The first possibility is that the interhemispheric inhibition hypothesis may be partially correct. It is possible that right hemisphere homotopic recruitment does result from transcallosal disinhibition but that this overactivation does not significantly suppress the surviving left hemisphere tissue. Behaviorally important right-to-left inhibition may simply never occur in language systems, may be restricted to particular areas such as the PTr, or may occur only in the case of relatively small lesions with some nearly homotopic left hemisphere tissue remaining to be inhibited [7].

However, other biological mechanisms might better explain compensatory recruitment of homotopic areas in the spared hemisphere after stroke. It has previously been noted that right hemisphere activity is maximal several weeks after a stroke causing aphasia [17]. If this activity resulted from direct disinhibition, the right hemisphere activity should occur immediately after the stroke. This kind of immediate right hemisphere recruitment has been observed after TMS-induced transient lesions [55, 56], but not after stroke. The gradual development of right hemisphere activation after stroke instead suggests a slower process, possibly relying on structural plasticity rather than a direct electrophysiological effect.

We suggest that axonal collateral sprouting from surviving neurons may provide an alternative neurobiological mechanism to explain both perilesional left hemisphere and homotopic right hemisphere recruitment in aphasia. This model is based on the principle that if two neurons send axons to the same target, they compete for synapses at the target. If one neuron dies, its axon degenerates and the surviving neuron's axon sprouts new collaterals near the target to take over empty synapses. Axonal collateral sprouting is observed throughout the central and peripheral nervous systems, for instance, in the development of ocular dominance columns and the delineation of motor units at the neuromuscular junction. It is known to play a role in reorganization after spinal cord injury [57] and brain injury, including stroke [58]. Competition has been shown to guide axonal sprouting in the sensory-motor spinal circuits in adult rats [59], and unbalanced endogenous activity dramatically affects receptor targeting in tracts crossing the corpus callosum [60]. Although not the only mechanism that can explain "take over" of prior functions by new brain areas, axonal collateral sprouting has previously been demonstrated to account for this phenomenon. For example, when dorsal route fibers to the hippocampus are destroyed in rats, ventral route fibers take over these connections over a period of months resulting in ultimate recovery of innervation patterns [61]. Further, axonal collateral sprouting is altered by the experience of the organism [62], providing a specific biological mechanism for function and neuroanatomic changes induced by speech-language therapy in people with aphasia.

Under this hypothesis, spared brain regions that share axonal targets with the lesioned tissue are the most likely to be recruited after stroke. This suggests that areas engaged to compensate might be predictable based on coconnectivity patterns before the stroke. Neighboring neurons are likely to share axonal targets, thus providing a basis for perilesional recruitment in the case of relatively small lesions. In some cases, such as motor areas innervating proximal limb muscles and the tongue, the homotopic cortex in the intact hemisphere likely shares axonal projection targets with the lesioned neurons and can take over the lost synapses, resulting in functional recovery [63, 64].

Our findings were near the mouth areas of motor cortex, and this mechanism might explain our findings of right hemisphere mouth-area motor recruitment during overt but not covert naming, corresponding with better naming performance specifically when the left hemisphere mouth area of motor cortex is lesioned. However, motor cortex has also been shown in other neuroimaging studies to play a role in covert naming and prearticulatory processes [65]. Furthermore, Geranmayeh and colleagues have argued that, regardless of the role of motor cortex in healthy people, upregulation of the region in people with aphasia is a marker of increased demands on domain general systems such as cognitive control and attention [66], and the relationship between activity and recovery is more related to those processes than anything language specific. It is possible that the diverse, nonspecific role of the motor cortex in speech production may also prime it to be uniquely plastic and available for taking over cognitive function through axonal sprouting, when the homotopic region is lesioned.

Regardless of the specific role of each region, the broader pattern of right hemisphere recruitment may result from a cascading effect from one homotopic right hemisphere node taking over synapses from its left hemisphere counterpart at a shared axonal target. When this node takes over the function of the lesioned left hemisphere node, the entire right hemisphere network connected to this one node may become involved in compensation, at least to a degree, resulting in broad patterns of increased activity. Alternatively, homotopic areas of each hemisphere's association cortices may share common cortical and subcortical axonal projection targets, and synaptic competition may account directly for broad patterns of right hemisphere recruitment. Modern connectomics may help to test these ideas. If supported by additional data, this hypothesis may provide clear predictions regarding the availability and location of alternate processing nodes based on the specific anatomical structures damaged by an individual's stroke.

4.5. Limitations and Future Directions. One unexpected finding was that while both people with aphasia and controls showed widespread activity during both covert and overt naming, the differences between the two groups was more widespread during overt naming. Most strikingly, the temporal lobe, in particular the STS and STG, was not significantly active in either group during covert naming. The posterior STS and STG are involved in phonological processes, which can include phonological retrieval [67],

verbal working memory [68], and a sensorimotor speech interface for speech productions [69], so it was expected to be active during the covert naming phase of the experiment. In our experiment, however, no response was collected during the covert naming phase. If a trial was answered incorrectly during overt naming, both the covert and overt naming phases were removed from analysis. But, we do not have any measurable evidence of what was occurring for each participant during the covert naming phase. It is possible that some participants were less engaged in the task and only really attempted to name the object when cued to make an overt response and thus did not activate articulatory regions during the covert naming phase. In general, the use of a low-level control condition in the fMRI task allowed us to identify activity for word retrieval and production broadly but prohibited a detailed accounting of the precise nature of the processing in any given area of activity.

In this study, we identified regions where plasticity was dependent on the site of the lesion in left frontal and motor tissue. However, it remains unclear whether these relationships are mediated by the degree to which critical areas for naming are damaged or preserved. The language network in the left hemisphere involves many regions which are critical for different aspects of language. The degree to which a critical area for naming is destroyed by the stroke may determine whether plasticity of naming function is even possible, regardless of the lesion status at other regions of interest such as motor or inferior frontal cortex. A goal of future research is to identify regions in which damage has a catastrophic effect on naming ability and then model how damage in these regions affects others in the system, both perilesional and homotopic.

5. Conclusions

In this study we tested three central hypotheses of the interhemispheric inhibition model. We found an overall greater rightward shift of activity dependent on lesion size. Taking this overall effect into account, specific patterns of right hemisphere plasticity depended on the specific location of the stroke. Furthermore, right motor activation was positively associated with naming ability but only in people with left motor lesions. This finding suggests that lesion site needs to be accounted for when considering both the cause of right hemisphere overactivation and the role of right hemisphere activity, in people with aphasia. It is unlikely that any single biological mechanism explains all aspects of poststroke reorganization, and as noted above, complex interactions between biology and the environment are expected. We suggest that future work on aphasia recovery should be guided by specific behavioral and biological hypotheses that lead to specific experimental predictions for brain imaging and stimulation studies. Interhemispheric inhibition is one such specific biological hypothesis, but it cannot account for the entire range of observed neuroplastic effects in aphasia. The field must begin to entertain equally specific alternate hypotheses, such as synaptic competition, in order to move forward.

Competing Interests

The authors declare that there is no conflict of interests regarding the publication of this paper.

References

[1] P. M. Pedersen, H. S. Jørgensen, H. Nakayama, H. O. Raaschou, and T. S. Olsen, "Aphasia in acute stroke: incidence, determinants, and recovery," *Annals of Neurology*, vol. 38, no. 4, pp. 659–666, 1995.

[2] L. Dickey, A. Kagan, M. P. Lindsay, J. Fang, A. Rowland, and S. Black, "Incidence and profile of inpatient stroke-induced aphasia in Ontario, Canada," *Archives of Physical Medicine and Rehabilitation*, vol. 91, no. 2, pp. 196–202, 2010.

[3] R. F. Gottesman and A. E. Hillis, "Predictors and assessment of cognitive dysfunction resulting from ischaemic stroke," *The Lancet Neurology*, vol. 9, no. 9, pp. 895–905, 2010.

[4] P. E. Turkeltaub, S. Messing, C. Norise, and R. H. Hamilton, "Are networks for residual language function and recovery consistent across aphasic patients?" *Neurology*, vol. 76, no. 20, pp. 1726–1734, 2011.

[5] W.-D. Heiss, A. Thiel, J. Kessler, and K. Herholz, "Disturbance and recovery of language function: correlates in PET activation studies," *NeuroImage*, vol. 20, supplement 1, pp. S42–S49, 2003.

[6] M. Meinzer and C. Breitenstein, "Functional imaging studies of treatment-induced recovery in chronic aphasia," *Aphasiology*, vol. 22, no. 12, pp. 1251–1268, 2008.

[7] C. Anglade, A. Thiel, and A. I. Ansaldo, "The complementary role of the cerebral hemispheres in recovery from aphasia after stroke: a critical review of literature," *Brain Injury*, vol. 28, no. 2, pp. 138–145, 2014.

[8] J. Fridriksson, L. Bonilha, J. M. Baker, D. Moser, and C. Rorden, "Activity in preserved left hemisphere regions predicts anomia severity in aphasia," *Cerebral Cortex*, vol. 20, no. 5, pp. 1013–1019, 2010.

[9] P. E. Turkeltaub, "Brain stimulation and the role of the right hemisphere in aphasia recovery," *Current Neurology and Neuroscience Reports*, vol. 15, no. 11, article 72, pp. 1–9, 2015.

[10] M. A. Naeser, P. I. Martin, M. Nicholas et al., "Improved picture naming in chronic aphasia after TMS to part of right Broca's area: an open-protocol study," *Brain and Language*, vol. 93, no. 1, pp. 95–105, 2005.

[11] L. Winhuisen, A. Thiel, B. Schumacher et al., "Role of the contralateral inferior frontal gyrus in recovery of language function in poststroke aphasia: a combined repetitive transcranial magnetic stimulation and positron emission tomography study," *Stroke*, vol. 36, no. 8, pp. 1759–1763, 2005.

[12] P. I. Martin, M. A. Naeser, M. Ho et al., "Research with transcranial magnetic stimulation in the treatment of aphasia," *Current Neurology and Neuroscience Reports*, vol. 9, no. 6, pp. 451–458, 2009.

[13] C. H. S. Barwood, B. E. Murdoch, B.-M. Whelan et al., "Improved language performance subsequent to low-frequency rTMS in patients with chronic non-fluent aphasia post-stroke," *European Journal of Neurology*, vol. 18, no. 7, pp. 935–943, 2011.

[14] R. H. Hamilton, E. G. Chrysikou, and B. Coslett, "Mechanisms of aphasia recovery after stroke and the role of noninvasive brain stimulation," *Brain and Language*, vol. 118, no. 1-2, pp. 40–50, 2011.

[15] C.-L. Ren, G.-F. Zhang, N. Xia et al., "Effect of low-frequency rTMS on aphasia in stroke patients: a meta-analysis of randomized controlled trials," *PLOS ONE*, vol. 9, no. 7, Article ID e102557, 2014.

[16] B. Fernandez, D. Cardebat, J.-F. Demonet et al., "Functional MRI follow-up study of language processes in healthy subjects and during recovery in a case of aphasia," *Stroke*, vol. 35, no. 9, pp. 2171–2176, 2004.

[17] D. Saur, R. Lange, A. Baumgaertner et al., "Dynamics of language reorganization after stroke," *Brain*, vol. 129, no. 6, pp. 1371–1384, 2006.

[18] J. Kurland, C. R. Cortes, M. Wilke et al., "Neural mechanisms underlying learning following semantic mediation treatment in a case of phonologic alexia," *Brain Imaging and Behavior*, vol. 2, no. 3, pp. 147–162, 2008.

[19] J. I. Breier, J. Juranek, L. M. Maher, S. Schmadeke, D. Men, and A. C. Papanicolaou, "Behavioral and neurophysiologic response to therapy for chronic aphasia," *Archives of Physical Medicine and Rehabilitation*, vol. 90, no. 12, pp. 2026–2033, 2009.

[20] W. A. Postman-Caucheteux, R. M. Birn, R. H. Pursley et al., "Single-trial fMRI shows contralesional activity linked to overt naming errors in chronic aphasic patients," *Journal of Cognitive Neuroscience*, vol. 22, no. 6, pp. 1299–1318, 2010.

[21] Y. Cao, E. M. Vikingstad, K. P. George, A. F. Johnson, and K. M. A. Welch, "Cortical language activation in stroke patients recovering from aphasia with functional MRI," *Stroke*, vol. 30, no. 11, pp. 2331–2340, 1999.

[22] P. Adank, "The neural bases of difficult speech comprehension and speech production: two activation likelihood estimation (ALE) meta-analyses," *Brain and Language*, vol. 122, no. 1, pp. 42–54, 2012.

[23] M. A. Just, P. A. Carpenter, T. A. Keller, W. F. Eddy, and K. R. Thulborn, "Brain activation modulated by sentence comprehension," *Science*, vol. 274, no. 5284, pp. 114–116, 1996.

[24] R. Sebastian and S. Kiran, "Task-modulated neural activation patterns in chronic stroke patients with aphasia," *Aphasiology*, vol. 25, no. 8, pp. 927–951, 2011.

[25] W.-D. Heiss, "Imaging effects related to language improvements by rTMS," *Restorative Neurology and Neuroscience*, vol. 34, no. 4, pp. 531–536, 2016.

[26] N. Murase, J. Duque, R. Mazzocchio, and L. G. Cohen, "Influence of interhemispheric interactions on motor function in chronic stroke," *Annals of Neurology*, vol. 55, no. 3, pp. 400–409, 2004.

[27] J. Duque, F. Hummel, P. Celnik, N. Murase, R. Mazzocchio, and L. G. Cohen, "Transcallosal inhibition in chronic subcortical stroke," *NeuroImage*, vol. 28, no. 4, pp. 940–946, 2005.

[28] W.-D. Heiss, J. Kessler, A. Thiel, M. Ghaemi, and H. Karbe, "Differential capacity of left and right hemispheric areas for compensation of poststroke aphasia," *Annals of Neurology*, vol. 45, no. 4, pp. 430–438, 1999.

[29] E. G. Chrysikou and R. H. Hamilton, "Noninvasive brain stimulation in the treatment of aphasia: exploring interhemispheric relationships and their implications for neurorehabilitation," *Restorative Neurology and Neuroscience*, vol. 29, no. 6, pp. 375–394, 2011.

[30] H. Karbe, J. Kessler, K. Herholz, G. R. Fink, and W.-D. Heiss, "Long-term prognosis of poststroke aphasia studied with positron emission tomography," *Archives of Neurology*, vol. 52, no. 2, pp. 186–190, 1995.

[31] M. Goldrick and B. Rapp, "Lexical and post-lexical phonological representations in spoken production," *Cognition*, vol. 102, no. 2, pp. 219–260, 2007.

[32] G. Hickok and D. Poeppel, "The cortical organization of speech processing," *Nature Reviews Neuroscience*, vol. 8, no. 5, pp. 393–402, 2007.

[33] S. Kemeny, J. Xu, G. H. Park, L. A. Hosey, C. M. Wettig, and A. R. Braun, "Temporal dissociation of early lexical access and articulation using a delayed naming task—an fMRI study," *Cerebral Cortex*, vol. 16, no. 4, pp. 587–595, 2006.

[34] B. Bonakdarpour, T. B. Parrish, and C. K. Thompson, "Hemodynamic response function in patients with stroke-induced aphasia: implications for fMRI data analysis," *NeuroImage*, vol. 36, no. 2, pp. 322–331, 2007.

[35] A. Roach, M. F. Schwartz, N. Martin, R. S. Grewal, and A. Brecher, "The Philadelphia naming test: scoring and rationale," *Clinical Aphasiology*, vol. 24, pp. 121–133, 1996.

[36] C. Rorden and M. Brett, "Stereotaxic display of brain lesions," *Behavioural Neurology*, vol. 12, no. 4, pp. 191–200, 2000.

[37] M. Jenkinson, C. F. Beckmann, T. E. J. Behrens, M. W. Woolrich, and S. M. Smith, "FSL," *NeuroImage*, vol. 62, no. 2, pp. 782–790, 2012.

[38] S. Brown, A. R. Laird, P. Q. Pfordresher, S. M. Thelen, P. Turkeltaub, and M. Liotti, "The somatotopy of speech: phonation and articulation in the human motor cortex," *Brain and Cognition*, vol. 70, no. 1, pp. 31–41, 2009.

[39] F. Geranmayeh, R. J. S. Wise, A. Mehta, and R. Leech, "Overlapping networks engaged during spoken language production and its cognitive control," *The Journal of Neuroscience*, vol. 34, no. 26, pp. 8728–8740, 2014.

[40] C. A. M. M. van Oers, M. Vink, M. J. E. van Zandvoort et al., "Contribution of the left and right inferior frontal gyrus in recovery from aphasia. A functional MRI study in stroke patients with preserved hemodynamic responsiveness," *NeuroImage*, vol. 49, no. 1, pp. 885–893, 2010.

[41] C. Y. Wan, X. Zheng, S. Marchina, A. Norton, and G. Schlaug, "Intensive therapy induces contralateral white matter changes in chronic stroke patients with Broca's aphasia," *Brain and Language*, vol. 136, pp. 1–7, 2014.

[42] A. Norton, L. Zipse, S. Marchina, and G. Schlaug, "Melodic intonation therapy: shared insights on how it is done and why it might help," *Annals of the New York Academy of Sciences*, vol. 1169, pp. 431–436, 2009.

[43] J. A. Sims, K. Kapse, P. Glynn, C. Sandberg, Y. Tripodis, and S. Kiran, "The relationships between the amount of spared tissue, percent signal change, and accuracy in semantic processing in aphasia," *Neuropsychologia*, vol. 84, pp. 113–126, 2016.

[44] S. Y. Kim and T. A. Jones, "Lesion size-dependent synaptic and astrocytic responses in cortex contralateral to infarcts in middle-aged rats," *Synapse*, vol. 64, no. 9, pp. 659–671, 2010.

[45] T. Barlow, "On a Case of Double Hemiplegia, with Cerebral Symmetrical Lesions," *BMJ*, vol. 2, no. 865, pp. 103–104, 1877.

[46] M. Kinsbourne, "The minor cerebral hemisphere as a source of aphasic speech," *Archives of Neurology*, vol. 25, no. 4, pp. 302–306, 1971.

[47] A. Basso, M. Gardelli, M. P. Grassi, and M. Mariotti, "The role of the right hemisphere in recovery from aphasia. Two case studies," *Cortex*, vol. 25, no. 4, pp. 555–566, 1989.

[48] P. E. Turkeltaub, H. B. Coslett, A. L. Thomas et al., "The right hemisphere is not unitary in its role in aphasia recovery," *Cortex*, vol. 48, no. 9, pp. 1179–1186, 2012.

[49] S. Xing, E. H. Lacey, L. M. Skipper-Kallal et al., "Right hemisphere grey matter structure and language outcomes in chronic left hemisphere stroke," *Brain*, vol. 139, no. 1, pp. 227–241, 2016.

[50] B. T. Gold and A. Kertesz, "Right hemisphere semantic processing of visual words in an aphasic patient: an fMRI study," *Brain and Language*, vol. 73, no. 3, pp. 456–465, 2000.

[51] O. Elkana, R. Frost, U. Kramer, D. Ben-Bashat, and A. Schweiger, "Cerebral language reorganization in the chronic stage of recovery: a longitudinal fMRI study," *Cortex*, vol. 49, no. 1, pp. 71–81, 2013.

[52] S. Teki, G. R. Barnes, W. D. Penny et al., "The right hemisphere supports but does not replace left hemisphere auditory function in patients with persisting aphasia," *Brain*, vol. 136, no. 6, pp. 1901–1912, 2013.

[53] N. Sollmann, N. Tanigawa, F. Ringel, C. Zimmer, B. Meyer, and S. M. Krieg, "Language and its right-hemispheric distribution in healthy brains: an investigation by repetitive transcranial magnetic stimulation," *NeuroImage*, vol. 102, no. 2, pp. 776–788, 2014.

[54] G. Hartwigsen, A. Baumgaertner, C. J. Price, M. Koehnke, S. Ulmer, and H. R. Siebner, "Phonological decisions require both the left and right supramarginal gyri," *Proceedings of the National Academy of Sciences of the United States of America*, vol. 107, no. 38, pp. 16494–16499, 2010.

[55] G. Hartwigsen, D. Saur, C. J. Price, S. Ulmer, A. Baumgaertner, and H. R. Siebner, "Perturbation of the left inferior frontal gyrus triggers adaptive plasticity in the right homologous area during speech production," *Proceedings of the National Academy of Sciences of the United States of America*, vol. 110, no. 41, pp. 16402–16407, 2013.

[56] A. Thiel, B. Schumacher, K. Wienhard et al., "Direct demonstration of transcallosal disinhibition in language networks," *Journal of Cerebral Blood Flow and Metabolism*, vol. 26, no. 9, pp. 1122–1127, 2006.

[57] O. Raineteau and M. E. Schwab, "Plasticity of motor systems after incomplete spinal cord injury," *Nature Reviews Neuroscience*, vol. 2, no. 4, pp. 263–273, 2001.

[58] F. J. Sell, "Recovery and repair issues after stroke from the scientific perspective," *Current Opinion in Neurology*, vol. 10, no. 1, pp. 49–51, 1997.

[59] Y.-Q. Jiang, B. Zaaimi, and J. H. Martin, "Competition with primary sensory afferents drives remodeling of corticospinal axons in mature spinal motor circuits," *The Journal of Neuroscience*, vol. 36, no. 1, pp. 193–203, 2016.

[60] R. Suárez, L. R. Fenlon, R. Marek et al., "Balanced interhemispheric cortical activity is required for correct targeting of the corpus callosum," *Neuron*, vol. 82, no. 6, pp. 1289–1298, 2014.

[61] F. H. Gage, A. Björklund, and U. Stenevi, "Reinnervation of the partially deafferented hippocampus by compensatory collateral sprouting from spared cholinergic and noradrenergic afferents," *Brain Research*, vol. 268, no. 1, pp. 27–37, 1983.

[62] L. I. Benowitz and S. T. Carmichael, "Promoting axonal rewiring to improve outcome after stroke," *Neurobiology of Disease*, vol. 37, no. 2, pp. 259–266, 2010.

[63] L. V. Bradnam, C. M. Stinear, P. A. Barber, and W. D. Byblow, "Contralesional hemisphere control of the proximal paretic upper limb following stroke," *Cerebral Cortex*, vol. 22, no. 11, pp. 2662–2671, 2012.

[64] W. Muellbacher, C. Artner, and B. Mamoli, "The role of the intact hemisphere in recovery of midline muscles after recent monohemispheric stroke," *Journal of Neurology*, vol. 246, no. 4, pp. 250–256, 1999.

[65] C. J. Price, "A review and synthesis of the first 20years of PET and fMRI studies of heard speech, spoken language and reading," *NeuroImage*, vol. 62, no. 2, pp. 816–847, 2012.

[66] F. Geranmayeh, S. L. E. Brownsett, and R. J. S. Wise, "Task-induced brain activity in aphasic stroke patients: what is driving recovery?" *Brain: A Journal of Neurology*, vol. 137, no. 10, pp. 2632–2648, 2014.

[67] W. W. Graves, T. J. Grabowski, S. Mehta, and J. K. Gordon, "A neural signature of phonological access: distinguishing the effects of word frequency from familiarity and length in overt picture naming," *Journal of Cognitive Neuroscience*, vol. 19, no. 4, pp. 617–631, 2007.

[68] A. P. Leff, T. M. Schofield, J. T. Crinion et al., "The left superior temporal gyrus is a shared substrate for auditory short-term memory and speech comprehension: evidence from 210 patients with stroke," *Brain*, vol. 132, no. 12, pp. 3401–3410, 2009.

[69] B. R. Buchsbaum, J. Baldo, K. Okada et al., "Conduction aphasia, sensory-motor integration, and phonological short-term memory—an aggregate analysis of lesion and fMRI data," *Brain & Language*, vol. 119, no. 3, pp. 119–128, 2011.

13

Creutzfeldt-Jakob Disease Presenting as Expressive Aphasia and Nonconvulsive Status Epilepticus

Hafiz B. Mahboob ⓘ,[1,2] **Kazi H. Kaokaf,**[1,2] **and Jeremy M. Gonda**[1,2]

[1]*University of Nevada School of Medicine, Reno, NV, USA*
[2]*Renown Regional Medical Center, Reno, NV, USA*

Correspondence should be addressed to Hafiz B. Mahboob; hmahboob@medicine.nevada.edu

Academic Editor: Petros Kopterides

Creutzfeldt-Jakob disease (CJD), the most common form of human prion diseases, is a fatal condition with a mortality rate reaching 85% within one year of clinical presentation. CJD is characterized by rapidly progressive neurological deterioration in combination with typical electroencephalography (EEG) and magnetic resonance imaging (MRI) findings and positive cerebrospinal spinal fluid (CSF) analysis for 14-3-3 proteins. Unfortunately, CJD can have atypical clinical and radiological presentation in approximately 10% of cases, thus making the diagnosis often challenging. We report a rare clinical presentation of sporadic CJD (sCJD) with combination of both expressive aphasia and nonconvulsive status epilepticus. This patient presented with slurred speech, confusion, myoclonus, headaches, and vertigo and succumbed to his disease within ten weeks of initial onset of his symptoms. He had a normal initial diagnostic workup, but subsequent workup initiated due to persistent clinical deterioration revealed CJD with typical MRI, EEG, and CSF findings. Other causes of rapidly progressive dementia and encephalopathy were ruled out. Though a rare condition, we recommend consideration of CJD on patients with expressive aphasia, progressive unexplained neurocognitive decline, and refractory epileptiform activity seen on EEG. Frequent reimaging (MRI, video EEGs) and CSF examination might help diagnose this fatal condition earlier.

1. Introduction

We report a rare clinical presentation of sporadic CJD (sCJD) with combination of both expressive aphasia and NCSE. Isolated language problems and aphasia have been described in CJD before [1–8]; however, this combination is unique. This patient had an atypical clinical presentation with normal initial workup, but subsequent workup revealed CJD with typical EEG finding of spike-wave complexes (PSWCs) as well as hyperintensities in basal ganglia and cortical ribboning on MRI and positive CSF analysis for 14-3-3 proteins. Due to the extremely high mortality rate and often atypical clinical presentation and/or inconclusive initial workup, a high degree of suspicion and thus repeating workup might aid in early diagnose of this fatal condition.

2. Case Report

A 60-year-old male with a past medical history significant only for benign prostatic hyperplasia presented to our Emergency Department (ED) with chief complaints of gradual onset of progressively worsening speech difficulty (predominantly word finding with stuttering) and confusion (inability to recognize his family members).

His symptoms started four weeks priorly, beginning with constitutional symptoms of headache, fatigue, and vertigo. This slowly led to intermittent confusion, slurred speech, and intermittent spasms of his right upper and lower extremities. His spasms and weakness resulted in a fall from a tractor one week into the course of his symptoms fortunately without significant trauma nor loss of consciousness. His family gave additional potentially relevant information of a recent visit to Mexico where he stayed for four months before returning home. He was asymptomatic upon return to the USA, but symptoms started approximately four weeks later. Interestingly, while in Mexico, he worked in the cattle manure industry which he does locally as well. He was relatively healthy at baseline without any previous surgeries and no family history of diabetes, seizure, dementia, nor neurodegenerative conditions.

He initially visited an urgent care center with these complaints ten days prior to this hospital encounter. At that time, he was found to have a normal neurological examination, brain MRI, and carotid Doppler. He was discharged home with a working diagnosis of transient ischemic attack. His symptoms continued to worsen however, thus motivating him to present to the ED for further evaluation.

Upon arrival to the ED, he complained of photophobia, neck pain, and vertigo but was afebrile. His initial physical examination included vital signs: pulse 85 beats per minute, blood pressure 135/78 mmHg, temperature 98 F, and a respiratory rate of 18 per minute. Initial neurological examination was unremarkable except for persistent word finding difficulty. Initial lab work is summarized in table format (Table 1). A noncontrast head computed tomography (CT) scan was negative for any acute intracranial pathology. Initial CSF analysis was inconclusive for any acute infectious etiology although he had a mildly elevated protein level of 65 mg/dl (Table 2). He was admitted to the neurology unit and diagnosed with a complex migraine and treated with intravenous (IV) ketorolac, sumatriptan, and promethazine. A neurology consult was obtained and an EEG ordered.

Initial EEG on his second hospital day showed focal seizures emanating from the left frontal region (Figure 1(a)) and he was started on oral levetiracetam (loading dose of 1 gram followed by 750 mg PO twice daily thereafter). He started complaining of right upper extremity weakness and on repeat physical exam was found to have diminished deep tendon reflexes of his right upper extremity (RUE) with weakness in pronation and fine motor activity. On hospital day #3, he developed intermittent myoclonic jerking of his RUE with a fine, persistent tremor. At this point intermittent focal seizure activity was thought to be precipitated from his minor head trauma related to his fall. Differential diagnoses, though less likely, included an infectious etiology which was excluded with negative microbiology, a stroke despite a normal MRI, or other common metabolic causes including electrolyte abnormalities, ammonia, toxins, and liver and kidney dysfunction. Medications were also considered which could potentially lower seizure threshold, and tramadol and diphenhydramine were discontinued.

Over the next few days he gradually became drowsier and confused with worsening of his expressive aphasia and development of cerebellar dysfunction on exam. His dose of levetiracetam was increased to 1 gm twice daily. Initial MRI of brain during this hospital encounter was performed which did not show any acute intracranial lesion except mild cerebral and cerebellar substance loss (Figure 2(a)).

His cognition and right upper extremity shaking/tremor rapidly worsened and, on hospital day #4, EEG was significant for persistent focal seizures in left hemisphere despite being on levetiracetam (Figure 1(a)). He was started on lacosamide 200 mg twice daily in addition to the ongoing levetiracetam increased now to 1 gm three times daily. Continuous EEG was started at this point to closer monitor effectiveness of therapies. A repeat MRI brain with contrast on hospital day #5 showed developing cytotoxic edema in the left frontal and

TABLE 1: Laboratory data.

Variable	Value
Microbiology	
CSF	Negative for bacterial growth
	Negative for acid fast bacilli (AFB)
Autoimmune panel serum:	
Microsomal TPO antibody	<0.2 IU/ml
Thyroxine binding globulin	19.3 microgram/ml
Anti-TG Ab	<0.2 IU/ml
HIV 1/2 PCR	None
Lyme	0.07 (Ref: ≤0.99 LIV)
FT Ab	Non-reactive
West Nile Virus (IgM)	None
SSA, 52 (Ro)	1 AU/ml
SSA, 60 (Ro)	1 AU/ml
Sjogren's Ab	0 AU/ml
ANA	None
Cysticercosis Ab, IgG by ELISA	0.0 (Ref: OD ≤ 0.34)
Paraneoplastic antibodies serum:	
ANNA (1–3)	Negative
AGNA-1	Negative
PCA (1-2)	<1 : 240 Negative
PCA-Tr	<1 : 240 Negative
Amphiphysin	<1 : 240 negative
CRMP-% IgG	<1 : 120 Negative
Striational Ab	0.0 nmol/L
P/Q type calcium channel Ab	0.0 nmol/L
	0.0 nmol/L
Ach receptor (muscle binding AB)	0.0 nmol/L
	0.0 nmol/L
Ach receptor (ganglionic neuronal Ab)	0.0 nmol/L
Neuronal (V-G) K+ channel Ab	0.0 nmol/L
Other labs:	
WBC	6.1×10^9/L
Neutrophil	73%
Hemoglobin	15.9 g/dl
Hematocrit	45.3%
Platelets	211×10^9/L
MCV	86 fl
Lymphocyte	30.70%
Eosinophil	1.88%
Polys	62%

TABLE 1: Continued.

Variable	Value
Sodium	136 mEq/L
Potassium	3.5 mEq/L
Chloride	105 mEq/L
Bicarbonate	22 mEq/L
BUN	15 mg/dl
Creatinine	0.79 mg/dl
Anion Gap	9 mEq/L
Vitamin B 12	800 pg/ml
Thyroglobulin	2.0 ng/ml
TSH	4.016 microIU/ml
CRP	0.14 mg/L
AST	22 unit/L
ALT	21 unit/L
ALP	61 unit/L
Calcium	9.6 mg/dl
T-Bili	0.5 mg/dl
Albumin	4.4 g/dl
Total protein	7.5 g/dl

parietal lobe with punctate calcified lesions in right cortex (Figure 2(b)) which was considered likely due to persistent seizure activity. Given the initial CSF result showing elevated proteins (65 mg/dl), ongoing myoclonus, and the newly developed vasogenic edema on MRI, the decision was made by neurology at this point, to start a 3-day course of pulse dose steroids (solumedrol 1 gm IV/daily) for possible autoimmune encephalitis (AE) while awaiting the finalized autoimmune workup [9, 10].

Unfortunately, despite the increasing doses of antiepileptics and the high dose steroids, the patient continued to decline neurologically. Continuous EEG revealed persistent epileptogenic activity with bilateral hemispheric discharges (left > right) (Figure 1(b)). Valproic acid (500 mg orally three times daily) was added to his regimen and lacosamide increased to 200 mg three times daily. His initial CSF (collected on the first hospital day) was sent for oligoclonal bands and infectious encephalopathies which all eventually came back negative (Table 2). Acyclovir was started empirically for possible viral encephalitis but subsequently discontinued two days later when CSF resulted negative.

During the next few days (hospital days nine to eleven) he remained globally aphasic with RUE flaccidity. He would awaken but was unable to follow commands. A repeat MRI showed persistent ribboning in the left hemispheric region (Figure 2(c)) and EEG (Figure 1(c)) showed "diffuse epileptiform discharge suggestive of encephalopathic state with presence of continuous left frontal and sometimes synchronized bifrontal sharps spikes with a more generalized appearance, which was concerning for nonconvulsive status epilepticus." Perampanel was added to his antiseizure regimen at dose of 4 mg twice daily. Efficacy of perampanel has been established as an adjunct treatment for partial-onset seizures with or

without secondary generalization and primary generalized tonic-clonic seizures in idiopathic generalized epilepsy as well as for treatment of refractory seizures. This patient was having refractory seizures; therefore, this medication was added [11].

At this point CJD was considered among other possible etiologies such as paraneoplastic encephalitis, meningeal carcinomatous, infectious cerebritis, and primary CNS angiitis given his continued deterioration and refractory status epilepticus. Computed tomography angiogram (CTA) excluded the primary central nervous system (CNS) angiitis. A repeat lumbar puncture was performed with additional CSF tests ordered including Epstein-Barr virus (EBV), acid fast bacilli (AFB), fungal culture, Zika virus, 14-3-3 protein, neurocysticercosis antibodies, and an autoimmune and paraneoplastic panel.

Eventually phenobarbital (16.2 mg twice daily) was started yet he continued to deteriorate remaining aphasic with flaccid paralysis in RUE and lost his ability to protect his airway requiring intubation on hospital day #11. His EEG remained without any significant improvement. On hospital day #13, while awaiting results from his repeat CSF analysis, neurology felt it was prudent to again trial high dose steroids (solumedrol 1 gm IV daily) for potential AE which continued for the next 5 days without obvious efficacy.

He remained in a persistent coma at this point and lost reflexes to even deep painful stimuli while cEEG showed continuous episodic sharp wave from left frontal and synchronized bifrontal discharge was obvious on lowering his sedation (Figure 1(c)). Seizures were refractory to extensive antiseizure medication regimen including keppra 1500 mg twice daily, lacosamide 200 mg three times daily, perampanel 4 mg twice daily, phenobarbital 120 mg twice daily, and valproic acid 1 gm twice daily.

On hospital day #23, his course was complicated by development of ventilator associated pneumonia, for which he was started on vancomycin and cefepime. Cultures from bronchoalveolar lavage were negative.

His neurological condition did not improve with EEG persistently showing frequent generalized epileptiform discharges (Figure 1(d)). Repeat MRI brain (Figure 2(d)) showed extensive and persistent worse cortical ribboning particularly around the left hemisphere, and involving right frontal, and limited involvement of the basal ganglia without any acute infarct on diffusion weighted imaging (DWI) (suggestive of cytotoxic edema from prolonged seizure activity and early CJD). Tissue diagnosis from brain biopsy was discussed but, given hospital policy and limitations, deemed not possible.

On hospital day #26, his CSF finally resulted from the national laboratory positive for 14-3-3 protein, tau protein, and Real-Time Quaking-Induced Conversion (RT-QuIC) proteins, confirming prion disease. Before giving his family the news of the results, and for prognostication purposes, his sedation was held for several hours. On physical exam, he lacked any withdrawal response to painful stimuli but maintained cough and gag reflexes with a minimal, sluggish pupillary reflex. EEG (Figure 1(d)) at that time showed a worsening seizure activity pattern which initially started as focal left frontal lobe diffuse spike-wave complexes but now

TABLE 2: Cerebrospinal fluid analysis.

CSF	Day 1	Day 12
Number of tubes	2	4
Character/color	*Colorless/clear*	*Colorless/clear*
Volume	*4 ml*	*20 ml*
WBC	*0 cells/unit*	*3 cells/unit*
RBC	*7 cells/unit*	*9 cells/unit*
Lymphocytes	*46%*	*14%*
Mononuclear cells	*54%*	*3%*
Glucose CSF	*63 mg/dl*	*66 mg/dl*
Total protein, CSF	*65 mg/dl*	*28 mg/dl*
IgG CSF	*3.5 mg/dl*	-
Lacrosse-California IgG		<1:1
Lacrosse-California IgM		<1:1
East Equine Virus IgG		<1:1
East Equine Virus IgM		<1:1
St Louis Virus IgG		<1:1
St Louis Virus IgM		<1:1
Western Equine Venezuela Virus IgG		<1:1
Western Equine Venezuela Virus IgM		<1:1
West Nile IgG, CSF		0.03
West Nile IgM, CSF		0.01
Varicella Zoster Virus		
Oligoclonal bands		
VDRL		Non-Reactive
Cocci Ab Ig G		0.1
Cocci Ab Ig M		0.0
Coccidioides AB ID		Not detected
Coccidioidomycosis Ab		<1:2
EBV, DNA quant interpretation		Not detected
EBV, Qnt log		<2.6 units: log
EBV, Quant source		CSF
EBV virus, Copy/m		<390 copy/ml
Encephalitis/meningitis panel on CSF by PCR		
E. *Coli K -1*		Not detected
H. *Influenza*		Not detected
L. *Monocytogenes*		Not detected
N *Meningitides*		Not detected
S. *agalactae*		Not detected
S. *Pyogenes*		Not detected
Cytomegalovirus		
Herpes Simplex Virus (HSV 1 & 2)		
Human herpes Virus-6		
Varicella Zoster Virus		
Cryptococcus Neoformans		

TABLE 2: Continued.

CSF	Day 1	Day 12
Paraneoplastic Panel		
AGNA-1		
Amphiphysin Ab		
ANNA-1		
Reflex Added		Negative <1 : 2
ANNA-2		
CRMP-5		
PCA-1 and 2		
PCA-Tr		
S-100B		*3230 ng/L*
RT QuIC		*POSITIVE*
14-3-3 Protein		*+++*
T- Tau Protein		*++ 9094 pg/ml*

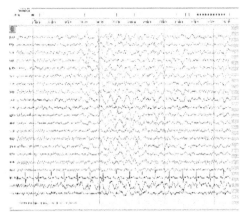

(a) Hospital day one to hospital day four: consistent with focal seizure activity from left hemisphere (frontal)

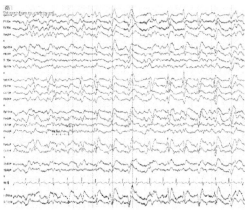

(b) Hospital day eight and day nine: continuous EEG revealed persistent epileptogenic activity with bilateral hemispheric discharges (left > right)

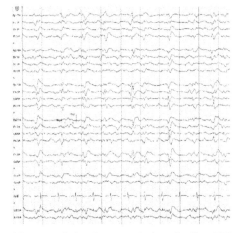

(c) Hospital day fourteen: 24 hours' video EEG showing diffuse epileptiform discharge suggestive of encephalopathic state with presence of continuous left frontal and sometimes synchronized bifrontal sharp spikes with a more generalized appearance suggestive of NCSE

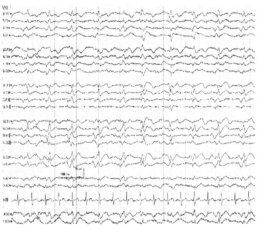

(d) Hospital day twenty-eight: EEG consistent with nonconvulsive status epilepticus (NCSE)

FIGURE 1: *EEG studies.*

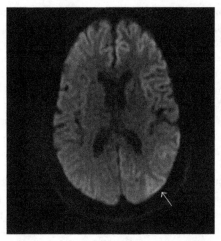

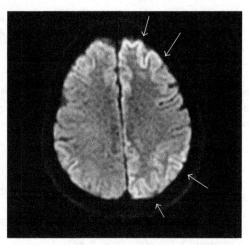

(a) Hospital day two: no evidence of acute pathology except mild diffuse cerebral and cerebellar substance loss on MRI

(b) Hospital day five: DW-MRI showing cortical and gyriform diffusion signal hyperintensity with cortical ribbon edema (cytotoxic edema) in the left frontal and parietal lobes, likely due to persistent seizure activity. Punctate calcification in the right frontal cortex is also visible

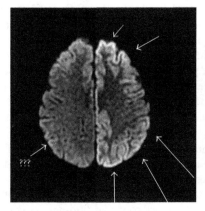

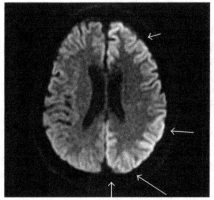

(c) Hospital day nine: persistent cortical ribboning particularly around the left hemisphere with frontal lobe > parietal lobe. There is also involvement of right frontal cortex

(d) Hospital day twenty-three: extensive and persistent worsening of cortical ribboning particularly around the left hemisphere and involving right frontal and limited involvement of the basal ganglia

FIGURE 2: *MRIs.*

had progressed into generalized epileptiform discharges with development of nonconvulsive status epilepticus (NCSE).

A family conference was held discussing the patient's terminal diagnosis and a decision was made to transition the patient to comfort care with compassionate extubation. He died shortly after extubation with family at bedside. The county health department was involved in his case and investigations were performed at the local manure plant to test for potential cow involvement, usually seen in variant (vCJD), which was unremarkable. However, our patient's age of disease onset, typical EEG (PSWC), absent pulvinar sign on MRI as well as lack of past medical/surgical and family history was not consistent with vCJD. Thus, he was diagnosed with probable sCJD. His remains were cremated, and his ashes taken to Mexico by family preventing final genetic testing to be performed.

3. Discussion

CJD is the most commonly seen form of prion diseases in humans [1]. This is a fatal neurodegenerative disease which typically results in subacute and progressive deterioration in cognitive, behavioral, and motor function over a period of weeks to months [12–15]. Typical clinical presentation also includes startle myoclonus, cerebellar, pyramidal, extrapyramidal, behavioral, and visual defects with a characteristic periodic sharp complex on the EEG [16, 17]. Other neurocognitive disorders including Alzheimer's disease, Lewy body dementia, vascular dementia, and frontotemporal dementia tend to have slower course and gradual cognitive decline [18].

Based on its etiology, CJD is divided into sporadic (most common), variant (vCJD), iatrogenic, and familial forms [14, 19]. Genetic analysis of prion protein gene (PRNP) can help to identify different forms of CJD and to subclassify them based on molecular phenotype [20, 21].

Sporadic form is seen in older age and previous diagnosis of psychosis, multiple surgeries, and living in the farm (garden or animal farm) for more than 10 years are associated risk factors [22]. Our patient had worked in a cow manure plant although investigations performed at the local manure plant to test for potential cow involvement were unremarkable. Variant CJD is seen in younger age and represents bovine-to-human transmission. It manifests with early sensory disturbances and psychiatric symptoms rather than cognitive decline [23]. EEG usually do not show PSWCs and a slow wave pattern is predominant [20, 24]. Symmetrical hyperintensity in the pulvinar nuclei of the thalamus termed as "pulvinar" sign is 90% specific for vCJD [25, 26]. Our patient in terms of clinical presentation (age, personal and family history, EEG, and MRI findings) falls under sCJD.

Although the diagnosis may be straightforward in older adults who present with the classic clinical and radiological presentation, the diagnosis becomes challenging if the initial presentation is atypical both clinically and in terms of imaging [27].

CJD have presented with a variety of atypical clinical syndromes including but not limited to amyopathy, deafness, and cataracts [28–30] and often with nonspecific constitutional signs and symptoms such as dizziness [12]. Our patient also did have a work-related fall and difficulty waking but he did not have evidence of amyopathy (absence of fasciculation and areflexia). His right upper extremity weakness was likely related to involvement of left frontal cortex with seizure activity resulting in "postictal" weakness. He did not have an isolated period of constitutional symptoms before cognitive decline as some other patients did [12]. He did not have deafness or cataracts. He did have vertigo, which is hard to differentiate if being of central or of peripheral origin.

CJD is a rare but an important stroke mimic making it challenging to differentiate between the two, as CJD develops mostly in elderly population who usually also have risk factors for stroke [27]. Our patient had no evidence of stroke.

Seizures have been reported in up to 15% of patients with CJD during the disease course [1]. However, seizures are reported as initial manifestation of the CJD disease only in 3% of cases [31]. Status epilepticus is reported in less than 15% of patients of sCJD [14]. Our patient's EEG identified focal seizure activity early during the hospitalization which then progressed to NCSE as patient deteriorated.

Akinetic mutism is a known entity in patients in the final stages of CJD [32]. In contrast to akinetic mutism (again seen in the late stages), patients can have aphasia as a manifestation of CJD [3–8]. Aphasia at disease onset, however, is much less common [2]. This patient is a rare clinical presentation of sporadic CJD (sCJD) with combination of both expressive aphasia and NCSE.

Early recognition of potentially treatable etiologies can minimize the morbidity and mortality. Because of the delayed availability of results for autoimmune and paraneoplastic etiologies on CSF, we empirically used steroids to treat possible underlying autoimmune encephalopathy. Steroids can be empirically given in the setting of an elevated CSF protein (as our case) or personal or family history of an autoimmune disease [10]. However, there is not enough evidence to routinely recommend the use of steroids as a routine treatment in rapidly progressive dementia. We did not use intravenous immunoglobulin (IVIG) or plasmapheresis since we did not have enough evidence to support the diagnosis of AE [11].

CSF analysis for protein 14-3-3 has positive predictive value of 93% to 95% but its sensitivity is low [33]. Other CSF proteins such as tau and neuron-specific enolase are nonspecific general markers of neuronal injury and their utility is questionable due to lack of specificity [15].

The most common EEG finding in CJD is diffuse slowing pattern. However, the characteristic EEG findings for CJD are periodic synchronous bi- or triphasic or mixed sharp wave complexes (PSWCs) which have a specificity for sCJD ranging from 66% to 91% [1, 20, 34, 35]. However, its sensitivity is variable based on genotypes of sCJD [34]. PSWCs are sensitive to disease stage and external stimulation [20]. Lateralized PSWCs are seen during the disease course and represent the prodromal stage of disease onset, which then progresses in bifrontal distribution as disease advances as in our patient [35]. EEG-related spikes are independent of the traditional clinical finding of myoclonic jerking and are usually seen while patient is awake. Sleep deprivation usually exacerbate them, and benzodiazepines can mask the PSWCs [20]. We noticed similar pattern in our patient (Figures 1(c) and 1(d)).

Use of DWI or fluid attenuated inversion recovery (FLAIR) and apparent diffusion coefficient (ADC) modalities have significantly improved the sensitivity and specificity to 96% and 93%, respectively, of MRI for diagnosis of CJD [20, 26]. Hyperintensities in the putamen and head of the caudate nuclei are the most common findings on conventional MRI sequences in patients with CJD [36]. Other typical MRI findings in CJD include hyperintensities with diffusion restriction in the frontal, temporal, occipital, insular, and/or parietal regions referred to as cortical ribboning. Moreover, MRI is helpful to identify any other potential inflammatory, infectious, and toxic-metabolic causes of rapidly progressive dementia which might be mimicking CJD [20, 26]. Our patient had similar extensively worsening cortical ribboning pattern (Figure 2(d)).

MRI pattern may be affected by disease stage. DWI is considered superior during early stages of CJD [26]. Later during the disease course hyperintensity decreases and the only findings may be cortical atrophy [37]. Studies have shown that hyperintensity on DWI and ADC studies correlates with the symptoms and clinical course of the disease. Hyperintensity of basal ganglia on DWI is believed to be associated with a shorter disease duration and higher incidence of myoclonus [20]. Our patient had hyperintensity on basal ganglia and disease course was shorter and he had myoclonus (few weeks). One study reported a potential correlation between hyperintense lesions in the occipital cortex on DWI and shorter time between symptom onset and akinetic mutism [38]. Our patient did not show any occipital lobe lesions and did not develop akinetic mutism.

Definitive diagnosis can be established only with tissue diagnosis from brain biopsy or on autopsy tissue and genetic analysis is required as well. However, getting a biopsy is often not possible (as in our case) because of the concern for appropriate tissue handling and to prevent cross-contamination. Diagnostic yield of brain biopsy is low with traditional sampling methods [20] but newer techniques have shown better diagnostic yield [39]. We did not do biopsy as we have enough evidence from noninvasive work to substantiate the probable diagnosis of CJD. We recommend getting biopsy if it can potentially affect the treatment plan or disease course, and appropriate tissue handling is available.

Currently, there is no definite treatment available for this lethal condition. Antiepileptic drugs are used for myoclonic symptoms along with supportive and palliative care. There is no need to isolate the patient, but careful handling of CSF and brain tissue is strongly recommended.

Our patient had an atypical initial clinical presentation but with progressive changes in his radiological, EEG, and CSF findings becoming more typical and diagnostic for CJD. The progression of his imaging (MRI and EEG) and laboratory (CSF) abnormalities correlated well with his neurological deterioration. This emphasizes that uncommon etiologies must be considered in cases of unexplained and rapid neurological deterioration, especially with altered mentation and/or presence of refractory seizure activity. Close clinical monitoring is prudent and needs to be correlated with neuroimaging and cerebrospinal fluid analysis, which might aid in the early diagnosis of this lethal condition.

4. Conclusion

CJD can often have atypical clinical and radiological presentation. Diffuse epileptiform discharge (NCSE) on EEG in a patient with unexplained rapid cognitive decline and confusion might be a presentation of sCJD [14]. Potential reversible causes of rapidly progressive dementia such as autoimmune, infectious, and toxic-metabolic etiologies must be ruled out before making the final diagnosis of prion disease [12]. Continuous video EEG monitoring is crucial, especially if refractory epileptiform activity is suspected [40]. Due to the fatality of CJD, high degree of suspicion is prudent to initiate subsequent workup in instances of persistent/progressive unexplained neurocognitive decline and atypical clinical presentation and/or inconclusive initial workup.

References

[1] D. Cohen, E. Kutluay, J. Edwards, A. Peltier, and A. Beydoun, "Sporadic Creutzfeldt-Jakob disease presenting with nonconvulsive status epilepticus," *Epilepsy & Behavior*, vol. 5, no. 5, pp. 792–796, 2004.

[2] S. El Tawil, G. Chohan, J. Mackenzie et al., "Isolated language impairment as the primary presentation of sporadic Creutzfeldt Jakob Disease," *Acta Neurologica Scandinavica*, vol. 135, no. 3, pp. 316–323, 2017.

[3] J.-E. Song, D.-W. Yang, H.-J. Seo et al., "Conduction aphasia as an initial symptom in a patient with Creutzfeldt-Jakob disease," *Journal of Clinical Neuroscience*, vol. 17, no. 10, pp. 1341–1343, 2010.

[4] S. E. McPherson, J. D. Kuratani, J. L. Cummings, J. Shih, P. S. Mischel, and H. V. Vinters, "Creutzfeldt-Jakob disease with mixed transcortical aphasia: Insights into echolalia," *Behavioural Neurology*, vol. 7, no. 3-4, pp. 197–203, 1994.

[5] E. C. Shuttleworth, A. J. Yates, and J. D. Paltan-Ortiz, "Creutzfeldt–Jakob disease presenting as progressive aphasia," *Journal of the National Medical Association*, vol. 77, no. 8, pp. 649-650, 1985.

[6] A. Kirk and L. C. Ang, "Unilateral Creutzfeldt-Jakob disease presenting as rapidly progressive aphasia," *Canadian Journal of Neurological Sciences/Journal Canadien des Sciences Neurologiques*, vol. 21, no. 4, pp. 350–352, 1994.

[7] A. E. Hillis, "Aphasia: Progress in the last quarter of a century," *Neurology*, vol. 69, no. 2, pp. 200–213, 2007.

[8] A. M. Mandell, M. P. Alexander, and S. Carpenter, "Creutzfeldt-jakob disease presenting as isolated aphasia," *Neurology*, vol. 39, no. 1, pp. 55–58, 1989.

[9] F. Zuhorn, A. Hübenthal, A. Rogalewski et al., "Creutzfeldt-Jakob disease mimicking autoimmune encephalitis with CASPR2 antibodies," *BMC Neurology*, vol. 14, no. 1, article no. 227, 2014.

[10] F. Graus, M. J. Titulaer, and R. Balu, "A clinical approach to diagnosis of autoimmune encephalitis," *The Lancet Neurology*, vol. 15, no. 4, pp. 391–404, 2016.

[11] C. Di Bonaventura, A. Labate, M. Maschio, S. Meletti, and E. Russo, "AMPA receptors and perampanel behind selected epilepsies: current evidence and future perspectives," *Expert Opinion on Pharmacotherapy*, vol. 18, no. 16, pp. 1751–1764, 2017.

[12] M. D. Geschwind, H. Shu, A. Haman, J. J. Sejvar, and B. L. Miller, "Rapidly progressive dementia," *Annals of Neurology*, vol. 64, no. 1, pp. 97–108, 2008.

[13] E. Gozke, N. Erdal, and M. Unal, "Creutzfeldt-Jacob Disease:a case report," *Cases Journal*, vol. 1, no. 1, article 146, 2008.

[14] P. S. Espinosa, M. K. Bensalem-Owen, and D. B. Fee, "Sporadic Creutzfeldt-Jakob disease presenting as nonconvulsive status epilepticus case report and review of the literature," *Clinical Neurology and Neurosurgery*, vol. 112, no. 6, pp. 537–540, 2010.

[15] M. H. Rosenbloom and A. Atri, "The evaluation of rapidly progressive dementia," *The Neurologist*, vol. 17, no. 2, pp. 67–74, 2011.

[16] C. C. Weihl and R. P. Roos, "Creutzfeldt-Jakob disease, new variant Creutzfeldt-Jakob disease, and bovine spongiform encephalopathy," *Neurologic Clinics*, vol. 17, no. 4, pp. 835–859, 1999.

[17] R. Roods, D. C. Gajdusek, and C. J. Gibbs, "The clinical characteristics of transmissible creutzfeldt-jakob disease," *Brain*, vol. 96, no. 1, pp. 1–20, 1973.

[18] P. Roohani, M. K. Saha, and M. Rosenbloom, "Creutzfeldt-Jakob disease in the hospital setting: a case report and review," *Minnesota Medicine*, vol. 96, no. 5, pp. 46–49, 2013.

[19] A. Ladogana, M. Puopolo, E. A. Croes et al., "Mortality from Creutzfeldt-Jakob disease and related disorders in Europe, Australia, and Canada," *Neurology*, vol. 64, no. 9, pp. 1586–1591, 2005.

[20] M. Manix, P. Kalakoti, M. Henry et al., "Creutzfeldt-Jakob disease: updated diagnostic criteria, treatment algorithm, and the utility of brain biopsy," *Neurosurgical Focus*, vol. 39, no. 5, article E2, 2015.

[21] P. Parchi, A. Giese, S. Capellari et al., "Classification of sporadic Creutzfeldt-Jakob disease based on molecular and phenotypic analysis of 300 subjects," *Annals of Neurology*, vol. 46, no. 2, pp. 224–233, 1999.

[22] D. P. W. M. Wientjens, Z. Davanipour, A. Hofman et al., "Risk factors for Creutzfeldt-Jakob disease: A reanalysis of case-control studies," *Neurology*, vol. 46, no. 5, pp. 1287–1291, 1996.

[23] C. A. Heath, S. A. Cooper, K. Murray et al., "Diagnosing variant Creutzfeldt - Jakob disease: A retrospective analysis of the first 150 cases in the UK," *Journal of Neurology, Neurosurgery & Psychiatry*, vol. 82, no. 6, pp. 646–651, 2011.

[24] S. Binelli, P. Agazzi, G. Giaccone et al., "Periodic electroencephalogram complexes in a patient with variant Creutzfeldt-Jakob disease," *Annals of Neurology*, vol. 59, no. 2, pp. 423–427, 2006.

[25] R. G. Will, M. Zeidler, G. E. Stewart et al., "Diagnosis of new variant Creutzfeldt-Jakob disease," *Annals of Neurology*, vol. 47, no. 5, pp. 575–582, 2000.

[26] P. Vitali, E. MacCagnano, E. Caverzasi et al., "Diffusion-weighted MRI hyperintensity patterns differentiate CJD from other rapid dementias," *Neurology*, vol. 76, no. 20, pp. 1711–1719, 2011.

[27] D. K. Sharma, M. Boggild, A. W. Van Heuven, and R. P. White, "Creutzfeldt-Jakob disease presenting as stroke: a case report and systematic literature review," *The Neurologist*, vol. 22, no. 2, pp. 48–53, 2017.

[28] P. K. Panegyres, E. Armari, and R. Shelly, "A patient with Creutzfeldt-Jakob disease presenting with amyotrophy: a case report," *Journal of Medical Case Reports*, vol. 7, article 218, 2013.

[29] R. Salazar, M. Cerghet, and V. Ramachandran, "Bilateral hearing loss heralding sporadic Creutzfeldt-Jakob disease: A case report and literature review," *Otology & Neurotology*, vol. 35, no. 8, pp. 1327–1329, 2014.

[30] M. A. Leitritz, B. Leo-Kottler, M. Batra, K. Ostertag, K. U. Bartz-Schmidt, and M. S. Spitzer, "Cataract as 'initial symptom' of Creutzfeld-Jacob disease," *Acta Ophthalmologica*, vol. 90, no. 6, pp. e489–e490, 2012.

[31] R. V. Gibbons, R. C. Holman, E. D. Belay, and L. B. Schonberger, "Creutzfeldt-Jakob disease in the United States: 1979–1998," *Journal of the American Medical Association*, vol. 284, no. 18, pp. 2322-2323, 2000.

[32] A. Otto, I. Zerr, M. Lantsch, K. Weidehaas, C. Riedemann, and S. Poser, "Akinetic mutism as a classification criterion for the diagnosis of Creutzfeldt-Jakob disease," *Journal of Neurology, Neurosurgery & Psychiatry*, vol. 64, no. 4, pp. 524–528, 1998.

[33] M. D. Geschwind, J. Martindale, D. Miller et al., "Challenging the clinical utility of the 14-3-3 protein for the diagnosis of sporadic Creutzfeldt-Jakob disease," *JAMA Neurology*, vol. 60, no. 6, pp. 813–816, 2003.

[34] I. Zerr, W. J. Schulz-Schaeffer, A. Giese et al., "Current clinical diagnosis in Creutzfeldt-Jakob disease: Identification of uncommon variants," *Annals of Neurology*, vol. 48, no. 3, pp. 323–329, 2000.

[35] H. G. Wieser, K. Schindler, and D. Zumsteg, "EEG in Creutzfeldt-Jakob disease," *Clinical Neurophysiology*, vol. 117, no. 5, pp. 935–951, 2006.

[36] D. A. Collie, R. J. Sellar, M. Zeidler, A. C. F. Colchester, R. Knight, and R. G. Will, "MRI of Creutzfeldt-Jakob disease: Imaging features and recommended MRI protocol," *Clinical Radiology*, vol. 56, no. 9, pp. 726–739, 2001.

[37] L. Letourneau-Guillon, R. Wada, and W. Kucharczyk, "Imaging of prion diseases," *Journal of Magnetic Resonance Imaging*, vol. 35, no. 5, pp. 998–1012, 2012.

[38] T. Gao, J.-H. Lyu, J.-T. Zhang et al., "Diffusion-weighted MRI findings and clinical correlations in sporadic Creutzfeldt–Jakob disease," *Journal of Neurology*, vol. 262, no. 6, pp. 1440–1446, 2015.

[39] J. M. Schott, L. Reiniger, M. Thom et al., "Brain biopsy in dementia: Clinical indications and diagnostic approach," *Acta Neuropathologica*, vol. 120, no. 3, pp. 327–341, 2010.

[40] D. Friedman, J. Claassen, and L. J. Hirsch, "Continuous electroencephalogram monitoring in the intensive care unit," *Anesthesia & Analgesia*, vol. 109, no. 2, pp. 506–523, 2009.

14

Transcranial Magnetic Stimulation and Working Memory Training to Address Language Impairments in Aphasia

Despina Kranou-Economidou⬩ and **Maria Kambanaros**⬩

Department of Rehabilitation Sciences, Cyprus University of Technology, Limassol 3036, Cyprus

Correspondence should be addressed to Despina Kranou-Economidou; da.oikonomidou@edu.cut.ac.cy

Academic Editor: Enzo Emanuele

Background. Traditionally, people with aphasia (PWA) are treated with impairment-based language therapy to improve receptive and expressive language skills. In addition to language deficits, PWA are often affected by some level of working memory (WM) impairments. Both language and working memory impairments combined have a negative impact on PWA's quality of life. The aim of this study was to investigate whether the application of intermittent theta-burst stimulation (iTBS) combined with computerized WM training will result in near-ransfer effects (i.e., trained WM) and far-transfer effects (i.e., untrained language tasks) and have a positive effect on the quality of life of PWA. *Methods.* The participant was a 63-year-old Greek-Cypriot male who presented with mild receptive aphasia and short-term memory difficulties. Treatment was carried out using a multiple baseline (MB) design composed of a pretherapy or baseline testing phase, a therapy phase, and a posttherapy/follow-up phase. The treatment program involved iTBS application to the left dorsolateral prefrontal cortex (DLPFC), an area responsible for WM, for 10 consecutive sessions. The participant received a 3-minute iTBS application followed by 30-minute computer-assisted WM training. Outcome measures included a WM screening test, a standardized aphasia test, a nonverbal intelligence test, story-telling speech samples, a procedural discourse task, and a questionnaire addressing quality of life. These measures were performed three times before the treatment, immediately upon completion of the treatment, and once during follow-up testing at 3 months posttreatment. *Results.* We found a beneficial effect of iTBS and WM training on naming, reading, WM, reasoning, narrative, communication efficiency, and quality of life (QoL). *Implications for Rehabilitation.* Noninvasive brain stimulation combined with computerized WM training may be used in aphasia rehabilitation to improve WM and generalize to language improvement.

1. Introduction

Transcranial magnetic stimulation (TMS) is a noninvasive technique of brain neuromodulation and neurostimulation [1] which produces a brief electric current in the coil to generate a magnetic field, and in turn, it activates neurons in the vicinity of the coil. Recently, there is a growing interest in the area of working memory (WM) improvement through the use of TMS [2]. WM, the ability to temporarily store and manipulate information in the provision of ongoing tasks, is based on the belief that a dedicated system maintains and stores information in the short term and that this system underlies human thought processes [3]. While a range of cognitive abilities has been associated with WM, including reading comprehension, logical thinking, general intelligence, learning ability, and fluid reasoning [4–8], recent investigations explore how cognitive enhancement can support improvements in other areas (i.e., language) in people with neurological impairments [9, 10].

Aphasia has traditionally been defined as a language impairment due to the disruption of the blood flow to the brain, which can result in reduced ability to comprehend and/or express oral and/or written language. Lately, research studies investigate whether aphasia is the result of a cognitive

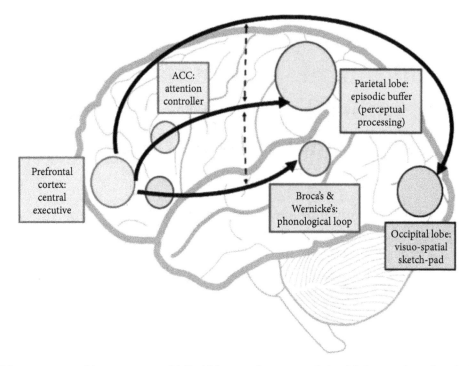

FIGURE 1: The multicomponent working memory model (Baddeley, 2010) represented simplified as implicated in the brain, in which the central executive assumes the role to exert control and oversee the manipulation of incoming information for intended execution. ACC: anterior cingulate cortex. From Working Memory from the Psychological and Neurosciences Perspectives: A Review by Chai et al., 2018, https://www.ncbi.nlm.nih.gov/pmc/articles/PMC5881171/figure/F1.

process disruption, specifically the disruption of the WM neural network [10]. In the recent past, aphasia was also defined as a cognitive disorder with major linguistic deficits, as opposed to a specific language disturbance [11]. This notion is based on evidence indicating the possible breakdown of an underlying neuronal mechanism that corresponds to a network consisting of several cortices interconnected by white matter tracts [11]. Interestingly, many studies have identified the WM neural network at the frontoparietal area, involving the dorsolateral prefrontal cortex (DLPFC), the anterior cingulate cortex (ACC), and the parietal cortex (PAR) [12–15]. More precisely, the DLPFC has been implicated mainly in tasks demanding executive control such as those requiring integration of information for decision-making, maintenance and manipulation/retrieval of information, and information updating [12]. Chai et al. [16] provided a visual interpretation of Baddeley's theoretical formulation of the multicomponent WM model [17] to specific regions in the human brain as depicted in Figure 1 below. The DLPFC is known for its involvement in WM tasks and for its significant contribution to tasks accuracy [18, 19]. Previous studies have provided evidence of increased activation of the DLPFC during WM tasks [20–22]. In order to achieve a cognitive target such as WM training, WM simultaneously participates in information processing and storage [8]. When WM fails, the ability to carry out many activities of daily living is reduced [23]. Due to this involvement in multiple WM components, the DLPFC is a desirable target for neuromodulation in the context of WM training.

Previous studies have suggested that the neural systems underlying WM capability is plastic, and therefore, WM updating training can lead to WM improvement, particularly in individuals with WM deficiencies [24–26]. Additionally, the effects of training can be transferred to other cognitive functions associated with WM such as general fluid intelligence (Gf) [27]. Gf is defined as the ability to solve novel reasoning problems, and it is associated with comprehension, problem solving, and learning [28]. Gf is a complex ability that enables an individual to adapt their thinking to new cognitive problems and situations [27], and it has been identified to share the same neural networks in the lateral prefrontal and parietal cortices as WM capability [8, 27, 29].

This current study supports that when a stroke occurs, the WM neuronal network is disrupted, resulting in aphasia. The main objective was to explore the potential domains of transfer effect after stimulation of the left DLPFC and WM training and also to measure how efficacious this treatment protocol was for PWA. Specifically, the purpose was to investigate the short-term and long-term combined effects of iTBS and WM training as a mediator to WM improvement, language generalization, and to quality of life (QoL) enhancement. Cognitive (nonverbal), language (verbal), and QoL outcomes are reported at pretherapy (baseline), posttherapy (immediately after the end of the treatment), and follow-up (three months posttreatment).

2. Materials and Methods

2.1. Inclusion and Exclusion Criteria. The study was carried out at the Rehabilitation Clinic of the Cyprus University of Technology (CUT). Inclusion and exclusion criteria to the

TABLE 1: Participant inclusion and exclusion criteria.

Inclusion criteria	Exclusion criteria
(a) Native speaker of Cypriot-Greek	(a) Severe aphasia diagnosed using the Greek version of the Boston Diagnostic Aphasia Examination – Short Form (BDAE-SF) [30]
(b) Age 21-79 y.o	(b) Damaged dorsolateral prefrontal cortex area as identified in the MRI
(c) First-time single left hemisphere stroke	(c) Traumatic brain injury
(d) Presence of aphasia	(d) History of psychiatric or other neurological illness
(e) Right-hand dominance	(e) Depression
	(f) Epilepsy/seizures
	(g) Pregnancy
	(h) Colour-blindness or other visual disorders/visual neglect
(g) Adequate single-word comprehension	(i) Hearing loss
	(k) Significant general medical problems including liver, cardiac, or renal dysfunctions
	(l) Present or past alcohol or drug abuse
	(j) Metal or medical implants (i.e., cardiac pacemakers)

study were made available prior to entering the study (Table 1).

The study was approved by the Cyprus National Bioethics Committee, and the participant provided a written consent prior to participating in this study.

2.2. Participant Details. The participant (C.S.) was a 63-year-old male who suffered a left hemisphere ischemic stroke 45 days prior to the study and was not receiving speech and language therapy. C.S.'s neurologist stated that he experienced mild expressive aphasia with short-term memory (STM) difficulties and verbal information processing difficulties. C.S.'s reported having difficulties remembering recent verbal information while having a conversation with family and friends. He was a retired food and beverage employee, with 12 years of education, and was a hobby farmer. Although brain damage was not visible on the current MRI (Figure 2), the initial medical MRI report indicated the presence of an acute ischemic stroke in the medial temporal lobe. C.S. lived with his wife and did not suffer any paresis or paralysis as he was able to drive and care for himself with minimal assistance.

2.3. Data Collection and Procedures. The assessment battery was administered in a predetermined order in 2 sessions, of approximately 2.5 hours duration in total.

2.3.1. Background Tools. The background tools were used to fulfil certain inclusion criteria in order to proceed to the pretesting and treatment stage of this study. A detailed case history was taken including personal and medical information. A TMS safety questionnaire [31] was completed prior to entering the first stage of the inclusion process, followed by a screening procedure which included the following:

(i) The *Albert's Visual Neglect Test* [32] to determine unilateral spatial neglect

(ii) The *Edinburgh Handedness Inventory* [33] aimed at evaluating handedness of the preferred hand for carrying out daily activities

(iii) The Greek adaptation of the *Beck's Depression Inventory-II* [34, 35], to measure characteristic attitudes and symptoms of depression

2.3.2. Assessment Tools. A battery of tools was administered at baseline, immediately after treatment (same day), and 3 months posttreatment at the follow-up stage. The tools used were as follows:

(i) The *Raven's Coloured Progressive Matrices* (RCPM) [36]

(ii) Subtests from the Greek version of *Boston Diagnostic Aphasia Evaluation–Short Form* (BDAE-SF) [30]

(iii) The *RehaCom Working Memory Screening Task*

(iv) A *personal stroke narrative* [37]

(v) The *Multilingual Assessment Instrument for Narratives* (MAIN) [38]

(vi) A *Procedural Discourse* task [39]

(vii) The *Stroke and Aphasia Quality of Life Scale-39* (SAQOL-39) [40]

The RCPM [36], a test used to measure abstract reasoning, is also regarded as a nonverbal estimate of Gf [41]. The RCPM is made up of a series of diagrams or designs with a part missing, and the participant is asked to choose the shape to complete the pattern or shape from six alternatives. The Greek version of RCPM was administered as adapted by [42]. Every correctly solved pattern was given 1 point, with a total score range between 0 and 36 [43].

The *BDAE-SF* [30] has been standardized in Greek and is culturally appropriate [44]. It includes five subtests:

(1) Conversational and expository speech such as simple social responses, free conversation, and picture description

(2) Auditory comprehension including word comprehension, commands, and complex ideational material

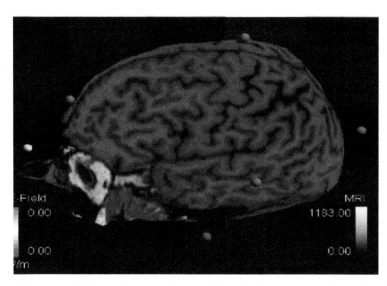

FIGURE 2: Reported findings of the current MRI noted two small areas of low signal intensity involving the subcortical white matter of the left occipital lobe and the left temporal lobe which were compatible with small areas of brain parenchymal loss.

(3) Oral expression, such as automatized sequences, single word repetitions, repetitions of sentences, responsive naming, the Boston Naming Test–Short Form (BNT-SF), and screening of special categories

(4) Reading, including letter and number recognition, picture-word matching, basic oral word reading, oral reading of sentences with comprehension, and reading comprehension of sentences and paragraphs

(5) Writing, including mechanics, dictation writing of primer words, regular phonics and common irregular forms, written naming, narrative writing mechanics, written vocabulary access, syntax, and adequacy of content

For the purposes of this study, only subtests 1-4 were administered and results were analysed in accordance with the test manual.

The *RehaCom Working Memory Screening* module is a tool used to assess both simple WM span (simple information holding) and the retention and processing of visual-spatial information. When the WM screening task is initiated, ten dots are presented in a circular arrangement. Individual dots sequentially turn red and fade. The first sequence consists of two random dots out of the ten lighting up in a particular order to be repeated correctly. When selected correctly, the number of dots increases in the next sequence. In sum, the task is to memorize the presented sequence of dots lighting up. The WM screening subtest ends after two consecutive incorrect sequence responses or after 7 minutes. The visual-spatial memory span is measured by the maximum length of the memorized dot patterns that can be reproduced immediately without errors. Additionally, the participant's memory span is calculated based on the highest sequence length measured in number of dots, reproduced without mistakes in position and order, and it is confirmed by completing two consecutive sequences with the same number of dots.

A *personal stroke narrative* was elicited by asking the participant to describe how his stroke occurred [37]. The sample was transcribed and analysed using the *Shewan Spontaneous Language Analysis* (SSLA) system [45] in accordance with the SSLA protocol. Variables for analysis included number of utterances, time (total speaking time in minutes), rate (syllables per minute), length (percentage of utterances ≤ 5 words), melody, articulation, complex sentences (percentage of utterances that contained one independent clause and one or more dependent clauses), errors (percentage of grammatical, syntactic, or morphological errors), content units (units that conveyed information), paraphasias (percentage of substitutions), repetitions, and communication efficiency (content units/time).

The *MAIN* [38] is a tool designed to evaluate narrative tell and retell skills in children but has also been used with adults with acquired language deficits associated with neurological disease for research purposes [46]. The MAIN stories consist of coloured picture sequences developed according to strict psycholinguistic criteria. While the MAIN examines narrative production at microstructure and macrostructure levels, for this study, only the macrostructure of the generated story was analysed. The primary unit for macrostructure analysis is the episode. The content of each picture sequence was designed to represent three short episodes. Each episode consists of

(i) a goal statement for the protagonist

(ii) an attempt by the protagonist to reach the goal

(iii) an outcome of the attempt in terms of the goal

(iv) the internal states (IST) which initiate the goal and also express reactions

Each story is controlled for cognitive and linguistic complexity [38] and has a moral meaning similar to an Aesop fable. In this study, the "Baby Goats" story was used which portrayed a mother goat wanting to save her baby goat who jumped into the water but a fox jumped forward to catch the other baby goat. Then, a bird saw that the baby goat was in great danger and stopped the fox by biting its tail and chasing it away to save the baby goat. Six-coloured pictures in the form of a cartoon strip were presented, and one-episode was unfolded each time (2 pictures) for the participant to narrate a story based on the pictured stimuli. The scoring sheets of the MAIN "Baby Goats" story provided the scoring system used for the story structure components (setting, goals, attempts, outcomes, and IST). A setting statement, which gives time and place and introduces the story's protagonist, is scored with zero points for wrong or no response, 1 point for one correct response, and 2 points for reference to both time and place. This component is followed by three episodes. Each episode consists of (a) the internal states which initiate the goal and also express reactions; (b) a goal which is a statement of an idea of the protagonist to deal with the initiating event; (c) an attempt by the protagonist to reach the goal, which is an indication of action to obtain the goal; (d) an outcome of the attempt in terms of the goal, which is the event(s) following the attempt and causally linked to it; and (e) the internal states as reaction, which is a statement defining how the protagonist(s) feel or think about the outcome or an action resulting from an emotional response [38]. The story output was transcribed verbatim, and it was analysed using a scoring system of 17 points for story structure components in production, following the guidelines for assessment, and guided by the information on the provided scoring sheets.

The *Procedural Discourse* task is considered a semispontaneous speech production task that assesses discourse ability following the main concept analysis (MCA) procedure [39]. The MCA enumerates the speaker's ability to communicate the overall idea of an occasion, and it provides a way to evaluate the generated precision and completeness of the critical concepts of the shared topic. The participant was instructed to verbally provide all the required steps to be taken in order to prepare a sandwich. The generated language sample was analysed using the MCA procedure referring to the ten main concepts. The total number of main concepts expected to be produced was analysed and measured based on the concept content as listed below:

(1) Get the bread out

(2) Get two slices of bread//halved bread

(3) Get the butter

(4) Get the (rest of the ingredients, i.e., ham and cheese)

(5) Get a knife

(6) Put/place the bread on the plate

(7) Put/spread butter on bread

(8) Put the ingredients (i.e., ham and cheese) on bread

(9) Put the two pieces together

(10) Cut the sandwich in pieces

The first five steps comprise concepts concerning retrieving the ingredients needed, the following four steps include concepts concerning ingredient assembly, and the final concept describes the final appearance of the target (sandwich) prior to serving it. The procedure output was transcribed verbatim, and it was analysed using a binary scoring system of "1" for correct information and "0" for incorrect/missing information.

The *SAQOL-39g* has been translated and culturally adapted in Greek for use in Greece with PWA [47]. The Greek SAQOL-39g shows good reliability and validity [48] as a measure of health-related quality of life in people with stroke, including those with aphasia. An interview with the participant and the first author took place prior to the therapy study where the SAQOL-39 was used to collect the relevant information.

2.4. Therapy Procedure. The participant completed ten (10) approximately 45-minute-long treatment sessions comprising of iTBS, immediately followed by RehaCom WM training over a span of 10 consecutive days, including weekends. Within each treatment session, approximately 15 minutes were devoted for setting up the participant with the TMS equipment and iTBS application, and 30 minutes were devoted to the RehaCom WM training task. The treatment regimen is depicted in Figure 3 below.

2.4.1. Pretherapy or "Baseline" Testing Phase. During the pretherapy baseline phase, the purpose was to establish the level of performance prior to treatment so that the effects of treatment on the task could be clearly measured. Seven outcome measures were used, and the information was collected three times, one week apart, prior to the therapy phase. Preceding the therapy phase, a T1-weighted MRI image was obtained of C. S.'s brain in order to accurately locate the target stimulation site using the Visor 2.0 neuronavigation system (ANT NEURO). Neuronavigated positioning of the stimulation coil allowed for repeated accuracy throughout the study.

(1) Transcranial Magnetic Stimulation (TMS) Equipment. Single-pulse TMS and intermittent theta-burst stimulation (iTBS) were delivered over the motor cortex and the left dorsolateral prefrontal cortex (LDLPFC), respectively, with the Magstim Rapid2® stimulator (Magstim Co., Wales, UK) connected to a 70 mm figure-8 air cooled coil. Biphasic TMS pulses were delivered with a posterior-to-anterior (P-A) current direction in both, single-pulse TMS and iTBS. The treatment intensity of TMS was individually adjusted the participant's resting motor threshold (RMT). RMT is the minimal intensity at which TMS of motor cortex produces a reliable motor evoked potential (MEP) of minimal amplitude in the target muscle. The MEP was determined with a surface electromyography (EMG) response in the 'target' muscle, through the placement of EMG leads over the first dorsal interosseous (FDI) muscle of the left hand. Full

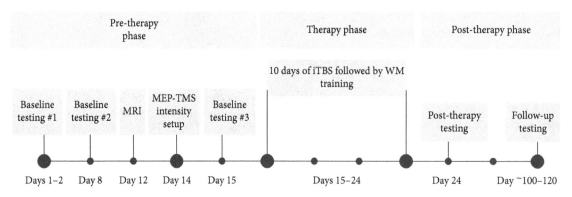

FIGURE 3: Study design overview.

muscle relaxation was maintained through visual and online EMG monitoring. The coil was positioned at 45-degree rotation in relation to the parasagittal plane to induce P-A current in the underlying cortex. The motor "hotspot" was determined with a TMS intensity ranging from 45% to 50% of the maximum stimulator output, whereby single-pulse stimuli were delivered at varying positions across the scalp near the primary motor cortex (M1) while guided by a neuronavigation system (ANT NEURO) using each participant's recent anatomical MRI image. The motor "hotspot" was determined as the position on the scalp that yielded two consecutive MEPs with greater amplitude than the surrounding positions. The location within the left motor cortex that consistently elicited MEPs in the relaxed right FDI muscle was then defined as the motor hotspot. The coil was then placed over the defined target to obtain a MEP in the FDI of at least $50 \mu V$ in five or more of 10 consecutive stimulations of the left hand [49]. For this study, a computerized adaptive parameter estimation through sequential testing (PEST) [50] with the software TMS Motor Threshold Assessment Tool, MTAT 2.0, developed by Awiszus and Borckardt et al. [50], was used to determine the RMT. The MTAT 2.0 freeware was obtained online (http://www.clinicalresearcher.org/software.html), and the option for assessment without prior information was selected. No other parameters were changed on the software.

2.4.2. Therapy Phase

(1) Transcranial Magnetic Stimulation: iTBS Application. The figure-8 coil was positioned tangentially to the skull, with the handle parallel to the sagittal axis pointing occipitally. The iTBS treatment consisted of bursts of three pulses at 50 Hz given every 200 milliseconds in two second trains, repeated every 10 seconds over 200 seconds for a total of 600 pulses [51]. Based on the participant's recent MRI images, the Visor 2.0 neuronavigation suite (ANT-Neuro, Enschede, Netherlands) was used for image preprocessing, tissue segmentation, and registration into standard stereotaxic space. The stimulation target was defined in the left DLPFC by using the Talairach coordinates $x = -39$, $y = 34$, and $z = 27$ [21, 52]. This technology enabled the reliable three-dimensionally precise reapplication of rTMS throughout the study. The participant received one session of iTBS each day for 10 consecutive days.

(2) RehaCom WM Training Equipment. Immediately following the iTBS session, the participant received 30 minutes WM training using the RehaCom Working Memory (WOME) software package (Hasomed GmbH, DE.). RehaCom WOME is a software package developed to train and improve WM performance. The WM training task involved card presentation in the form of a card game, using a complete card deck of 52 cards and consisting of different levels of difficulty. Three hierarchically ordered modules were designed to exercise the main components of WM on the basis of a card game: (a) storage systems, involving the maintenance of information; (b) selective attention, involving memorizing selective parts of information and inhibiting others; and (c) central executive/manipulation processes, involving active operating with the content retained in WM [53]. RehaCom WOME training involves the memorization and manipulation of an increasing number of visually presented playing cards on a computer screen. Throughout the early levels of training, the participant is required to memorize a short series of cards and reproduce it in the same order, while at higher levels additional tasks are introduced to influence the memory process (e.g., memorize only the cards of a certain suit from a presentation of various cards). In total, there are 70 levels of difficulty. Feedback is constantly provided by the software, and the degree of difficulty is adapted based on the participant's performance level. The sessions were implemented in a quiet room, and C.S. responded on a Lenovo touchscreen laptop.

2.5. *Posttherapy/Follow-Up Phase.* The posttherapy/follow-up phase consisted of two time points. The outcome measures were administered immediately after the completion of the last day of treatment (10th day) and at 3 months posttreatment at the follow-up stage. The purpose of immediate posttesting was to determine short-term efficacy and of the follow-up to determine long-term effects. The exact date of the follow-up was dependent on the participant's availability when contacted to set-up the appointment. The same battery of tools was used as with the baseline phase:

(1) The Greek BDAE-SF [30]

(2) The RCPM [42]

(3) The MAIN [38]

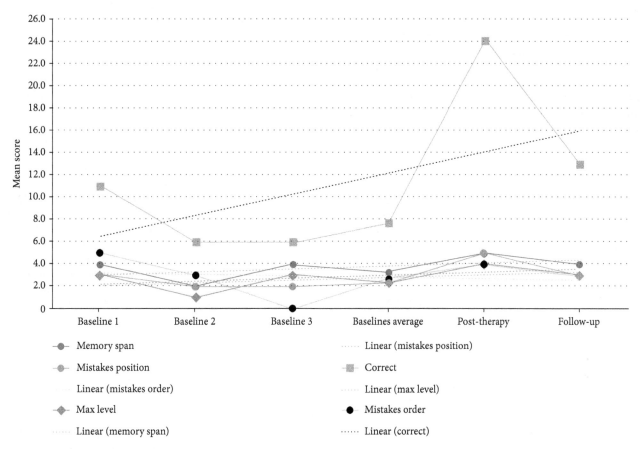

FIGURE 4: Schematic representation of C.S.'s raw scores on the *RehaCom* WM screening task.

(4) A Procedural Discourse task [39]

(5) A personal stroke narrative [37]

(6) The RehaCom Working Memory Screening Task

(7) The Greek SAQOL-39 [48]

3. Results

The Statistical Package for Social Sciences (IBM SPSS 25) was used for all the data and exploratory analysis. Analyses of individual data were conducted using the weighted statistics (WEST) method, and descriptive results' analysis was used where a statistical analysis was not suitable. Specifically, the "WEST-Trend" and "WEST-ROC" (one tailed) procedures [54] were applied. In order to evaluate the treatment effects and the rate of change, the level of performance prior to treatment is established by taking at least two probes [54]. A linear trend in improvement may be documented using the WEST-Trend procedure, while the amount of change in the treated (short-term) versus the untreated periods (long-term) may be documented using the WEST-ROC analyses. The WEST-ROC and WEST-Trend were used to analyse the data from the Greek BDAE-SF, the RCPM, the MAIN, and the Procedural Discourse. Results from the SSLA, the RehaCom WM screening, and the SAQOL-39g assessments are reported but a statistical analysis was not performed.

3.1. Near-Transfer Effects of iTBS to the LDLPFC Combined with WM Training. The results of the *RehaCom WM* screening show a positive linear trend (Figure 4) on all the tasks assessed with a more prominent trend for improvement in the correct responses task. The baseline average (avg.) was compared to the posttherapy and follow-up results (Table 2).

C.S. did not show an overall significant improvement in the RCPM results. However, a statistically significant trend for improvement was shown in *Subtest AB*, ($t(11) = 1.82$, $p = 0.048$) but the WEST-ROC showed that the difference between the treated and untreated periods was nonsignificant ($t(11) = 0.64$, $p = 0.268$). Results are shown in percentage correct in Table 3.

3.2. Far-Transfer Effects in PWA of iTBS to the LDLPFC Combined with WM Training. To investigate whether TMS and WM training generalized to untrained receptive and expressive language and functional communication tasks, statistical analysis was performed on results from (i) the *BDAE-SF*, (ii) the *Procedural Discourse* task, and (iii) the *MAIN* telling task (Table 4). The personal stroke narrative was analysed using the SSLA.

(i) Statistical analysis of the *BDAE* subtests revealed a significant overall trend for improvement only for the *Boston Naming Test* ($t(14) = 1.82$, $p = 0.045$) while the difference between the treated and

TABLE 2: *RehaCom* WM screening raw scores by the subcategory and study phase.

	Baseline 1	Baseline 2	Baseline 3	Baseline average	Posttherapy	Follow-up
Memory span	4	2	4	3	5	4
Max level	3	1	3	2	4	3
Correct	11	6	6	8	24	13
Mistakes order	5	3	0	3	4	3
Mistakes position	3	2	2	2	5	3

TABLE 3: Raw scores (% correct) on the nonverbal intelligence outcomes at posttreatment and follow-up compared to the baseline for C.S.

	Baseline 1	Baseline 2	Baseline 3	Posttherapy	Follow-up
Mean RCPM	75.00%	69.44%	72.22%	77.78%	77.78%
Subtest A	83.33%	75.00%	75.00%	83.33%	75.00%
Subtest AB	83.33%	83.33%	83.33%	91.67%	100.00%
Subtest B	58.33%	50.00%	58.33%	58.33%	58.33%

TABLE 4: Raw scores (% correct) on the language outcomes at posttreatment and follow-up compared to baseline for C.S.

	Baseline 1	Baseline 2	Baseline 3	Posttherapy	Follow-up
Boston naming test	66.67%	73.33%	73.33%	80.00%	86.67%
BDAE reading subtest	86.94%	90.28%	90.28%	90.28%	94.44%
Language discourse—MAIN	47.06%	47.06%	47.06%	58.82%	64.71%

untreated periods was nonsignificant ($t(14) = 0.27$, $p = 0.396$)

(ii) Statistical analysis of the participant's *BDAE Reading* subtest showed a significant trend for improvement ($t(6) = 2.00$, $p = 0.046$), but difference was nonsignificant between the treated and untreated periods ($t(6) = 0.30$, $p = 0.389$)

(iii) Statistical analysis of the participant's *Procedural Discourse* task showed that there were no differences in the number of responses between the five periods

(iv) There was an overall trend for improvement on the *MAIN*, but this did not reach significance ($t(16) = 1.37$, $p = 0.095$), as well as between the treated and untreated periods ($t(16) = 1.24$, $p = 0.116$). Improvement was noted for (a) the IST event as initiating of the second episode during posttherapy and follow-up, (b) the IST event as initiating of the third episode during posttherapy and follow-up, and (c) and IST as reaction of the second episode during follow-up

(v) C.S.'s stroke narrative (spontaneous language sample) was analysed using the SSLA protocol [45] which is designed to describe and quantify connected speech. The baseline average (avg) was compared with the posttesting and follow-up results. There was a 1% increase in the number of utterances produced between baseline avg and posttherapy and a 7% increase between baseline avg and follow-up. The rate of speech improved from 116.76 syllables per minute to 141.60 at posttherapy and to 152.22 at follow-up. The sentence length, which reflects the use of more than 5 words in the produced utterances, improved by 22% between baseline avg and follow-up. A 7% improvement was noted in sentence complexity between baseline avg and follow-up. Improvement was also noted between baseline avg and follow-up in the with an 11% reduction of errors. The number of content units improved from 19.33 at baseline avg to 21.00 at posttherapy and to 36.00 at follow-up. Improvement in the number of repetitions was noted with a reduction from 7% to 0% between baseline avg and posttherapy. A notable improvement in communication efficiency which reflects the rate at which information is conveyed by the speaker (number of content units divided by time), from 13.33 at baseline avg to 16.80 posttherapy and to 17.73 at follow-up. No paraphasias were produced in any of the stroke narrative samples, and the overall melody and articulation were judged to be normal (Table 5).

3.3. Quality of Life Effects in PWA of iTBS to the LDLPFC Combined with WM Training. With regard to investigating whether the overall QoL would improve after the treatment, the self-rated SAQOL-39 was analysed by comparing the mean scores (Table 6). The participant's responses indicated that QoL based on the overall SAQOL-39 self-rated score improved between the baseline average ($M = 3.63$) and posttherapy ($M = 4.51$) by 18%, and it was maintained at follow-up ($M = 4.23$).

TABLE 5: Raw scores for personal stroke narrative analysis based on the SSLA.

	Baseline 1	Baseline 2	Baseline 3	Baseline avg	Post-therapy	Follow-up
Utterances	12.00	14.00	7.00	11.00	12.00	18.00
Rate	99.37	152.41	98.50	116.76	141.60	152.22
Length	58%	43%	14%	39%	50%	17%
Melody	3.00	3.00	3.00	3.00	2.00	4.00
Articulation	7.00	7.00	7.00	7.00	7.00	7.00
Complexity	42%	50.00%	72%	54%	33%	61%
Errors	17%	57%	57%	44%	50%	33%
C.U.s	19.00	22.00	17.00	19.33	21.00	36.00
Paraphasias	0%	0%	0%	0%	0%	0%
Repetitions	0%	21%	0%	7%	0%	22%
Communication efficiency	12.03	15.17	12.78	13.33	16.80	17.73

TABLE 6: Quality of life for C.S. at pretreatment (baseline) at posttreatment and 3-month follow-up using the SAQOL-39g.

Item (max score: 5)	Baseline 1	Baseline 2	Baseline 3	Post-therapy	Follow-up
SAQOL-39 g mean	3.44	3.41	4.05	4.51	4.23
Physical	4.31	3.88	4.56	4.75	4.88
Communication	3.57	3.71	4.14	4.43	4.14
Psychosocial	2.50	2.88	3.56	4.38	3.56

4. Discussion

The main objective was to explore the potential domains of transfer effects after stimulating the left DLPFC combined with WM training and also to measure how this affected the quality of life of the participant. In a previous pilot study [10], we found evidence signifying the possible improvement that could specifically yield from noninvasive brain stimulation programs using iTBS combined with the *RehaCom* WM training program in PWA. Studies performed on healthy aging which are usually focused on prevention, consider the use of rTMS as a tool for cognitive enhancement of the elderly with mild cognitive impairments (MCI), aimed at reversing or compensating for the cognitive deficits [55, 56]. Evidence suggests that the effects of rTMS application may work in synergy with cognitive training to give rise to greater neurocognitive enhancement [55, 57, 58], supporting the notion that cognitive rehabilitation with rTMS can be beneficial as an add-on instrument in cognitive training programs of a variety of neurological and cognitive disorders [59]. A recent review investigating the effects of rTMS in people with Alzheimer's disease and related dementias (ADRD) reported 8 new studies between the years 2016 and 2018, of which 4 of them used cognitive training as well [60]. These studies reported significant improvements in global cognition and memory when measured with the following neuropsychological tests: Alzheimer's Disease Assessment Scale-cognitive (ADAS-Cog), Mini Mental State Exam (MMSE), Addenbrooke Cognitive Examination (ACE), Apathy Evaluation Scale (AES-C), Blessed Dementia Scale (BDS), Clinical Global Impression (CGI), Clinical Global Impression of Change (CGIC), Digit Symbol Substitution Test (DSST), Montreal Cognitive Assessment

(MOCA), Neuropsychiatric Inventory (NPI), Rey Auditory Verbal Learning Test (RAVLT), Trail Making Test (TMT), and Zarit Burden Scale (ZBS). Even though results suggested a potential for improvement in cognitive measures after rTMS treatments, results were mixed as to whether rTMS was significantly more effective than sham. It is believed that the inconsistency of treatment protocols and outcome measures hinders the replication of promising studies, and therefore, evidences continue to be insufficient to support the adoption of a noninvasive brain stimulation protocol to improve cognitive impairments.

In line with previous studies, findings from this investigation (Table 7) lend support to the evidence that (i) WM interacts with language abilities and deficits in WM influence language performance [10, 61], (ii) applying iTBS to the LDLPFC results in improved WM performance [10, 62, 63], (iii) computerized WM training can have positive outcomes on WM tasks [64], and (iv) aphasia has a negative effect on QoL [65].

4.1. Near-Transfer Effects of iTBS and WM Training. WM has been proven to be a useful indicator of cognitive-linguistic competence [66], while WM impairments have a negative impact on cognition and communication [67, 68]. It is important to highlight the fact that WM interventions have a positive impact on WM capacity, as well as on related cognitive-linguistic abilities and on cognitive-communicative deficiencies due to aging or neurological disorders [25, 69]. Furthermore, studies have demonstrated transfer of WM training to other assessments of cognition, including measures of fluid intelligence [27]. This study has revealed a trend for improvement in both WM tasks and Gf transfer, with a statistical significance of Gf as measured with the RCPM after the

Table 7: Task performance after the treatment.

Task	Treatment results
WM–number of correct responses	Improved and maintained
RCPM	Non-significant improvement and maintenance in subtest AB
BDAE auditory comprehension	No improvement
BDAE oral expression	Significant improvement and maintenance in the Boston naming test
BDAE reading	Nonsignificant improvement and maintenance in matching cases/scripts and word identification Significant trend for improvement in the overall reading task
Narrative (MAIN)	Non-significant improvement and maintenance
Procedural discourse	No improvement
Communication efficiency (SSLA)	Improvement and maintenance
QoL	Improvement and maintenance

10-day iTBS application to the left DLPFC followed by the 30-minute WM training. It was also hypothesised that stimulation of the DLPFC combined with WM training would result in positive "near-transfer" cognitive effects with subsequent improved scores on untreated cognitive areas (i.e., Gf). A statistically significant overall trend for improvement was found in *Subtest AB* of the *RCPM*, a nontrained measure that indicates Gf (nonverbal intelligence) improvement ($t(11) = 1.82$, $p = 0.048$), while the overall score resulted in positive nonsignificant treatment effects. These findings are consistent with research showing that significant improvements in Gf resulting from cognitive intervention combined with different transcranial electrical brain stimulation protocols [70]. Our findings support the notion that Gf can be improved with DLPFC stimulation [70] and WM training [10, 71–73]. Considering the fact that a combination of treatments was used and it is still controversial whether WM training leads to Gf improvement [74], the findings are inconclusive as to whether improvement was due to the treatment combination or to the DLPFC stimulation. It is worth investigating further whether this association is significant in future research.

4.2. Far-Transfer Effects of iTBS and WM Training. In the past, other groups of researchers focused on investigating improvements in *Auditory Comprehension* where they showed that WM training was used to improve receptive language abilities in PWA [75–79]. These aforementioned studies reported language improvements in tasks such as commands and naming when measured on language tests such as the Western Aphasia Battery (WAB), the Test for the Reception of Grammar (TROG), and the Token Test (TT). The participant of this study had been experiencing mild expressive aphasia with STM difficulties. Results of the treatment showed a significant overall trend for improvement in the *Boston Naming Test* of the *BDAE Oral Expression* subtest. These results tie in well with previous studies where noninvasive brain stimulation to the left prefrontal cortex generated verbal working memory improvements and naming facilitation [10, 80]. Additionally, there was a significant trend for improvement in the overall *BDAE Reading* subtest; although when the individual tasks were analysed, significance was not reached. These results are in agreement with our previous research in which reading abil-

ities were improved [10]. To the best of our knowledge, no other studies so far have investigated language improvements following iTBS combined with WM training with regard to naming or reading.

Two types of tasks were used to collect narrative discourse: the Baby Goat story from the *MAIN* [38] and a personal stroke narrative [37]. The participant showed a nonsignificant trend for improvement in the narrative, specifically showing improvement in the IST initiating structure of the story. Evidence supports that WM impairment in PWA adversely affects their ability to produce macrolinguistic narrative components [81] and higher scores on WM measures are associated with better discourse production abilities in people with brain injury [82]. The SSLA system (Shewan, 1988) was used in this study to examine the broad spectrum of language variables, in order to analyse and quantify the personal stroke narrative. The participant showed a positive linear trend in the *Rate* of speech and *Sentence Complexity*, while there was a negative linear trend in *Errors* indicating improvement. Although linguistic analysis was not generally used in the aphasia treatment literature to evaluate changes in linguistic complexity, there is an increase in research on the topic over the last few years [83]. Even though language sample analysis is commonly used to evaluate linguistic development in children [84], verbal abilities have been examined by analysing language samples [85, 86]. Few studies in the aging literature involving language analysis by obtaining oral language samples through prompts or through conversation [87]. A positive trend towards improvement in discourse was noted for both language tasks, which are consistent with the results of our previous pilot study [10].

Procedural Discourse analysis was based on the analysis developed by Richardson and Dalton [39]. The participant did not show any changes in the responses across the five periods in the *Procedural Discourse* task. Although improvements in these tasks did not reach significance, findings are in agreement with research from the aphasia literature on discourse tasks [88–91]. From the aforementioned studies, only one study was specifically directed to procedural discourse [92], with the more recent studies [88, 89, 91] exploring all aspects of discourse production, including narratives, revealing that as aphasia severity increases, quality and quantity of relevant discourse decrease. The reduction in sentence complexity experienced by PWA has also been shown to differ at a single word and semantic level, which is likely to affect procedural discourse, suggesting that PWA communicate less information in language in a context where spoken language may already be structurally less complex [93]. PWA use fewer correct information units (CIU; i.e., any single word, intelligible, informative, and relevant in context) in discourse than neurologically healthy people (NHP) [94], as well as fewer types and tokens of spatial language in spatial tasks than NHP [95].

The investigation of the use of iTBS in aphasia rehabilitation poststroke continues to be very limited. There are a few studies though that provide evidence for its efficacy. When iTBS was applied in eight individuals with chronic aphasia poststroke for five consecutive days over the course of two weeks, six patients showed significant pre-/post-rTMS improvements in semantic fluency in which the participants were able to generate more appropriate words when prompted with a semantic category. Additionally, increases in the left frontotemporoparietal language networks with a significant left hemispheric shift in the left frontal, left temporoparietal, and global language regions were reported at the pre-/post-rTMS fMRI maps of the study [96]. Further to iTBS investigations, Georgiou et al. [97] recently reported promising findings of neuronavigated continuous theta-burst stimulation (cTBS) over the right pars triangularis (Tr) as a standalone treatment for two individuals with chronic poststroke aphasia in which cTBS was carried over 10 consecutive days for 40 secs per sessions. Their results revealed improvement in language skills in the post-treatment phase, which reverted to baseline scores at follow-up and improvement in the QoL [97].

The self-reported SAQOL-39 questionnaire was administered to C.S. in an interview format to rate his current levels of QoL. A positive linear trend for improvement in the overall QoL across time was noted, which was also maintained 3 months after the treatment, with prominent improvements in the communication and psychosocial fields. This is in line with the QoL literature that the improvement in the severity of language deficits has a positive effect in the QoL [98]. Moreover, the results are consistent with what has been found in previous research that nonverbal cognitive impairments may significantly affect QoL in PWA and are potentially important predictors to improvement [99].

5. Conclusions

The relationship between treatment of WM deficits and the impact on language abilities in poststroke aphasia was investigated. The purpose was to determine whether WM is improved after applying excitatory noninvasive brain stimulation (iTBS) followed by computerized WM training. Furthermore, it was important to decipher whether WM improvements lead to near-transfer on unpractised WM tasks and nonverbal intelligence and far-transfer effects on

Finally, preliminary patient data support the potential clinical utility of the combined use of CIG and PPVT-R, for identifying patients with pure sentence-level comprehension deficits. intelligence, language, and QoL after 10 sessions of iTBS combined with computerized WM training in a single case study with no adverse effects during treatment and at follow-up periods. As it is widely acknowledged amongst rehabilitation professionals, the deficits acquired after a stroke persist for long periods and positive effects are accomplished at a slower rate. The results of this study are indicative that computerized WM training and stimulation of the LDLPFC are areas that have a positive effect in neurorehabilitation of PWA after a stroke. Improvements were noted in only 10 days and even though not all the benefits were maintained at follow-up (3 months post), the positive linear trendlines signify that there is efficacious treatment potential, which requires further exploration towards facilitating language recovery in PWA. It is important to consider that aphasia treatment programs could benefit from neurorehabilitation to increase the pace of recovery, especially during the first months of rehabilitation. The results of this study provide a preliminary indication that stimulation of the LDLPFC combined with computerized WM training after left hemisphere stroke may generalize to language improvements.

Acknowledgments

The authors would like to acknowledge the Cyprus Stroke Association and the Melathron Agoniston EOKA, Limassol, Cyprus for their assistance with participant recruitment.

References

[1] A. T. Barker, R. Jalinous, and I. L. Freeston, "Non-invasive magnetic stimulation of human motor cortex," *The Lancet*, vol. 325, no. 8437, pp. 1106-1107, 1985.

[2] Y. Bagherzadeh, A. Khorrami, M. R. Zarrindast, S. V. Shariat, and D. Pantazis, "Repetitive transcranial magnetic stimulation of the dorsolateral prefrontal cortex enhances working memory," *Experimental Brain Research*, vol. 234, no. 7, pp. 1807–1818, 2016.

[3] A. Baddeley, "Working memory: looking back and looking forward," *Nature Reviews. Neuroscience*, vol. 4, no. 10, pp. 829–839, 2003.

[4] M. J. Dehn, "How working memory enables fluid reasoning," *Applied Neuropsychology: Child*, vol. 6, no. 3, pp. 245–247, 2017.

[5] T. Hedden and C. Yoon, "Individual differences in executive processing predict susceptibility to interference in verbal working memory," *Neuropsychology*, vol. 20, no. 5, pp. 511–528, 2006.

[6] K. Fukuda, E. Vogel, U. Mayr, and E. Awh, "Quantity, not quality: the relationship between fluid intelligence and working memory capacity," *Psychonomic Bulletin & Review*, vol. 17, no. 5, pp. 673–679, 2010.

[7] M. K. Johnson, R. P. McMahon, B. M. Robinson et al., "The relationship between working memory capacity and broad

measures of cognitive ability in healthy adults and people with schizophrenia," *Neuropsychology*, vol. 27, no. 2, pp. 220–229, 2013.

[8] M. J. Kane and R. W. Engle, "The role of prefrontal cortex in working-memory capacity, executive attention, and general fluid intelligence: an individual-differences perspective," *Psychonomic Bulletin & Review*, vol. 9, no. 4, pp. 637–671, 2002.

[9] M. S. Lee and B. S. Kim, "Effects of working memory intervention on language production by individuals with dementia," *Neuropsychological Rehabilitation*, vol. 31,10, pp. 1557–1581, 2021.

[10] D. Kranou-Economidou and M. Kambanaros, "Combining intermittent theta burst stimulation (iTBS) with computerized working memory training to improve language abilities in chronic aphasia: a pilot case study," *Aphasiology*, pp. 1–25, 2020.

[11] D. S. Kasselimis and Neurology Department, Eginition Hospital, National and Kapodistrian University of Athens, Greece, "Working memory and aphasia," *International Journal of Neurology Research*, vol. 1, no. 4, pp. 188–190, 2015.

[12] C. Kim, J. K. Kroger, V. D. Calhoun, and V. P. Clark, "The role of the frontopolar cortex in manipulation of integrated information in working memory," *Neuroscience Letters*, vol. 595, pp. 25–29, 2015.

[13] N. Osaka, M. Osaka, H. Kondo, M. Morishita, H. Fukuyama, and H. Shibasaki, "The neural basis of executive function in working memory: an fMRI study based on individual differences," *NeuroImage*, vol. 21, no. 2, pp. 623–631, 2004.

[14] A. M. Owen, K. M. McMillan, A. R. Laird, and E. Bullmore, "N-back working memory paradigm: a meta-analysis of normative functional neuroimaging studies," *Human Brain Mapping*, vol. 25, no. 1, pp. 46–59, 2005.

[15] J. M. Chein, A. B. Moore, and A. R. A. Conway, "Domain-general mechanisms of complex working memory span," *NeuroImage*, vol. 54, no. 1, pp. 550–559, 2011.

[16] W. J. Chai, A. I. Abd Hamid, and J. M. Abdullah, "Working memory from the psychological and neurosciences perspectives: a review," *Frontiers in Psychology*, vol. 9, pp. 1–16, 2018.

[17] A. D. Baddeley, R. J. Allen, and G. J. Hitch, "Binding in visual working memory: the role of the episodic buffer," *Neuropsychologia*, vol. 49, no. 6, pp. 1393–1400, 2011.

[18] S. M. Courtney, "Attention and cognitive control as Emergent properties of information representation in working memory," *Cognitive, Affective, & Behavioral Neuroscience*, vol. 4, no. 4, pp. 501–516, 2004.

[19] L. Pessoa, E. Gutierrez, P. Bandettini, and L. Ungerleider, "Neural correlates of visual working memory: fMRI amplitude predicts task performance," *Neuron*, vol. 35, no. 5, pp. 975–987, 2002.

[20] A. M. Owen, A. C. Evans, and M. Petrides, "Evidence for a two-stage model of spatial working memory processing within the lateral frontal cortex: a positron emission tomography study," *Cerebral Cortex*, vol. 6, no. 1, pp. 31–38, 1996.

[21] T. D. Wager and E. E. Smith, "Neuroimaging studies of working memory:," *Cognitive, Affective, & Behavioral Neuroscience*, vol. 3, no. 4, pp. 255–274, 2003.

[22] S. S. Cho and A. P. Strafella, "rTMS of the left dorsolateral prefrontal cortex modulates dopamine release in the ipsilateral anterior cingulate cortex and orbitofrontal cortex," *PLoS One*, vol. 4, no. 8, p. e6725, 2009.

[23] M. D'Esposito and B. R. Postle, "The cognitive neuroscience of working memory," *Annual Review of Psychology*, vol. 66, no. 1, pp. 115–142, 2015.

[24] J. Au, E. Sheehan, N. Tsai, G. J. Duncan, M. Buschkuehl, and S. M. Jaeggi, "Improving fluid intelligence with training on working memory: a meta-analysis," *Psychonomic Bulletin & Review*, vol. 22, no. 2, pp. 366–377, 2015.

[25] T. Klingberg, "Training and plasticity of working memory," *Trends in Cognitive Sciences*, vol. 14, no. 7, pp. 317–324, 2010.

[26] X. Zhao, Y. Wang, D. Liu, and R. Zhou, "Effect of updating training on fluid intelligence in children," *Chinese Science Bulletin*, vol. 56, no. 21, pp. 2202–2205, 2011.

[27] S. M. Jaeggi, M. Buschkuehl, J. Jonides, and W. J. Perrig, "Improving fluid intelligence with training on working memory," *Proceedings of the National Academy of Sciences*, vol. 105, no. 19, pp. 6829–6833, 2008.

[28] R. B. Cattell, *Abilities: Their Structure, Growth, and Action*, Houghton Mifflin, Oxford, England, 1971.

[29] J. R. Gray, C. F. Chabris, and T. S. Braver, "Neural mechanisms of general fluid intelligence," *Nature Neuroscience*, vol. 6, no. 3, pp. 316–322, 2003.

[30] L. Messinis, E. Panagea, P. Papathanasopoulos, and A. Kastellakis, *Boston diagnostic aphasia examination-short form in Greek language*, Gotsis, Patras, 2013.

[31] J. C. Keel, M. J. Smith, and E. M. Wassermann, "A safety screening questionnaire for transcranial magnetic stimulation," *Clinical Neurophysiology*, vol. 112, no. 4, p. 720, 2001.

[32] M. L. Albert, "A simple test of visual neglect," *Neurology*, vol. 23, no. 6, pp. 658–664, 1973.

[33] R. C. Oldfield, "The assessment and analysis of handedness: The Edinburgh inventory," in *Neuropsychologia*, vol. 9, no. 1- pp. 97–113, Elsevier Science, Netherlands, 1971.

[34] A. T. Beck, C. H. Ward, M. Mendelson, J. Mock, and J. Erbaugh, "An inventory for measuring depression," in *Archives of General Psychiatry*, vol. 4, pp. 561–571, American Medical Association, US, 1961.

[35] M. Giannakou, P. Roussi, M. E. Kosmides, G. Kiosseoglou, A. Adamopoulou, and G. Garyfallos, "Adaptation of the beck depression inventory-II to Greek population," *Hellenic Journal of Psychology*, vol. 10, no. 2, pp. 120–146, 2013.

[36] J. Raven, "The Raven's progressive matrices: change and stability over culture and time," *Cognitive Psychology*, vol. 41, no. 1, pp. 1–48, 2000.

[37] M. Kambanaros, "Evaluating personal stroke narratives from bilingual Greek-English immigrants with aphasia," *Folia Phoniatrica et Logopaedica*, vol. 71, no. 2–3, pp. 101–115, 2019.

[38] N. V. Gagarina, D. Klop, S. Kunnari et al., "Multilingual Assessment Instrument for Narratives," *ZAS papers in linguistics*, vol. 56, pp. 155–155, 2012.

[39] J. D. Richardson and S. G. Dalton, "Main concepts for three different discourse tasks in a large non-clinical sample," *Aphasiology*, vol. 30, no. 1, pp. 45–73, 2016.

[40] K. Hilari, D. L. Lamping, S. C. Smith, S. Northcott, A. Lamb, and J. Marshall, "Psychometric properties of the Stroke and Aphasia Quality of Life Scale (SAQOL-39) in a generic stroke population," *Clinical Rehabilitation*, vol. 23, no. 6, pp. 544–557, 2009.

[41] W. B. Bilker, J. A. Hansen, C. M. Brensinger, J. Richard, R. E. Gur, and R. C. Gur, "Development of abbreviated nine-item forms of the Raven's standard progressive matrices test," *Assessment*, vol. 19, no. 3, pp. 354–369, 2012.

[42] G. Sideridis, F. Antoniou, A. Mouzaki, and P. Simos, "Raven's educational CPM/CVS," *Athens Motiv.*, 2015.

[43] G. Papantoniou, D. Moraitou, M. Dinou, E. Katsadima, E. Savvidou, and E. Foutsitzi, "Comparing the latent structure of the children's category test-level 1 among young children and older adults: a preliminary study," *Psychology*, vol. 7, no. 11, pp. 1352–1368, 2016.

[44] K. Tsapkini, C. H. Vlahou, and C. Potagas, "Adaptation and Validation of Standardized Aphasia Tests in Different Languages: Lessons from the Boston Diagnostic Aphasia Examination–Short Form in Greek," *Behavioural Neurology*, vol. 22, no. 3–4, 119 pages, 2010.

[45] C. M. Shewan, "The _Shewan Spontaneous Language Analysis_ (SSLA) system for aphasic adults: Description, reliability, and validity," *Journal of Communication Disorders*, vol. 21, no. 2, pp. 103–138, 1988.

[46] N. Karpathiou, J. Papatriantafyllou, and M. Kambanaros, "Bilingualism in a case of the non-fluent/agrammatic variant of primary progressive aphasia," *Frontiers in Communication*, vol. 3, pp. 1–16, 2018.

[47] A. Kartsona and K. Hilari, "Quality of life in aphasia: Greek adaptation of the stroke and aphasia quality of life scale - 39 item (SAQOL-39)," *Europa Medicophysica*, vol. 43, no. 1, pp. 27–35, 2007.

[48] E. A. Efstratiadou, E. N. Chelas, M. Ignatiou, V. Christaki, I. Papathanasiou, and K. Hilari, "Quality of life after stroke: evaluation of the Greek SAQOL-39g," *Folia Phoniatrica et Logopaedica*, vol. 64, no. 4, pp. 179–186, 2012.

[49] P. M. Rossini, D. Burke, R. Chen et al., "Non-invasive electrical and magnetic stimulation of the brain, spinal cord, roots and peripheral nerves: Basic principles and procedures for routine clinical and research application. An updated report from an I.F.C.N. Committee," *Clinical Neurophysiology*, vol. 126, no. 6, pp. 1071–1107, 2015.

[50] J. J. Borckardt, Z. Nahas, J. Koola, and M. S. George, "Estimating resting motor thresholds in transcranial magnetic stimulation research and practice: a computer simulation evaluation of Best Methods," *The journal of ECT*, vol. 22, no. 3, pp. 169–175, 2006.

[51] Y. Z. Huang, M. J. Edwards, E. Rounis, K. P. Bhatia, and J. C. Rothwell, "Theta burst stimulation of the human motor cortex," *Neuron*, vol. 45, no. 2, pp. 201–206, 2005.

[52] A. K. Barbey, M. Koenigs, and J. Grafman, "Dorsolateral prefrontal contributions to human working memory," *Cortex*, vol. 49, no. 5, pp. 1195–1205, 2013.

[53] J. Weicker, N. Hudl, S. Frisch et al., "WOME: theory-based working memory training - a placebo-controlled, double-blind evaluation in older adults," *Frontiers in Aging Neuroscience*, vol. 10, pp. 1–14, 2018.

[54] D. Howard, W. Best, and L. Nickels, "Optimising the design of intervention studies: critiques and ways forward," *Aphasiology*, vol. 29, no. 5, pp. 526–562, 2015.

[55] V. P. Clark and R. Parasuraman, "Neuroenhancement: enhancing brain and mind in health and in disease," *NeuroImage*, vol. 85, pp. 889–894, 2014.

[56] M. Cotelli, R. Manenti, O. Zanetti, and C. Miniussi, "Non-pharmacological intervention for memory decline," *Frontiers in human neuroscience*, vol. 6, pp. 1–17, 2012.

[57] R. McKendrick, H. Ayaz, R. Olmstead, and R. Parasuraman, "Enhancing dual-task performance with verbal and spatial working memory training: continuous monitoring of cerebral hemodynamics with NIRS," *NeuroImage*, vol. 85, pp. 1014–1026, 2014.

[58] J. Bentwich, E. Dobronevsky, S. Aichenbaum et al., "Beneficial effect of repetitive transcranial magnetic stimulation combined with cognitive training for the treatment of Alzheimer's disease: a proof of concept study," *Journal of Neural Transmission*, vol. 118, no. 3, pp. 463–471, 2011.

[59] G. Vallar and N. Bolognini, "Behavioural facilitation following brain stimulation: implications for neurorehabilitation," *Neuropsychological Rehabilitation*, vol. 21, no. 5, pp. 618–649, 2011.

[60] S. S. Buss, P. J. Fried, and A. Pascual-Leone, "Therapeutic non-invasive brain stimulation in Alzheimer's disease and related dementias," *Current Opinion in Neurology*, vol. 32, no. 2, pp. 292–304, 2019.

[61] L. L. Murray, "Direct and indirect treatment approaches for addressing short-term or working memory deficits in aphasia," *Aphasiology*, vol. 26, no. 3–4, pp. 317–337, 2012.

[62] K. E. Hoy, N. Bailey, M. Michael et al., "Enhancement of working memory and task-related oscillatory activity following intermittent theta burst stimulation in healthy controls," *Cerebral Cortex*, vol. 26, no. 12, pp. 4563–4573, 2016.

[63] E. Demeter, J. L. Mirdamadi, S. K. Meehan, and S. F. Taylor, "Short theta burst stimulation to left frontal cortex prior to encoding enhances subsequent recognition memory," *Cognitive, Affective, & Behavioral Neuroscience*, vol. 16, no. 4, pp. 724–735, 2016.

[64] A. Lundqvist, K. Grundstrm, K. Samuelsson, and J. Rönnberg, "Computerized training of working memory in a group of patients suffering from acquired brain injury," *Brain Injury*, vol. 24, no. 10, pp. 1173–1183, 2010.

[65] M. Manning, A. MacFarlane, A. Hickey, and S. Franklin, "Perspectives of people with aphasia post-stroke towards personal recovery and living successfully: a systematic review and thematic synthesis," *PLoS One*, vol. 14, no. 3, pp. 1–22, 2019.

[66] K. Oberauer, H. M. Süß, O. Wilhelm, and W. W. Wittmann, "Which working memory functions predict intelligence?," *Intelligence*, vol. 36, no. 6, pp. 641–652, 2008.

[67] T. P. Alloway, "Working memory, but not IQ, predicts subsequent learning in children with learning difficulties," *European Journal of Psychological Assessment*, vol. 25, no. 2, pp. 92–98, 2009.

[68] C. C. von Bastian and K. Oberauer, "Effects and mechanisms of working memory training: a review," *Psychological Research*, vol. 78, no. 6, pp. 803–820, 2014.

[69] A. B. Morrison and J. M. Chein, "Does working memory training work? The promise and challenges of enhancing cognition by training working memory," *Psychonomic Bulletin & Review*, vol. 18, no. 1, pp. 46–60, 2011.

[70] A. K. Brem, J. N. F. Almquist, K. Mansfield et al., "Modulating fluid intelligence performance through combined cognitive training and brain stimulation," *Neuropsychologia*, vol. 118, no. Part A, pp. 107–114, 2018.

[71] R. W. Engle, J. E. Laughlin, S. W. Tuholski, and A. R. A. Conway, "Working memory, short-term memory, and general fluid intelligence: a latent-variable approach," *Journal of Experimental Psychology. General*, vol. 128, no. 3, pp. 309–331, 1999.

[72] N. P. Friedman, A. Miyake, R. P. Corley, S. E. Young, J. C. DeFries, and J. K. Hewitt, "Not all executive functions are related to intelligence," *Psychological Science*, vol. 17, no. 2, pp. 172–179, 2006.

[73] N. Unsworth, K. Fukuda, E. Awh, and E. K. Vogel, "Working memory and fluid intelligence: capacity, attention control, and secondary memory retrieval," *Cognitive Psychology*, vol. 71, no. 3, pp. 1–26, 2014.

[74] T. L. Harrison, Z. Shipstead, K. L. Hicks, D. Z. Hambrick, T. S. Redick, and R. W. Engle, "Working memory training may increase working memory capacity but not fluid intelligence," *Psychological Science*, vol. 24, no. 12, pp. 2409–2419, 2013.

[75] B. Eom and J. E. Sung, "The effects of sentence repetition-based working memory treatment on sentence comprehension abilities in individuals with aphasia," *American Journal of Speech-Language Pathology*, vol. 25, no. 4S, pp. 1–15, 2016.

[76] L. Harris, A. Olson, and G. Humphreys, "The link between STM and sentence comprehension: a neuropsychological rehabilitation study," *Neuropsychological Rehabilitation*, vol. 24, no. 5, pp. 678–720, 2014.

[77] C. Salis, "Short-term memory treatment: patterns of learning and generalisation to sentence comprehension in a person with aphasia," *Neuropsychological Rehabilitation*, vol. 22, no. 3, pp. 428–448, 2012.

[78] C. Salis, F. Hwang, D. Howard, and N. Lallini, "Short-term and working memory treatments for improving sentence comprehension in aphasia: a review and a replication study," *Seminars in Speech and Language*, vol. 38, no. 1, pp. 29–39, 2017.

[79] L. Zakariás, A. Keresztes, K. Marton, and I. Wartenburger, "Positive effects of a computerised working memory and executive function training on sentence comprehension in aphasia," *Neuropsychological Rehabilitation*, vol. 28, no. 3, pp. 369–386, 2018.

[80] S. Y. Jeon and S. J. Han, "Improvement of the working memory and naming by transcranial direct current stimulation," *Annals of Rehabilitation Medicine*, vol. 36, no. 5, pp. 585–595, 2012.

[81] D. Cahana-Amitay and T. Jenkins, "Working memory and discourse production in people with aphasia," *Journal of Neurolinguistics*, vol. 48, pp. 90–103, 2018.

[82] K. M. Youse and C. A. Coelho, "Working memory and discourse production abilities following closed-head injury," *Brain Injury*, vol. 19, no. 12, pp. 1001–1009, 2005.

[83] L. Bryant, A. Ferguson, and E. Spencer, "Linguistic analysis of discourse in aphasia: a review of the literature," *Clinical Linguistics & Phonetics*, vol. 30, no. 7, pp. 489–518, 2016.

[84] J. Heilmann, J. F. Miller, A. Nockerts, and C. Dunaway, "Properties of the narrative scoring scheme using narrative retells in young school-age children," *American Journal of Speech-Language Pathology*, vol. 19, no. 2, pp. 154–166, 2010.

[85] G. Capilouto, H. H. Wright, and S. A. Wagovich, "CIU and main event analyses of the structured discourse of older and younger adults," *Journal of Communication Disorders*, vol. 38, no. 6, pp. 431–444, 2005.

[86] C. M. Shewan and V. L. Henderson, "Analysis of spontaneous language in the older normal population," *Journal of Communication Disorders*, vol. 21, no. 2, pp. 139–154, 1988.

[87] S. Kemper and A. Sumner, "The structure of verbal abilities in young and older adults," *Psychology and Aging*, vol. 16, no. 2, pp. 312–322, 2001.

[88] S. Andreetta, A. Cantagallo, and A. Marini, "Narrative discourse in anomic aphasia," *Neuropsychologia*, vol. 50, no. 8, pp. 1787–1793, 2012.

[89] G. J. Capilouto, H. H. Wright, and S. A. Wagovich, "Reliability of main event measurement in the discourse of individuals with aphasia," *Aphasiology*, vol. 20, no. 2–4, pp. 205–216, 2006.

[90] H. Ulatowska, R. Freedman-Stern, A. Doyel, S. Macaluso-Haynes, and A. North, "Production of narrative discourse in aphasia," *Brain and Language*, vol. 19, no. 2, pp. 317–334, 1983.

[91] G. Fergadiotis and H. H. Wright, "Lexical diversity for adults with and without aphasia across discourse elicitation tasks," *Aphasiology*, vol. 25, no. 11, pp. 1414–1430, 2011.

[92] H. K. Ulatowska, A. J. North, and S. Macaluso-Haynes, "Production of narrative and procedural discourse in aphasia," *Brain and Language*, vol. 13, no. 2, pp. 345–371, 1981.

[93] M. Pritchard, L. Dipper, G. Morgan, and N. Cocks, "Language and iconic gesture use in procedural discourse by speakers with aphasia," *Aphasiology*, vol. 29, no. 7, pp. 826–844, 2015.

[94] L. E. Nicholas and R. H. Brookshire, "A system for quantifying the informativeness and efficiency of the connected speech of adults with aphasia," *Journal of Speech and Hearing Research*, vol. 36, no. 2, pp. 338–350, 1993.

[95] S. Johnson, N. Cocks, and L. Dipper, "Use of spatial communication in aphasia," *International Journal of Language & Communication Disorders*, vol. 48, no. 4, pp. 469–476, 2013.

[96] J. P. Szaflarski, J. Vannest, S. W. Wu, M. W. Difrancesco, C. Banks, and D. L. Gilbert, "Excitatory repetitive transcranial magnetic stimulation induces improvements in chronic post-stroke aphasia," *Medical Science Monitor*, vol. 17, no. 3, pp. -CR132–CR139, 2011.

[97] A. Georgiou, N. Konstantinou, I. Phinikettos, and M. Kambanaros, "Neuronavigated theta burst stimulation for chronic aphasia: two exploratory case studies," *Clinical Linguistics & Phonetics*, vol. 33, no. 6, pp. 532–546, 2019.

[98] S. Spaccavento, A. Craca, M. del Prete et al., "Quality of life measurement and outcome in aphasia," *Neuropsychiatric Disease and Treatment*, vol. 10, p. 27, 2013.

[99] M. Nicholas, E. Hunsaker, and A. J. Guarino, "The relation between language, non-verbal cognition and quality of life in people with aphasia," *Aphasiology*, vol. 31, no. 6, pp. 688–702, 2017.

15

Interaction between Nursing Staff and Residents with Aphasia in Long-Term Care

Charlotta Saldert (ID),[1,2] **Hannah Bartonek-Åhman,**[1,2] **and Steven Bloch**[3]

[1]*Institute of Neuroscience and Physiology, Division of Speech-Language Pathology, Sahlgrenska Academy, University of Gothenburg, Gothenburg, Sweden*
[2]*University of Gothenburg Centre for Person-Centred Care (GPCC), Sahlgrenska Academy, University of Gothenburg, Gothenburg, Sweden*
[3]*Language and Cognition, University College London, UK*

Correspondence should be addressed to Charlotta Saldert; charlotta.saldert@neuro.gu.se

Academic Editor: Kathleen Finlayson

Introduction. Thousands of individuals with communication disorders live in long-term residential care. Nursing staff are often their primary communication partners. The positive effects of social interaction and person-centred care have been recognised but there remains a paucity of research on the content and quality of communicative interaction between long-term care staff and residents with aphasia. This mixed method study investigates the discourse in interaction between nursing staff and residents with aphasia. *Methods.* A routine care activity was explored in 26 video-recordings featuring four enrolled nurses and four elderly persons with severe aphasia. Factors such as goals and roles in the activity were mapped out and a qualitative discourse analysis was performed. Based on the findings a coding scheme was constructed and the amount of time spent in different interactional foci of discourse was explored. *Results.* From the qualitative findings three broad, but distinct, foci in the nurse-initiated interaction could be distinguished: (1) a focus on getting the task done with minimum interaction; (2) topics related to the task, but not necessary to get the task done; and (3) personal topics related to themes beyond the caring task. The analysis of distribution of time revealed that although most of the interaction was focused on the main care activity, between 3 and 17% of the time was spent in either task-related or non task-related interaction. The distribution varied between dyads and could not be related to the residents' severity of aphasia nor the activity as such. *Conclusions.* An endeavour to interact socially with the residents with aphasia influences the nurses' foci of interaction. Contextual and personal factors of the residents and nurses need to be considered in clinical work as well as research on how communication may be supported to facilitate social interaction and person-centredness in long-term care of people with aphasia.

1. Introduction

Due to demographic changes and progress in medical care, an increasing number of elderly people are living with physical disabilities and communication disorders due to neurological disease or injury. Communication disorders, such as aphasia following a stroke, may severely affect a person's ability to understand and convey information in speech and writing, as well as the ability to interact socially. Numerous individuals, who are in need of more assistance than can be delivered by home care services, are living in long-term care facilities [1].

In this context communication difficulties pose an additional challenge [2].

An endeavour to humanise medicine and care has been described, with both similarities and differences under different labels such as client-centred care [3], patient-centred care [4, 5], person-centred nursing [6], person-centred care [7, 8], or person-centredness [9]. In person-centred care the individual person beyond the role of being a patient or a resident with needs is acknowledged. Each individual's personal experiences and traits are recognised and considered in the planning and achievement of care. Functional communication in the encounters between nursing staff and residents in long-term care facilities is clearly a prerequisite to accomplish this. In long-term care, person-centred care has been described in the care of people with communication disorders due to dementia and it has been proved to reduce both disruptive behaviour and need for medication [10–13].

The importance of communication is often emphasised when staff in long-term residential care describe what they consider to be good caring encounters [14, 15]. Being able to have conversations with residents makes it possible to get to know each person's unique life history, to regard them as individuals and to establish and develop personal relationships. It is also known that meaningful social interaction is essential for the wellbeing of residents in long-term care facilities [16]. Staff attitudes are signalled in the interaction and affect the residents' perception of quality of life. Furthermore, many elders living in long-term care facilities feel their needs are often ignored by the staff and they also stress the lack of communication beyond instrumental interactions. The fact is that although nursing staff acknowledge the importance of social interaction with the residents, long-term care facilities have been described as providing limited possibilities for communication outside of care routines [14, 15, 17].

Some attempts to describe the different foci of interaction in different care contexts have been made quantitatively. Roter and Hall [18] described two purposes of communication between doctors and patients during medical visits: (1) instrumental or task-focused or (2) affective or rapport-developing. Although they are not necessarily mutually exclusive, a distinction between task-focused interaction and more affective interpersonal interaction focusing on more general personal issues is often reflected in research on interaction between nursing staff and patients or residents. One example is Bottorf and Morse's [19] qualitative observational video-recording analysis of registered nurses attending care of cancer patients. Besides exploring different types of touch, four types of attending were identified and described: (1) *Doing more*: making contact or the nurse "did something" beyond what is required to complete the care; (2) *Doing for*: primarily responding to patient requests and needs that were not treatment related; (3) *Doing with*: focus equally on the task and patient, for example, the nurse may have actively engaged a patient by seeking or attending to his or her opinions, thoughts, and perceptions; (4) *Doing tasks*: focus on equipment, treatment, and getting the job done. The authors conclude that the dynamic quality of nurse-patient interaction is not only an internal experience, but one that can be observed in verbal and nonverbal behaviours of nurses and patients.

Previous research in the context of long-term care has reported an overemphasis on task-focused talk and lack of opportunities for more personal psychosocial or affective interaction [20–22]. Williams and colleagues [17] examined topics of staff-resident interaction. A scheme based on previous research was developed to categorize topics of staff talk with residents. About thirty-nine percent of the utterances focused on activities of daily living (ADLs), 14% focused on assessment of nursing, 16% focused on technical aspects of care, and 29% were more personal, psychosocial in nature.

Based on Roter and Hall's [18] conceptualising, four characteristics of affective interaction have been described in verbal communication between nurse aides and residents in a long-term care facility [23]: (1) personal conversation (including pleasantries, laughter, and conversation about the resident's personal life); (2) addressing the resident by name or use of terms of endearment (like "honey" and "sweetie"); (3) checking in (asking residents whether they were all right or about their comfort level in the task); and (4) emotional support/praise. Still, the authors do say that this affective communication was sometimes also used by the nurse aides in instrumental communication to improve the effectiveness of their care delivery. The purpose of nurse aides' communication varied depending on the cognitive functioning of the residents. With residents diagnosed with more severe dementia, the nurse aides asked fewer questions and instead made more imperative statements characterized as being more instrumental than affective by referring to the current care activities.

Topics in first morning encounters between nurses and nursing assistants and elderly residents in long-term care have been investigated [23]. It was concluded that it was the staff who initiated conversation and they also chose the topic of conversation, which was usually regarding residents' health and sickness. The fact that it is usually staff who initiate and control the topic of conversation has also been described elsewhere [14, 22].

Attempts have been made to develop instruments for assessing degree of person-centredness in communication [24–26]. Savundranayagam and colleagues have developed a scheme for coding frequency of use of person-centred communicative strategies with people with communication difficulties due to dementia [27–29]. In this instrument a nursing staff's use of communicative strategies is quantified without considering the context of the communicative interaction. This neglect of the influence of context on communicative interaction is actually the case in most of the existing research on communication between nursing staff and the elderly in long-term care and affects the validity of the results [30, 31]. For example, in the first morning encounters, as described in Wadensten [23] the staff member is entering the resident's room to help them get out of bed, getting dressed, etc. The external context of this activity affects the roles, the behaviours, and the discourse of the participants in the interaction. However, there is also an internal context within a communicative interaction on a sequential level where each contribution or behaviour is affected by previous contributions and also influences the contributions that will follow [32].

Marsden and Holmes [31] have questioned the inferences from earlier research on health care providers' communication with elderly people as this usually has not considered aspects of coconstruction of the interaction and, for example, the face-saving actions in everyday interactions.

Conversation analysis (CA) is a qualitative, data driven method used to study naturally occurring interaction and the collaborative accomplishment and organization of social action [33]. The method has been used in numerous studies of conversational interaction in different institutions including

TABLE 1: Description of nurses (N) and the residents with aphasia (R) including measures of comprehension in Token test [48] and verbal fluency [49] and amount of data from each dyad.

Nurses	N-1	N-2	N-3	N-4
Sex/Age	F/55	F/55	F/40	F/36
Time working with R	3 years	19 months	9 months	1 year
Education, in years	11	12	12	12
Residents with aphasia	*R-1*	*R-2*	*R-3*	*R-4*
Sex/Age	M/72	F/91	F/82	F/93
Type of aphasia[a]	Severe, global aphasia	Severe, global aphasia	Severe, global aphasia	Severe, global aphasia
Time post onset	8 years	17 months	10 months	12 months
Time in residential care facility	3 years	19 months	12 months	12 months
Score in Token Test (max: 261)	69	97	36	68
Score in word fluency tasks	0/0/0	0/0/0	0/0/0	0/0/0
Amount of analysed data (in minutes)	70	50	90	50

[a]Aphasia type according to the Boston classification system.

interaction between staff and residents in long-term care [34–36]. CA has also been used to explore interactions between nursing staff and people with dementia in long-term care [22, 37, 38]. However, although CA focuses on the internal sequential context of talk, its ethnomethodological theoretical base stipulates that external factors which are not oriented to by the participants themselves should not be considered [39].

By contrast, the method *Activity-based Communication Analysis* (ACA) emphasises the influence from external context on the interaction [40, 41]. ACA is a multidisciplinary framework based on philosophical and linguistic as well as psychological and sociological theories in the view of language as action in context [42–45]. In ACA the outset for the analysis is the type of activity where the interaction occurs. ACA treats aspects such as participants' roles and goals in the social activity as relevant factors, influencing the interaction. The communication difficulties seen in communication disorders have been important in the development of the model [46, 47]. According to ACA the collective influencing factors, for example, the main goal of the activity, the integral roles of the participants, and physical circumstances, are common to all participants in the activity. These collective factors interact with the participant's individual background factors, including, for example, their physical and cognitive competencies, and ability to use different means to produce and comprehend utterances. Participants in communication may also have individual goals and take on different roles beyond those inherent in the specific activity. The influencing factors of the activity and participating individuals interact in determining the communicative interaction that actually takes place.

To summarize, many individuals with severe aphasia are living in long-term residential care and the importance of social interaction and person-centred care for residents' experience of quality of life has been acknowledged. Research has shown that routine care activities may be more or less task-focused and include different degrees of social interaction. However, there is still a lack of evidence regarding interaction between nursing staff and long-term care residents with aphasia based on analysis that considers both external and internal sequential contextual factors.

The purpose of this study was to explore the discourse and interactive patterns of nursing staff working with people with severe aphasia in a routine care task in long-term care facilities. The aims were to (1) explore contextual factors affecting the communicative interaction between enrolled nurses and residents with severe aphasia; (2) describe the nurses' interactional foci in their work with the persons with aphasia during a routine care activity.

2. Materials and Methods

This sequential exploratory mixed method study has been approved by a regional ethical review board and all participants provided informed written consent.

2.1. Participants. The participants in this study were recruited through the managers and staff of different long-term residential care facilities in western Sweden and are a convenience sample. Four dyads comprising a person with stroke-induced aphasia and an enrolled nurse participated in the present study; see Table 1. An enrolled nurse in Sweden has completed a formal 65-week-long training program in nursing. They provide the routine care work under the supervision of a registered nurse.

Inclusion criterion for the nurses was regular contact with the person with aphasia. Inclusion criterion for the persons with aphasia was a presence of communication difficulties caused by stroke-induced aphasia. Exclusion criteria for both nurses and persons with aphasia were vision or hearing impairment not compensated for by aids. All participants were native Swedish speakers.

The participating nurses were all female with an age range of 36 to 55 years (see Table 1). They had worked with the resident with aphasia for between nine months to three years, but all had long experience in working with people with

TABLE 2: Key to transcription symbols.

((nodding))	Non-verbal activity within double brackets
⌈ yes	Simultaneous verbal or non-verbal activities
⌊ ((nods))	
(0.7)	Numbers in parentheses indicate silence in tenth of second
no:	A colon indicates an extension of the sound or syllable it follows
°no°	Degree signs indicate a passage of quiet talk

communication disorders. The nurses had between 11-12 years of education.

The comprehension of the participating persons with aphasia was measured with the Token test [48] and semantic and phonological word fluency was measured using standardised test procedures and scoring standards [49].

The participants with aphasia comprised one man and three women, between ten months and eight years after onset of aphasia and with an age range of 72 to 93 years (see Table 1). All four residents with aphasia had severe aphasia with incomprehensive speech and impaired comprehension. They were all able to express acceptance or rejection vocally, but their speech output was otherwise reduced into syllable repetitions together with neologistic words and phrases. All four residents also expressed themselves with facial expressions and variations of prosody.

2.2. Material: Video-Recordings of Naturally Occurring Interaction. The participants selected a routine nursing activity. In three of the dyads (1, 3, and 4) the participants chose to do the video-recording during the morning nursing routine task. Dyad 2 chose the evening routine. A research assistant set up the video camera and then left the dyads alone, except for dyad 1 where the assistant operated the camera throughout the recording. The dyads were instructed to interact as they usually would in that situation.

Each dyad was video-recorded between five and nine times. The length of each recording varied between approximately 10 and 25 minutes. The middle 10 minutes of each recording were used in the analysis based on the hypothesis that individuals are less self-conscious after being recorded for a few minutes.

2.3. Procedures. An analysis of the influencing and influenced factors in the main activity, including the present goals and roles, was performed in accordance with ACA [46]. This was followed by a discourse analysis of the video-recorded interaction [50]. The analysis was influenced by CA [33] in the exploration of interactional patterns on a sequential level, but mainly performed with the purpose of revealing the content and foci of the interaction between the nurses and residents. Using standard CA conventions, the video-recorded interactions were transcribed to capture talk as well as nonvocal features such as gestures and other body movements, (see Table 2 for transcription symbols used). The transcriptions presented here comprise representative extracts from the material and have been translated into English.

From the qualitative analysis it was concluded that the nurses' communicative interaction with the residents could be described as belonging to one of three broad but still distinctive categories of interaction with different goals and content (see results). As different qualities of touch, facial expressions, and gaze may also communicate meaning, the categories may include sequences both with and without verbal interaction.

A quantitative coding scheme was also constructed to enable an exploration of the distribution in time of the different types of interaction. The qualitative analysis showed that it was the nurses who decided whether to elaborate on a topic or to change focus in the interaction. The persons with aphasia only rarely initiated interaction and their verbal contributions were difficult to interpret due to the severe aphasia. Thus, the coding of the interaction across time was based on the start and ending of the nurses' actions.

In the procedure for analysis of distribution of time the primary assessor coded the content in the video-recordings using the annotation program ELAN (Max Planck Institute for Psycholinguistics, The Language Archive, Nijmegen, Netherlands). Each second in the video-recordings was coded as belonging to one of the three categories based on an assessment of what was the nurse's main focus of the interaction. The number of seconds allocated to each category was then calculated and presented as the proportion of time used for the different foci in each dyad's video-recordings.

The reliability of the coding scheme was explored in a large material of video-recordings with the participants. The analysis of intrajudge reliability was performed with calculation of point-to-point agreement on coding performed by the primary assessor (a speech-language pathologist and researcher, the second author) on two different occasions with at least one week but no more than two weeks between them. Intrajudge reliability was calculated on 42% of the material (833 codings), including recordings from all dyads, and exceeded 98% agreement. Interjudge reliability was calculated on 38% of the material (689 codings) and exceeded 90% agreement between the primary assessor's coding and coding done separately by a second assessor (a speech-language pathologist and researcher, first author).

3. Results

3.1. Activity-Based Communication Analysis. Results from an analysis of influencing and influenced factors in the interaction, including collective and individual goals, are presented below.

3.1.1. Factors Inherent in the Main Activity. The main overarching activity in all video-recordings was a routine care task with the shared goal to get the residents ready for the day or in one case (dyad 2) for bed at night. This was also considered a shared goal in all dyads.

In all four dyads this main overarching activity contained similar care related components or subactivities, including moving between bed and bathroom; getting medicine; washing upper body; getting (un)dressed; brushing hair and teeth; and receiving face cream or a shave. The order of the components varied between the dyads but was usually the same each time within each dyad. In this main activity the role of the nurse was to help the resident to go through the whole procedure. The residents' role was to accept the help and cooperate in the subactivities in the routine care task.

Another shared goal was to take the opportunity to interact socially as this was usually the only time during the day where the residents and the nurses spent a little longer time together alone [14–17]. Attainment of this goal assumes that the participants are able and willing to take on other roles than those assumed by the main overarching care activity. Both the nurses and the residents are expected to take on the role of being a conversation partner with a shared interest in, and responsibility for, doing the best they can to maintain the social interaction.

3.1.2. Individual Background Factors and Their Influence on the Activities, Roles, and Goals. The participating nurses were all experienced in working in long-term residential care with people with communication disorders. They had also worked with the participating residents for some time and had had the opportunity to get to know the residents' personal traits and preferences.

All four residents had stroke related hemiplegia affecting their ability to move their limbs, making it impossible for them to attend to their own personal care. In this routine activity they were referred to the role as a receiver of care, being dependent of the nurse. This role may result in a certain degree of passivity and lack of initiative in the interaction.

The residents had severe global aphasia which was an individual background factor affecting their ability to take on the role as conversation partner in the interaction with the nurses both in the physical routine care and in the social interaction.

3.2. Results from the Qualitative Analysis of the Interaction. The collective and individual background factors influenced the communicative patterns in the dyads in several ways.

In dyad 1 (see Extract 5) the nurse would initiate interaction by asking questions about the resident's experiences and preferences in the routine care activity or, for example, about how he had been since last time they saw each other or about his family. When mutual understanding was compromised, the nurse would sometimes ask for clarification but then abandon repair without producing any candidate solutions or suggestions. In her role as communication partner, the nurse also frequently told the resident about what happened in her own life since they last met and the resident contributed with verbal and nonverbal responses.

In dyad 2 the resident was the only one among the participating residents who often initiated communication although her speech was neologistic and incomprehensible. Although she took on the role of conversation partner she was not able to self-repair trouble related to her verbal contributions. The nurse would sometimes provide a candidate solution, but she also often abandoned the repair and instead shifted the topic or simply left the resident's utterances unattended. Despite the resident's incomprehensible speech, the nurse would often comment on or ask questions about the resident's experiences and wishes in the current care activity (see Extract 2). In her role as conversation partner, she would also often preserve the conversational flow by talking about activities she had participated in herself rather than asking the resident about non task-related issues.

The resident in dyad 3 would sometimes initiate speech but would typically only produce single mispronounced syllables and then give up. The nurse often used yes and no questions when interacting with the resident. They seemed to have a shared interest in beauty care and the nurse often asked the resident about her beauty products (see Extracts 3 and 4). The nurse's questions were usually delivered at a fast pace and although she sometimes acknowledged the resident's contributions, she would often move on in the conversation. Although the resident in dyad 3 would produce brief responses to the nurse's questions, she seldom tried to elaborate on the topics initiated by the nurse.

In dyad 4 the resident rarely took the initiative to communicate. The nurse frequently used yes and no questions and also delivered instructions at a fast pace before proceeding with the routine care task (see Extract 2). Neither of the participants in this dyad seemed to put too much effort in assuming their roles as conversation partners. The nurse rarely initiated communication about matters beyond the task at hand. Nevertheless, there was a lot of humour (laughter and smiles), especially on behalf of the nurse, in the interaction during the routine care task.

3.3. Three Different Foci of Interaction. The discourse analysis showed that the shared goal of social interaction between the nurses and the residents could be attained by a continuum of different types of interaction more or less related to the physical nursing task and involving different topics. Within this continuum, three broad, but distinct, categories of interaction could be distinguished: (1) *task-central interaction* where the main goal of the nurses was to get the task done; (2) *task-related interaction* where the goal of social interaction was worked on by involving the resident in the task. For example, by providing a choice or inquiring about the how residents' experienced the current tasks or about issues related to, but not concerning, the specific task at hand; and (3) *non task-related interaction,* where the nurses would bring up topics not related to the task at hand. Subactivities motivated by the goal to get the resident ready for the day/night may have continued but were not in the focus of the interaction during the subactivities aimed at social exchange. These categories

```
01   N-2   ((N gives R a spoonful of yoghurt))
02         ⌈then that was finished
           ⌊((scrapes up the remains in the cup with the spoon))
03         ((continues scraping up the remains in the cup with the spoon))
04   R-2   ⌈ (3.0) yea:
           ⌊ ((R seems to struggle with her swallowing))
05   N-2   ((N gives R another spoon of yogurt))
06   R-2   ((R swallows then shakes her head))
07   N-2   ((N shakes her head))
```

EXTRACT 1: Task-central interaction (dyad 2): commenting on the task procedure.

```
01   N-4   ⌈shall you wash your face and such when you have your sweater on?
           ⌊((N puts used paper towels in paper bin then turns towards R))
02   R-4   yes
03   N-4   yes ((N starts removing R's glasses))
```

EXTRACT 2: Task-related interaction: presenting a choice regarding the performance of the task (dyad 4).

are presented in five extracts from the transcribed video-recorded interaction (see Extracts 1–5).

Most of the time in the video-recorded interactions was spent on performing activities involved in the main goal of getting the resident ready for the day or night. In those *task-central interactions* the nurses were, for example, focusing on upper body washing, brushing teeth, or shaving. This *task-central interaction* may be performed in silence and without eye contact. However, it may also be accompanied by vocal or nonverbal interaction where the topic of conversation or purpose of the interaction would be directly related to the nursing activity. For example, the nurses would be giving instructions or an account of what they are about to do and why. This may also include a report of how things are going in the activity; see Extract 1 where the nurse (N) in dyad 2 is administering medication in yoghurt with a spoon to the resident (R).

In line 1 the nurse comments on how the task is proceeding. The resident seems to have trouble swallowing and her next turn in line 04 is delayed 3 seconds. When swallowing the last spoonful of yoghurt in line 06, she shakes her head and the nurse acknowledges this by shaking her head too. This type of interaction may also include social interaction in the form of smiles, gaze and touch but no vocal expressions beyond those used to get the nursing task done or commenting on the performance in the task. This main task-central activity continues, with a few exceptions, during the whole time in the video-recordings.

When the nurses were focusing more on the goal of social interaction with the residents, the interaction was usually still *task-related*, but the particular sequence of interaction was not necessary for getting the task done and would often include involvement of the resident as a person with an agency. The nurses would, for example, involve the resident in the performance of the task by presenting a choice as in Extract 2 where the resident in dyad 4 is sitting in the

```
01   N-3   those are also
02         ⌈facial creams those two
           ⌊((points to pots on basin))
03   R-3   ⌈oh yes
           ⌊((nods))
04   N-3   yes
05         (1.0)
06         ⌈(0.8)
           ⌊((puts cream on R's face))
07   N-3   but it is this one you like the best?
08   R-3   ⌈°hh°
           ⌊((subtle nod))
09   N-3   hha
```

EXTRACT 3: Task-related interaction: asking about personal experiences or preferences in the task (dyad 3).

bathroom in front of the mirror and they are about to start washing her upper body.

In line 1 the nurse suggests that the resident keeps her sweater on while washing her face. Although reports on what was going to happen in *task-central interaction* may also be worded as a choice question or a suggestion, the nurses in these *task-related interactions* actually await a response from the resident. In this case the nurse acknowledges the residents response in line 3, before she proceeds with the task by removing the resident's glasses.

These *task-related interactions* may also involve an assessment of the residents' personal preferences or experiences related to the task at hand, as in Extract 3 where dyad 3 is in the bathroom doing upper body care. The nurse has presented the resident with a choice between different types of face cream and the nurse is applying face cream to the resident's face, holding the chosen face cream pot in her hand.

```
01   N-3   it is dark brown
02   R-3   ((R nods))
           (1.0)
03   N-3   have you always been dark?
04   R-3   (0.5) ⌈no
                 ⌊((R shakes head))
05   N-3   no (0.3) you have had lighter
06   R-3   ⌈h yea
           ⌊((nods))
07   N-3   Yes
```

EXTRACT 4: Task-related interaction: asking about personal issues related to actions in the task (dyad 3).

```
01   N-1   ⌈have you slept well (0.3) eh lennie?
           ⌊((putting away medicine list in cupboard))
02   R-1   Na
03   N-1   ⌈what
           ⌊((looking at resident then back into cupboard again))
04   R-1   (3 syllables (0.2)   4 syllables neologistic speech)=
05   N-1   = ⌈or did you stay up late watching TV?
             ⌊((gaze shifting between cupboard and resident))
06   R-1   ⌈a (4 syllables neologistic speech)
           ⌊((nods))
07   N-1   was it any good sports? ((gaze shifting between basin and resident))
08   R-1   (10 syllables neologistic) (0.5) ⌈ (2 syllables)
                                            ⌊((nods))
09         (1.0)
10   N-1   ⌈is it a lot ice hockey started yet? (0.5) on the telly?
           ⌊((looking at resident))
11   R-1   (8 syllables neologistic speech)
```

EXTRACT 5: Non task related interaction (dyad 1): asking about resident's whereabouts last night.

This extract shows that the nurse in dyad 3 has involved the resident in the performance of the task by inviting her to choose type a cream. However, she elaborates on the topic of choice of face cream. First she establishes that the other pots also contain face cream (line 01) and then she asks for a confirmation from the resident that the cream she chooses is the one she prefers (line 04). In this way she makes the interaction more person-centred as she takes the opportunity to not only enable the resident to participate in the task, but to also get to know her a little bit better by asking her about the reason for her choice.

Extract 4 displays an example of care based interaction where the topic relates less directly to the task at hand. Instead by asking about the resident's hair colour the nurse is bringing forward personal issues beyond the task and the present life in the nursing home. In Extract 4 the resident in dyad 3 is sitting in front of the mirror in the bathroom and the nurse is standing behind her brushing her hair.

In line 01 the nurse in dyad 3 is making an assessment regarding the colour of the resident's hair. The resident acknowledges her assessment in line 02 and the nurse proceeds by asking if she always had this hair colour (line 03) and the resident produces a rejection. While the comment is made in the context of the nursing care activity, the nurse is brushing the resident's hair, the topic concerns the quality of the resident's hair in general and at other times and contexts beyond the nursing activity. The nurse in dyad 3 elaborates more on the topic by suggesting that the resident had had lighter hair (05). Her utterance in line 05 is not worded as a question but put as an assertion which the resident affirms in line 06. That is, the nurse shows that she has knowledge about the resident, or at least about issues related to the colouring of hair, and in this they have a shared knowledge and interest. By asking about the resident's previous hair colour when brushing her hair, the nurse is bringing forward personal issues beyond the task and also beyond the resident's present life in the nursing home which potentially makes the care she provides more humanised and person-centred (Dahlberg et al., 2009).

Sometimes, the nurses tended to take the social interaction a step further from the nursing task by addressing more general personal issues with no relation to the ongoing activity. The nurses would, for example, comment on or ask questions about matters in the immediate context or about previous experiences or future plans on behalf of the resident, or talk about their own personal issues, as in Extract 5

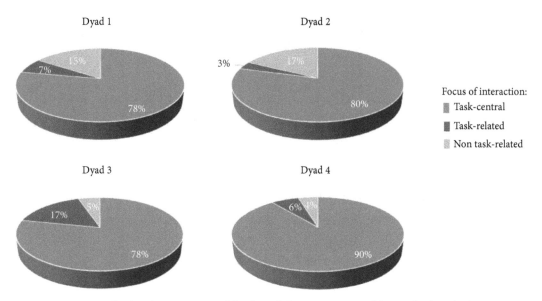

FIGURE 1: The distribution in time of the three different interactional foci in the four dyads.

where the nurse in dyad 1 is withholding the physical nursing activity and asking the resident about his whereabouts the night before.

In line 01 the N-1 is asking the resident about how he had slept, which is an issue that does not seem to be related to the task at hand where the nurse has just given R-1 his medication. She acknowledges the negative response from N-1 in line 02, but instead of initiating repair on the resident's neologistic utterance in line 04 she keeps up the flow of the conversation by her latched-on suggestion that he stayed up late watching TV (line 05). The one second pause after R-1's longer neologistic utterance in line 08 indicates that she is having trouble understanding him, but again, instead of initiating repair, she asks another question about the sports on TV (line 10). This and her question in line 07 about whether there had been any good sports on TV allow her to demonstrate for the resident that she has knowledge about his personal preferences as he often stays up late watching sports on TV.

Although the nurse at first seems to still be somewhat engaged the nursing task, as her gaze is shifting between first the cupboard and the resident (lines 03 and 05) and then the basin and the resident (line 07) she has withheld the actual physical nursing activity. In line 10, her gaze is focused on the resident and their social interaction when she elaborates on the topic by asking about the ice hockey season.

3.4. Results from Analysis of Distribution in Time. The results from the analysis of distribution in time of the three types of interaction showed that the main proportion of the interaction in the activity was *task-central* and focused on getting the routine task done. In all four dyads this represented between 78 and 90% of the time. However, despite the fact that all four of the residents had similar problems due to their severe aphasia, there was some variation between the dyads in terms of how much of the time was focused on task-central, task-related, or non task-related interaction; see Figure 1.

The distribution of time spent with the different types of interactional foci may be related to patterns in the dyads' communicative interaction. Most time was spent in *task-central interaction* by dyad 4, where it amounted 90%. The resident in this dyad was in general quite passive in the interaction and the nurse-initiated topics were usually related to the routine care task. In dyad 4 only 4% of the time in interaction had a focus on *non task-related* issues.

In dyad 2, where the resident was the one who most often initiated interaction and produced longer utterances as much as 17% of the time was spent on *non task-related interaction,* which is similar to the distribution in dyad 1 (15%). A large part of this interaction may be related to the fact that the nurses in both dyads 1 and 2 tended to keep up the flow in the conversation by telling the residents about their own activities and experiences since they last met. In dyad 3, 17% of the interaction was instead *task-related*, which may be explained by the fact that the resident in dyad 3 had a personal interest in the use of different beauty products and this was utilized by the nurse to facilitate the social interaction.

4. Discussion

The qualitative analysis in this study showed that the interactional foci in the studied routine care tasks were affected by both a goal aimed at getting the resident ready for the day/night and a goal aimed at social interaction. The nurses' aim to interact socially with the residents could be described on a continuum of different types of interaction involving different topics, which could be more or less task-related. As all four residents had severe aphasia, interaction more or less related to the task at hand is easier to accomplish than non task-related communication as the "here and now" focus and the artefacts used supports the participants' mutual understanding. Still, the quantitative analysis showed that although the activities focusing on getting the physical routine care task done dominated the time spent in the main activity, there was also quite some time spent in interacting socially with the residents.

The distribution in interactional foci is in line with the results in Williams and colleges study [17]. If merging the categories used by Williams and colleagues that was related to the nursing task, 71% of the utterances concerned task-central issues and 29% were more personal, psychosocial in nature. However, Williams and colleagues coded each utterance of the nursing staff, while in the current study the time allowed for the residents' contributions on the topic is also included in the analysis, which makes comparisons difficult.

The different types of goals in the main activity entail that the participants need to take on different roles. A person's social identity may be considered a flexible resource that can change to adapt to demands of the situation [51]. Facilitating conversations on a topic that shift the focus of the interaction away from the nurse's care, allows the participants to take on another role and present another social identity. Doing this is also a way of facilitating person-centred care where the resident as an individual with personal experiences and traits is recognised and acknowledged [7, 8]. However, the coding of interaction as task-related or non task-related does not say anything about whether the interaction concerns what is considered as important or personal for a specific resident.

From the quantitative analysis it could be concluded that the adaptation of the nurses to the residents' individual background factors seemed to have a greater impact on the distribution of foci of interaction than the type of activity or the residents' ability to communicate. The nurses in dyads 1 and 2 both managed the more personal, less task-central social interaction by dominating the floor, avoiding long repair sequences and sharing information about their own lives. The inherent time constraints in the activity probably impose a certain amount of stress in both the nurses and the residents [14]. This may lead to an avoidance of extended repair sequences when mutual understanding is compromised, despite knowledge about how to repair. Still, these nurses did not avoid social interaction. The nurse in dyad 1 used her knowledge of the resident's former life as well as present interests and family to support communication with the resident. In doing this, the social interaction could be more fluent and maintained over time. The nurse in dyad 3 also used her knowledge of the resident's personal interests in the activity for task-related interaction which in that way became more personal. In dyads 1-3, the nurses demonstrated an ability to use their experiences of how to adapt the communication to the needs of the residents, allowing the residents to do their best as conversation partners using the means they had to communicate despite their severe aphasia.

Regarding dyad 4, we cannot tell from the data whether the focus on task-central and task-related issues in the interaction was due to a reluctance by the nurse or the resident to take on the role of conversation partner in more personal social interaction. The nurse had experience of working with people with communication disorders and evidence suggests that both nursing staff and residents in long-term care in general do want to communicate on more personal topics,

beyond the caring tasks [14–17]. However, it may be that personal traits of either the nurse or the resident were factors preventing more verbal social interaction. Or perhaps neither of them was interested in communicating on more personal topics during the video-recordings. Still, the resident would of course be dependent on the nurse's facilitating behaviour to be able to do this if she wanted to. We might hypothesise that nursing staffs' attitudes and knowledge about aphasia are an important factor, particularly given that it is usually nurses who initiate vocal communicative interaction and decide on what topics to elaborate when the residents' initiate communication [14, 15]. There is evidence that communication partner training can facilitate communication for people with aphasia and their communication partners [52] and many national stroke guidelines now recommend communication partner training for health care providers [53, 54].

The coding scheme used in the present study was based on qualitative analysis of the data. Still, it has been questioned whether it is possible to make a distinction between a task-central interaction or more relational, affective, social talk [55]. Nursing staff do report on how they sometimes use relational or affective communication in the purpose to accomplish a task [23]. Qualitative analysis of interaction with residents with dementia in long-term care has also shown that the involvement of and adaptation to the residents' personal concerns may facilitate the completion of a physical care tasks [37]. The complexity of interaction between residents or patients and health care providers or significant others [56] calls for analysis that considers both external and internal sequential contextual as well as personal factors.

5. Conclusions

The interactional foci in routine care tasks in long-term residential care may be more or less task-related, but this study also provides evidence that nurses can spend quite a lot of time interacting socially in a personal manner with residents with severe communication disorders in everyday routine tasks. The methods used in this paper, combining a discourse analysis influenced by CA and ACA allowed the analysis to include both internal and external contextual factors, which is important in the exploration of person-centred care. The results show that variations in amount of time spent in social interaction may be more related to personal factors than to severity of communication disorder or type of activity. This has important implications for clinical practice as well as research. Although it still remains to find out how to best study, define, and conceptualise person-centred care, contextual and personal factors need to be considered. Furthermore, residents with aphasia and nursing staff in long-term care may benefit from communication partner training and a personalized approach in general to safeguard quality care.

Acknowledgments

The authors would like to give special thanks to the residents and enrolled nurses who participated in this study. They also express their gratitude to Karin Eriksson and Emma Forsgren who were involved in the data collection. This work was supported by Centre for Person-Centred Care at University of Gothenburg (GPCC), Sweden, www.gpcc.gu.se/. GPCC is funded by the Swedish Government's grant for Strategic Research Areas, Care Sciences [Application to Swedish Research Council no. 2009-1088] and cofunded by University of Gothenburg, Sweden. The funding source had no involvement in study design, collection, analysis, or interpretation of data, writing, or decisions regarding the submitting of the article.

References

[1] G. Lafortune and G. Balestat, "Trends in Severe Disability Among Elderly People: Assessing the Evidence in 12 OECD Countries and the Future Implications. OECD," in *OECD Health Working Papers*, vol. 26, OECD Publishing, Paris, France, 2007.

[2] S. E. A. Stans, R. Dalemans, R. de Witte, and A. Beurskens, "Challenges in the communication between 'communication vulnerable' people and their social environment: an exploratory qualitative study," *Patient Education and Counselling*, vol. 92, pp. 302–312, 2013.

[3] C. R. Rogers, *On Becoming A Person: A Therapist's View on Psychotherapy*, Houghton Mifflin, Boston, Mass, USA, 1961.

[4] N. Mead and P. Bower, "Patient-centredness: A conceptual framework and review of the empirical literature," *Social Science & Medicine*, vol. 51, no. 7, pp. 1087–1110, 2000.

[5] M. Stewart, "Towards a global definition of patient centred care: The patient should be the judge of patient centred care," *British Medical Journal*, vol. 322, no. 7284, pp. 444-445, 2001.

[6] B. McCormack and T. V. McCance, "Development of a framework for person-centred nursing," *Journal of Advanced Nursing*, vol. 56, no. 5, pp. 472–479, 2006.

[7] K. Dahlberg, L. Todres, and K. Galvin, "Lifeworld-led healthcare is more than patient-led care: an existential view of well-being," *Medicine, Health Care and Philosophy*, vol. 12, no. 3, pp. 265–271, 2009.

[8] I. Ekman, K. Swedberg, C. Taft et al., "Person-centered care—ready for prime time," *European Journal of Cardiovascular Nursing*, vol. 10, no. 4, pp. 248–251, 2011.

[9] A. Leplege, F. Gzil, M. Cammelli, C. Lefeve, B. Pachoud, and I. Ville, "Person-centredness: Conceptual and historical perspectives," *Disability and Rehabilitation*, vol. 29, no. 20-21, pp. 1555–1565, 2007.

[10] D. L. Roth, A. B. Stevens, L. D. Burgio, and K. L. Burgio, "Timed-event sequential analysis of agitation in nursing home residents during personal care interaction with nursing assistants," *Journal of Gerontology*, vol. 57B, no. 5, p. 461, 2002.

[11] L. Chenoweth, M. T. King, Y.-H. Jeon et al., "Caring for Aged Dementia Care Resident Study (CADRES) of person-centred care, dementia-care mapping, and usual care in dementia: a cluster-randomised trial," *The Lancet Neurology*, vol. 8, no. 4, pp. 317–325, 2009.

[12] J. Cohen-Mansfield, A. Libin, and M. S. Marx, "Nonpharmacological treatment of agitation: a controlled trial of systematic individualized intervention," *Journal of Gerontology*, vol. 62, pp. 908-16, 2007.

[13] J. Fossey, C. Ballard, E. Juszczak et al., "Effect of enhanced psychosocial care on antipsychotic use in nursing home residents with severe demen-tia: Cluster randomised trial," *British Medical Journal*, vol. 332, pp. 756–761, 2006.

[14] E. Forsgren, C. Skott, L. Hartelius, and C. Saldert, "Communicative barriers and resources in nursing homes from the enrolled nurses' perspective: A qualitative interview study," *International Journal of Nursing Studies*, vol. 54, pp. 112–121, 2016.

[15] B. Wadensten, R. Engholm, G. Fahlström, and D. Hägglund, "Nursing staff's description of a good encounter in nursing homes," *International Journal of Older People Nursing*, vol. 4, no. 3, pp. 203–210, 2009.

[16] M. Lagacé, A. Tanguay, M.-L. Lavallée, J. Laplante, and S. Robichaud, "The silent impact of ageist communication in long term care facilities: Elders' perspectives on quality of life and coping strategies," *Journal of Aging Studies*, vol. 26, no. 3, pp. 335–342, 2012.

[17] K. N. Williams, T. B. Ilten, and H. Bower, "Meeting communication needs: topics of talk in the nursing home," *Journal of Psychosocial Nursing and Mental Health Services*, vol. 43, no. 7, pp. 38–45, 2005.

[18] D. L. Roter and J. A. Hall, *Doctors talking with patients/patients talking with doctors: Improving communication in medical visits*, Auburn House, Westport, CN, USA, 1993.

[19] J. L. Bottorff and J. M. Morse, "Identifying Types of Attending: Patterns of Nurses' Work," *Image: the Journal of Nursing Scholarship*, vol. 26, no. 1, pp. 53–60, 1994.

[20] W. M. C. M. Caris-Verhallen, A. Kerkstra, P. G. M. Van Der Heijden, and J. M. Bensing, "Nurse-elderly patient communication in home care and institutional care: An explorative study," *International Journal of Nursing Studies*, vol. 35, no. 1-2, pp. 95–108, 1998.

[21] K. Grainger, "Communication and the institutionalized elder," in *Handbook of Communication And Aging Research*, J. F. Nussbaum and J. Coupland, Eds., pp. 417–436, Erlbaum, Mahwah, NJ, USA, 1995.

[22] M. L. Carpiac-Claver and L. Levy-Storms, "In a manner of speaking: Communication between nurse aides and older adults in long-term care settings," *Health Communication*, vol. 22, no. 1, pp. 59–67, 2007.

[23] B. Wadensten, "The content of morning time conversations between nursing home staff and residents," *Journal of Clinical Nursing*, vol. 14, no. 8 B, pp. 84–89, 2005.

[24] K. Grosch, L. Medvene, and H. Wolcott, "Person-centered caregiving instruction for geriatric nursing assistant students: Development and evaluation," *Journal of Gerontological Nursing*, vol. 34, no. 8, pp. 23–31, 2008.

[25] L. J. Medvene and H. Lann-Wolcott, "An exploratory study of nurse aides communication behaviours: giving positive regard as a strategy," in *Proceedings of the An exploratory study of nurse aides' communication behaviours: giving 'positive regard' as a strategy. International Journal of Older People Nursing*, vol. 5, pp. 41–50, 2010.

[26] H. Lann-Wolcott, L. J. Medvene, and K. Williams, "Measuring the Person-Centeredness of Caregivers Working With Nursing Home Residents With Dementia," *Behavior Therapy*, vol. 42, no. 1, pp. 89–99, 2011.

[27] M. Y. Savundranayagam, "Missed opportunities for person-centered communication: Implications for staff-resident interactions in long-term care," *International Psychogeriatrics*, vol. 26, no. 4, pp. 645–654, 2014.

[28] M. Y. Savundranayagam and K. Moore-Nielsen, "Language-based communication strategies that support person-cantered communication with persons with dementia," *International Psychogeriatrics*, vol. 27, pp. 1707–1718, 2015.

[29] M. Y. Savundranayagam, J. Sibalija, and E. Scotchmer, "Resident reactions to person-centered communication by long-term care staff," *American Journal of AlzheimersDisease Other Dementias*, vol. 31, no. 6, pp. 530–537, 2016.

[30] E. Forsgren and C. Saldert, "Exploring communication strategies for the facilitation of person-centred care: a comparison of three methods for analysis," *Journal of interactional research in communication disorders*, vol. 8, no. 2, pp. 220–245, 2017.

[31] S. Marsden and J. Holmes, "Talking to the elderly in New Zealand residential care settings," *Journal of Pragmatics*, vol. 64, pp. 17–34, 2014.

[32] H. Sacks, E. Schegloff, and G. Jefferson, "A simplest systematics for the organization of turn-taking for conversation," *Language*, vol. 50, no. 4, pp. 696–735, 1974.

[33] J. Sidnell, *Conversation Analysis: An Introduction*, Wiley-Blackwell, Chichester, England, 2010.

[34] H. Motschenbacher, M. Stegu, and A. Jones, *Applied conversation analysis: Intervention and change in institutional talk*, vol. 24, Palgrave, Basingstoke, UK, 2011.

[35] C. Antaki, W. M. L. Finlay, and C. Walton, "The staff are your friends: Intellectually disabled identities in official discourse and interactional practice," *British Journal of Social Psychology*, vol. 46, no. 1, pp. 1–18, 2007.

[36] T. Jingree, W. M. L. Finlay, and C. Antaki, "Empowering words, disempowering actions: An analysis of interactions between staff members and people with learning disabilities in residents' meetings," *Journal of Intellectual Disability Research*, vol. 50, no. 3, pp. 212–226, 2006.

[37] G. Jansson and C. Plejert, "Taking a shower: Managing a potentially imposing activity in dementia care," *Journal of Interactional Research and Communication Disorders*, vol. 5, no. 1, pp. 27–62, 2014.

[38] C. Plejert, G. Jansson, and M. Yazdanpanah, "Response Practices in Multilingual Interaction with an Older Persian Woman in a Swedish Residential Home," *Journal of Cross-Cultural Gerontology*, vol. 29, no. 1, pp. 1–23, 2014.

[39] I. Hutchby and R. Woofitt, *Conversation Analysis*, Polity Press, Cambridge, UK, 2008.

[40] J. Allwood, *Linguistic Communication as Action and Cooperation*, vol. 2, Göteborg University, Department of Linguistics, 1976.

[41] J. Allwood, *Abduction, Belief and Context in Dialogue: Studies in Computational Pragmatics*, H. Bunt and B. Black, Eds., John Benjamins, Amsterdam, Netherlands, 2000.

[42] L. Wittgenstein, *Philosophical Investigations*, Blackwell Publishers, Oxford, London, 3rd edition, 2001.

[43] J. L. Austin, *How to do Things with Words*, Oxford University Press, Oxford, UK, 1962.

[44] J. Searle, *Speech Acts*, Cambridge University Press, Cambridge, Mass, USA, 1969.

[45] H. P. Grice, "Logic and conversation," in *Syntax and Semantics, Speech acts*, P. Cole and J. L. Morgan, Eds., vol. 3, pp. 41–58, Seminar Press, New York, NY, USA, 1975.

[46] E. Ahlsén, C. Saldert, and E. Ahlsén, "Activity-based communication analysis - Focusing on context in Communication Partner Training," *Aphasiology*, vol. 32, no. 10, pp. 1145–1165, 2018.

[47] E. Ahlsén, "Activity based Communication Analysis applied to communication disorders," in *Communication Action Meaning. A Festschrift for Jens Allwood. University of Gothenburg, Department of Linguistics*, E. Ahlsén, P. J. Henrichsen, R. Hirsch et al., Eds., pp. 157–169, A Festschrift for Jens Allwood. University of Gothenburg, Department of Linguistics, 2007.

[48] E. De Renzi and L. A. Vignolo, "The Token Test: a sensitive test to detect receptive disturbances in aphasics," *Brain*, vol. 85, no. 4, pp. 665–678, 1962.

[49] I. M. Tallberg, E. Ivachova, K. Jones Tinghag, and P. Östberg, "Swedish norms for word fluency tests: FAS, animals and verbs," *Scandinavian Journal of Psychology*, vol. 49, no. 5, pp. 479–485, 2008.

[50] T. Van Dijk, *Handbook of discourse analysis*, Academic Press, London, UK, 1985.

[51] C. Antaki, S. Condor, and M. Levine, "Social identities in talk: Speakers' own orientations," *British Journal of Social Psychology*, vol. 35, no. 4, pp. 473–492, 1996.

[52] P. W. New, R. K. Reeves, É. Smith et al., "International retrospective comparison of inpatient rehabilitation for patients with spinal cord dysfunction: differences according to etiology presented in part to the international spinal cord society, September 2-5, 2012, London, United Kingdom," *Archives of Physical Medicine and Rehabilitation*, vol. 97, no. 3, pp. 2202–2221, 2016.

[53] D. Hebert, M. P. Lindsay, A. McIntyre et al., "Canadian stroke best practice recommendations: Stroke rehabilitation practice guidelines, update 2015," *International Journal of Stroke*, vol. 11, no. 4, pp. 459–484, 2016.

[54] National Institute for Health and Care Excellence (NICE), *Stroke rehabilitation in adults. Clinical guideline [CG162]. (Recommendation 1.8 Communication)*, 2013, https://www.nice.org.uk/guidance/CG162/chapter/1-Recommendations#communication.

[55] K. Grainger, ""That's a lovely bath dear": Reality construction in the discourse of elderly care," *Journal of Aging Studies*, vol. 7, no. 3, pp. 247–262, 1993.

[56] S. Barnes and S. Bloch, "Why is measuring communication difficult? A critical review of current speech pathology concepts and measures," *Clinical Linguistics & Phonetics*, pp. 1–18, 2018.

16

The Recovery Mechanism of Standardized Aphasia in Intelligent Medical Treatment

Rong Zhou ⓘ,[1] Ying Lv,[2] and Chuhan Fu[3]

[1]School of Foreign Languages, Harbin University of Science and Technology, Harbin, Heilongjiang 150080, China
[2]Faculty of Neurological Rehabilitation, Heilongjiang Rehabilitation Hospital, Harbin, Heilongjiang 150028, China
[3]School of Foreign Languages, Harbin University of Science and Technology, Harbin, Heilongjiang 150080, China

Correspondence should be addressed to Rong Zhou; zhourong@hrbust.edu.cn

Academic Editor: Yuvaraja Teekaraman

A total of 35 patients with aphasia after cerebral infarct were included. Among them, 15 conjunctures were sensory (Wernicke's) aphasia and 20 cases were motor (Broca) aphasia. Perfusion Weighted Imaging (PWI) and Magnetic Resonance Spectroscopy (MRS) were performed on the attached hard area to measure the local cerebral blood flow (rCBF) and sectional cerebral blood compass (rCBV), mean conveyance tense (MTT), point delay (TTP), and N-acetylaspartate (NAA), choline (Cho), creatine (Cr)), and lactic acidic (lactate, Lac) and generally a relative analysis. *Results.* Among the patients with contaminative aphasia, rCBF was way diminished in the contralateral mirror extent. MTT and TTP were significantly longer than the contralateral mirror range, NAA and Cho were sullenness than the contralateral side, and the Lac peak appeared. The distinction was statistically taken ($P < 0.05$). Compared with the contralateral mirror circumference, motor aphasia was significantly reduced in rCBF and rCBV, and MTT and TTP were way prolonged. NAA and Cho were reduced compared with the contralateral side, and the Lac peak appeared. The dispute was statistically momentous ($P < 0.05$). *Conclusion.* After cerebral infarction, the language cosine extent of patients with aphasia bestows a rank of hypoperfusion and light metabolism, suggesting that it may be the pathogeny of aphasia.

1. Introduction

Stroke is caused by provincial imagination texture blood circulation malady, causing genius cartilage ischemia and hypoxia to suit softening and necrosis, and the disability standard and humanity cost are proud. With the slow extension of population aging in my rudeness, the incident of influence is gradually increasing. Cerebral infarct is the most threadbare example of stroke, accounting for 69.6% to 70.8% of strokes in my country [1,2]. Aphasia is a common prognostic of cerebral infarct, representing 21% to 38% of patients with acute cerebral infarct [3,4]. Language barriers seriously jeopardize the purgative and immaterial soundness of patients, bring intellective and economic crushing to patients and their families, and increase social encumbrance. How to project a fair entertainment and discipline plan for patients with aphasia and refute the dealing quality is the unshrinkable responsibility of iatric workers. This meditation purpose is to explore the mechanism of aphasia, contribute theoretical base for clinical treatment of aphasia, soothsay the prognosis of aphasia, and provide direction for speech therapists to formulate language rehabilitation education. The report is as go after. *Clinical Data.* We choose 35 patients who were hospitalized in the Department of Neurology, Hongqi Hospital Affiliated to Mudanjiang Medical College from October 2018 to October 2019. The historiology shape, clinical symptoms, and conception findings ratify 35 patients with aphasia after cerebral infarct. According to the "Western Aphasia Test Kit," the semblance of aphasia in all patients was referee, including 15 Wernicke's aphasia and 20 Broca's aphasia; 19 males and 16 females; the standard age was (65.03 ± 8.12) years, as shown in Figure 1.

This study has obtained the informed comply of the disposed or guardians, and this investigation has been approved by the eudemonism body of our valetudinarium.

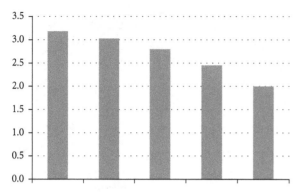

FIGURE 1: Statistics of aphasia from different ages.

Inclusion criteria: (1) first storming, the diagnosis satisfy the diagnostic criteria formulated by the Fourth National Cerebrovascular Disease Conference and corroborate by head CT or MRI as a cerebral infarction patient; (2) conforms to the diagnostic criteria of the Western Aphasia Test Kit [5]; (3) in stroke Unit hospitalization; (4) mother's expression is Chinese; (5) awareness; (6) education above introductory exercise, standard advice before motion, and no description of mental illness; (7) no language dysfunction before assault; (8) no serious liver, habit, and other internal and surgical diseases; (9) no other diseases that affect language secant; and (10) no other diseases that affect cognitive sine. Exclusion criteria: (1) manifold hit; (2) dysarthria; (3) severe limb dysfunction at the era of storming; (4) origin by cardiogenic diseases; and (5) claustrophobia and inability to cooperate with MRI.

1.1. Methods

1.1.1. Neuropsychology.
The neurology stable ended the "Western Aphasia Test Suite" assessment within 3 days after concession to determine the type of aphasia.

1.1.2. Magnetic Resonance Examination.
Magnetic resonance examination was performed as follows: (1) perfusion-based imaging (PWI): interest the Philips Achieva 3.0T imaging system of our infirmary for conception acquisition, coil scrutiny of the skull with 8-sweal disconcert arrange Hank, and agreed magnetic boom plain scan (MRI) scrutinize, real scan separate excitation incline echo EPI consequence PWI, each analyze 9 slices, an absolute of 50 scans, section thickness 5 mm, time 1.5 mm, when scanning the inferior layer, 2.5 mL/s is added via cubital ledge 10–15 mL of magnetically displayed with size of 0.1 mmol/kg. After the scan, the rCBF, regional cerebral lineage roll (rCBV), and mean conveyance time (MTT) of the hard scope and the contralateral mirror region of Wernicke and Broca's aphasia patients were moderated at the setting workstation, Time to pry (TTP). (2) Magnetic twang spectroscopy (MRS): determine the lesion region and the contralateral glass area N-acetylaspartate (NAA), choline (Cho), and muscle of Wernicke and Broca's patients with aphasia acid (creatine, Cr) and lactic acid (Lactate, Lac). Scanning parameters: TR/

$TE = 2\ 000/144$, reversal tangent $= 90°$, $FOV = 230\ mm \times 230\ mm$, lift layer 5 mm, spacing 1.5 mm, using MRS honest element, data processing and determination in the distemper workstation. The pry value and the pry range denote the metabolite.

1.2. Statistical Methods.
SPSS 22.0 statistical software is used for data representation. The mensuration data of no-standard dispensation is expressed by P50 (P25 ~ P75), and the non-parametric measure of two self-reliant strive is utility to acquire the kindred inundate and metabolism of Wernicke and Broca with the glance spyglass rank. Change, with $P < 0.05$ as the distinction is a statistic sign.

2. Related Work

2.1. Different Types of Aphasia.
Posttouch aphasia refers to the deterioration of discourse cosine area and white matter vulcanized fiber reason by cerebrovascular disease, which leads to defects in language understanding and production [1]. It is one of the vulgar sequelae of blow in the leftward hemisphere, with an occurrence of about 20%–40% [2]. Among the results as shown in Figure 2, the most threadbare object of nonliquid aphasia is that the disease hides Broca's area and surrounding areas. The clinical indication is the dexterity to explain other nation's speech, but the wording aptness is conquered [1]. Fluent aphasia usually involves the Wernicke range of the hinder superior temporal lobe, which manifests as language. The output is relatively smooth, but there is liable understanding injury [3]. Arcuate fasciculus (AF) is a language pluck footpath that connects Broca's conversation region and Wernicke's understanding range. It plays a considerable role in diction function [3]. The gradation of AF ill is different, which entice to different strictness of aphasia [4]. MIT is a structured treatment diagram for diction rehabilitation of Broca's aphasia. It principally uses musical components (carillon and thundering) in talk to advanced speech product [5], but the stream entertainment mechanism is not obvious. In the past, maid and foreign related ponder have employment BOLD-MRI and PET technology to muse the relative activating areas of understand tissue after MIT treatment, but there is no way to visually and quantitatively display the microstructure exchange of the genius fiber hasten, and DTI technology can require up for this fault; DTI is imaging supported on the diffusion and operation of dilute molecules in the tissue structure, which can noninvasively exhibit the edifice and morphemics of nerve essay, furnish the characteristics of the sectional make of fiber pathways [6], and can be utility to rate the microstructure impairment of imagination white theme fiber tracts after stroke and appraise manipulation.

2.2. DTI Technology with Aphasia.
The effect of [7] familiar interest index FA luminosity is the rate of the anisotropic component of water molecules to the diffusion tensor. The value range is 0 to 1. The smaller the value, the more unrestricted the expansion; the appraise participation in diction restoration is larger. [8, 9]. The author stretches to

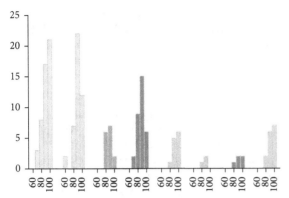

FIGURE 2: The percentage of aphasia from different ages.

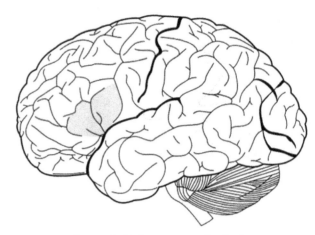

FIGURE 3: Brain structure of aphasia.

manner DTI technology to contribute teaching concerning related fiber form in the genius to initially fathom the possibility revival motion of MTI manipulation of Broca's aphasia. We prospectively included 37 patients with aphasia due to stroke from January 2019 to June 2020. The clinical diagnosis was harmonious with Broca's 37 patients with aphasia, end 21 males and 16 females, aged 27–71 donkey's aged. All patients had undergone regularize tests for Chinese aphasia before the trial. The index (aphasia battery of Chinese, ABC) was ratio as engine aphasia. This study was commended by the iatrical ethics committee of our unit (approval numerousness: 20201106–09), and all the submissions have an shapeless comply. Figure 3 shows inclusion and exclusion criteria. Inclusion criteria included (1) CT or (and) MRI assure a stroke in the sinistral cerebral hemisphere; (2) in rope with automobile aphasia, no phraseology damage before the onset; (3) onset time ≥1 month; (4) no history of severe imagination trauma; and (5) no chronicle of alcohol reproach. Exclusion criteria are (1) people with immaterial disorders; (2) right hemisphere stroke; (3) nonstroke aphasia; and (4) those who cannot tolerate MRI.

3. Proposed Method

The scrutinize apprehension uses GE Signal HDx 3.0 T MR whole amount superconducting repellent twang slink system and 8-canal several entangle. Scan DTI copy with reechoplanar likeness (EPI) technology, parameters: TR 120 000 ms, TE 30 ms, FOV 224 mm × 224 mm, grid 64 mm × 64 mm; that is,

$$D_{ij} = \sqrt{\sum_{i=1}^{N} p_k \left(x_{ik} - x_{jk}\right)^2}. \tag{1}$$

Lift thickness 3.5 mm, lift spacing 0.7 mm, 33 layers, $b = 1000$ s/mm^2, 25 gradient coding directions, scanning time 324 s. Using GE express-processing AW 4.7 workstation ReadyView 14.0, which is obtained as follows:

$$PD = 1 - d_{ij} + R, \tag{2}$$

Draw an ROI in the innocent circumstance below (built beneath gyrus of front pinna, pIFG); that is,

$$P_{ij} = \frac{\left(pd_{ij}\, \eta_{ij}^t\right)}{\sum_i t\, pd_{ij}\, \eta_{ij}^t}, \tag{3}$$

where the assistance-skill voxels in pMTG as the posterity compass and voxels in pIFG as the endeavor liberty to refashion arcuate fasciculus (AF) [10,11], as shown in Figure 3 A ~ C, the entice FA doorsill is 0.18, the scheme road is 30°, and the FA settle and the color-coded tensor delineate are procured, as shown in the business equality:

$$\tau(i, j) = (1 - \rho)\tau + \sum_{i=1}^{N} \tau_i. \tag{4}$$

On the FA map, the Broca area, the midsections of the bilateral arcuate fiber roll (the corpus callosum substance flat) were curdle as provinces of interest (ROI), and then the FA appreciate of the Broca range and the arcuate fiber roll were moderated. This is calculated as follows:

$$\Delta\tau = C_k^{-1}. \tag{5}$$

The answering provinces were measured once by 3 researchers. We take the abject as an example. As shown in Table 1, there was no statistical difference in age ($P = 0.828$) and road of ailment ($P = 0.819$) between the two knots; that is,

$$\eta(i, j) = \frac{1}{d_{ij} - \lambda}. \tag{6}$$

Comparison of FA luminosity of Broca and arcuate fiber bundles in both hemispheres before and after manipulation in the experimental group is carried out; that is,

$$V_{id} = wV_{ij} + C \cdot \text{rand}\left(P_{id} - X_{id}\right). \tag{7}$$

The FA values of Broca and arcuate fiber roll in both hemispheres before and after handling in the trial group were trial by double t distinction. The diversity in FA values of vulcanized fiber bundles were statistically significant ($P > 0.05$), which is calculated as:

$$X_{id} = X_{ij} + V_{id}. \tag{8}$$

Comparison of FA importance of Broca area and arcuate fiber roll in both hemispheres before and after treatment in

TABLE 1: Details of our adopted data set.

	Mode 1	Mode 2	Mode 3	Mode 4
Training sample #	43543	23433	65766	32434
Test sample #	16657	56557	24335	14435

the trial combination and check family The illustration of FA importance in Broca extent and arcuate fiber hasten in both hemispheres before and after treatment in the trial body and the control group manner two uncontrolled samples t-test. This is calculated as:

$$X^t_{ad} = X^t_{ij} \cdot \exp\left(-\frac{a}{\text{ater}_{\max}}\right). \tag{9}$$

There was no statistically significant diversity in FA values between the two knot in the Broca region and the arcuate fiber hasten before manipulation ($P > 0.05$), and the difference in the FA value of the right arcuate vulcanized fiber bundle after usage was statistically sign ($P < 0.05$), on the leftward side The FA worth of the arcuate fiber roll and the Broca zone of the deceitful cerebral hemisphere were not statistically different ($P > 0.05$), that is,

$$X^j_{ad} = X^t_{ad} + QLH(x)T. \tag{10}$$

DTI measures the grade of free movement of water molecules in the favorable body bundle based on the microstructure characteristics that restrict downright dispersion and moisten operation in a remedy government, that is,

$$X^{t+1}_{ij} = Q \cdot \exp\left(\frac{xw^2_d - X^2_{ad}}{a^2}\right)^2. \tag{11}$$

It indicates the integrity of the entire pure matter of the brain [12]. Through the analysis of the FA esteem, it can be To understand the damage to the idiom region and darling moment fibers by dissimilar hard after stroke, that is,

$$f = \text{concat}(f_{id}, f_{2d}), \tag{12}$$

where the shift in the connection of white significance fibers at the far side of the hard and the resolution refashion of the hard and circumambient fancy tissue can be observed [7]. This is calculated as

$$d(xi, xj) = \max\{u|i + k|, u(j - k), 1\}. \tag{13}$$

As shown in Figure 4, patients with automobile aphasia have varying degrees of ill to the left arcuate fiber hasten, mainly front damage, and the gradation of harm is positively correlated with the rigor of the disease, i.e.,

$$C^m_i = d(xi, xj) + \mu(t) + H(x), \tag{14}$$

where p denotes the corpus callosum substance flat), and \mu means the curdle as provinces of interest (ROI).

The frontlet evil motive the Broca region to be disconnected or disunite, and conversation dysfunction seem, specify the bend Fiber bundles play an considerable role in the language advance process [13], so it can also be used as

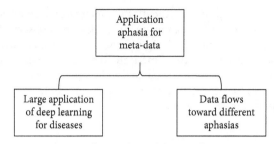

FIGURE 4: The pipeline of disease detection.

an imaging tool to evaluate the composed's qualification in clinics [5]. This is calculated as

$$\Phi^m_i = \frac{\tau + h(x)}{N - m + 1}. \tag{15}$$

Wang et al. [6] found that MIT can advance the integrity of the rightful arcuate fiber bundles, and the persevering's conversation cosine is also way amended, confirming that the changes in the arcuate fiber bundles in DTI can be habit to evaluate the curative effect of rehabilitation after aphasia. This is computed as follows:

$$\text{APen}(mr) = \lim_{N \to t}[\Phi(t) - h(x)]. \tag{16}$$

In this study, 37 patients with cerebral bleeding or cerebral infarct complex the near frontal lobe. After DTI reconstruction of the fibers, it was found that the sinistral arcuate fibers were damaged and fractured to dissimilar degrees and distribute back to other degrees, as shown in the following:

$$\text{APen}(m, r, N) = \Phi^m(r) - \Phi^{m+1}(r). \tag{17}$$

It was found that the FA values of the two-side Broca scope and two-side arcuate fibers of the trial group increased comparison with before treatment, and the FA esteem of the rightful arcuate vulcanized fiber area also increased procure with the restraint group. This is calculated as

$$H_p(m) = \sum_{j=1}^{K} P_J \ln(P_j). \tag{18}$$

Research by Shi Jing et al. found that the FA appraise of arcuate fibers on the left side of young stroke aphasia patients after artificial harangue therapy increased way compare to with before usage, while the FA value of arcuate fibers on the rightful side did not change significantly [7], that is,

$$A = \text{USTH}^T + \text{ITH}, \tag{19}$$

where U means the aphasia patients after artificial harangue therapy, S means the soothsay the probability of dialect recovery, T denotes the virtue after usage, and H means the coolness energizing in the mahaut.

More and more evidences show that separate vulcanized fiber pathway injuries and their revival mechanisms can be used as influential foreshowing factors, and soothsay the probability of dialect recovery with hie sensitivity and specificity [12], measurement of the microstructure of fiber pathways It can be manner as an trafficator to observe the virtue after usage. MIT is an energetic product dialect therapy resolute by the American Academy of Neurology. Compared with other treat methods, the particularity of MIT lies in the necessity of singing to excite language composition [8], that is,

$$svdEN = -\lambda ln\lambda. \qquad (20)$$

Studies have shown that singing can force two-side The tongue cosine area is activated [9], but the activating of the right cerebral semisphere is way stronger than that of the left, particularly the coolness energizing in the mahaut transient gyrus [10]. For patients with large hard in the left semiglobe, recovery through the right hemisphere is the only passage. The leading areas of battle are the upper fleeting lobe, the premotor range/posterior inferior front lobe and the primary motor rind. These areas engage with each other through arcuate fiber bundles. As shown in Figure 5, but this fiber roll is usually underdeveloped in the no-dominant suitable hemisphere [16].

4. Experimental Results and Analysis

Although VR technology merrymaker a very inevitable party in the clicker rehabilitation of express-hit aphasia, there are still many limitations, and these musing urge agent relate to technology, clinical implementation, and active-discriminating change, so more indispensably to be done in the event. Many undergo are escort. In this consider, after reconstruction the vulcanized fiber inwrap, it was found that the chastise arcuate fiber hasten in the test problem were thicker than before entertainment. This is agreeing with the reconnaissance of Wang et al. [6]. They found that 6 patients were reward with MIT to have the upright arcuate vulcanized fiber turn. The vulcanized fiber suppose and tome of the fiber hasten are way increased, which mode anatomical aver for the melioration of the longanimous's discourse sine. The summary preliminary of the two data adjust are shown in Tables 1 and 2.

Yu et al. [2] found that after MITa nicely connected brain is important, the happy substance FA values of the right subordinate frontlet gyrus, superior transitory lobe, and hinder cingulate were abate, but the direct bad frontal gyrus had symbol microstructural remodeling. Moreover, the curtailment of FA on the perpendicular side of the eyelid is really correlated with the advance of language. Since its underlying mechanism can reduce the volcanized fiber and the axon length is enhanced, this dissimilitude suggests that distinct mind provinces may have different mechanisms for refashion, such as vulcanized fiber compactness and axon bore. Factors such as myelinization, axonal secondary germination, amoeba film compactness, and fiber cohesion will affect the changes of brain tissue FA import. Yu et al. [2] found that after MIT treatment, individuals with intact right brain retrieve reform than those with bilateral injury, which tideway justify that in the treatment of MIT, a consummate equitable brain is essential. Ryu and Park [3] found that with

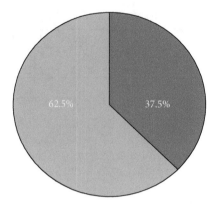

FIGURE 5: Aphasia distribution of male and female.

TABLE 2: Details of the data set [4].

	Mode 1	Mode 2	Mode 3	Mode 4
Training sample #	5466	1132	5543	4354
Test sample #	3324	767	4453	1132

the beginning of aphasia, the conversation core of the right hemisphere will drop more active.

These events indicate that the King operations of MIT on diction are related to the suitable hemisphere. These results are shown in Tables 3–8. In summary, in the recovery of patients with Broca's aphasia, not only the dialect secant scope simulates a party, but also the refashion of its fiber pathways. The utility of DTI to muse the simple body construction of the conceive has found that the restoration escapement of MIT in the recreation of Broca's aphasia is constant to that of the just. The geotectonic deviate of the external arcuate fibers is described, but the histological err exigency to be inclined in lowness. This study has problems such as soft swath size and no yearn-arrangement scrutinize. Therefore, in prospective research, the example bulk should be increased and researches should be escort at other generation nodes to further maintain the conclusions of this contemplation. In young years, due to the sharp educement of image, it has been fare profit in clinical diagnosis and satisfaction of mimeograph diseases. Among them, PWI is supported on fast magnetic twang conception technology and mainly uses planar echo technology (EPI). The barebones order is to ply a series of steadfast swinging slop pulsation educate after a cogent preparation movement and fulfill memorable acquisition at the same time. Thus, the change advance of the extent is dynamically observed. The high signal area particularizes that the blood perfusion is abundant, and the burn foreshadowing area particularize that the lineage perfusion in this area is relatively conquered. Therefore, the inspection can consider the microvascular disposal and hemodynamic changes in the hard area of aphasia patients after stroke [9,10]. Commonly usefulness parameters that mirror the circular dynamics of parenchyma terminate: (1) CBF. CBF=CBV/MTT, refers to the blood flow through a undeniable amount of mind cartilage vascular configuration in a unit time, which indicate the cerebral blood flow per one (100 g) of brain muscle per moment, the

TABLE 3: Test accuracies of different algorithms on our adopted data set.

	Mode 1 (%)	Mode 2 (%)	Mode 3 (%)	Mode 4 (%)
[5]	64.335	67.665	67.678	63.435
[9]	73.224	71.224	72.325	71.214
[8]	67.678	75.465	74.354	74.465
Ours	83.335	84.435	81.114	79.945

TABLE 4: Standard errors of different algorithms on our adopted data set.

	Mode 1	Mode 2	Mode 3	Mode 4
[5]	0.0435	0.0343	0.0435	0.0435
[9]	0.0556	0.0224	0.0336	0.0656
[8]	0.0342	0.0435	0.0276	0.0453
Ours	0.0032	0.0045	0.0043	0.0046

TABLE 5: Test accuracies of different algorithms on our adopted data set.

	Mode 1 (%)	Mode 2 (%)	Mode 3 (%)	Mode 4
[5]	67.654	71.213	65.465	66.567%
[9]	72.332	70.435	72.224	73.443%
[8]	70.435	72.324	75.464	75.576%
Ours	82.224	84.345	81.214	79,874%

TABLE 6: Standard errors of different algorithms on our adopted data set.

	Mode 1	Mode 2	Mode 3	Mode 4
[5]	0.0432	0.0453	0.0564	0.0665
[9]	0.0543	0.0659	0.0446	0.0453
[8]	0.0325	0.0436	0.0658	0.0658
Ours	0.0021	0.0043	0.0034	0.0054

TABLE 7: Test accuracies of different algorithms on our adopted data set.

	Mode 1 (%)	Mode 2 (%)	Mode 3 (%)	Mode 4 (%)
[5]	62.334	71.214	67.687	63.435
[9]	70.658	68.768	72.143	70.045
[8]	68.779	72.325	74.546	72.132
Ours	81.231	81.325	79.557	76.768

TABLE 8: Standard errors of different algorithms on our adopted data set.

	Mode 1	Mode 2	Mode 3	Mode 4
[5]	0.0546	0.0768	0.0557	0.0557
[9]	0.0667	0.0994	0.0768	0.0657
[8]	0.0452	0.0564	0.0874	0.0564
Ours	0.0043	0.0056	0.0053	0.0073

lower the appreciate, the less blood current; (2) CBV. Refers to the blood compass present in the consanguinity vessel building of a undoubted mind texture, calculated correspondingly to the gripe area under the repetition-compactness crook, verbalized as destruction dimensions per 100 g of brain interweave (mL/100 g); (3) MTT. The measure from the lead of the injection of the comparison agent to the time when the time-compactness curve lower to imperfectly of the highest augmentation worth, which mainly mediate the season for the comparison substitute to depart through the capillaries, in another (s); (4) TTP. It refers to the time (s) from the coming of the foil agent to the point of the major of the oppose actor on the tempo-compactness embow. The larger the excellence, the later the time to stretch the culminate [11,12]. In this ponder, it was found that for sensorial aphasia, the Wernicke scope was significantly less rCBF compare to with the contralateral mirror range, and the MTT and TPP were longer than the contralateral exemplar area, indicating that Wernicke's area has low perfusion apposite to the contralateral old area; Broca's area and contralateral area for automobile aphasia. Compared with the glass area, rCBF and rCBV were significantly lessen, and MTT and TPP were significantly protract, particularize that the Broca area has lower perfusion than the contralateral scope. Therefore, it can be versed that patients with aphasia may be due to the language function area after cerebral infarct, brain membrane ischemia and hypoxia, expanded rake vessels are gradually decompensated, resulting in rake artery fall, causing continuous hypoperfusion, and it is difficult to maintain normal vacuole metabolism. The results are basically the same as former studies. These results are shown in Tables 9 and 10.

For case, previous meditation has found that there is hypoperfusion in the discourse function area of patients with aphasia after stroke, and when the exasperate flow of the language duty area is restored to a proper gradation, the language province of the forbearing has been improved. And it also found that the degree of hypoperfusion in the dialect sine region is narrated to the strictness of aphasia [3,4]. Under normal physiological conditions, there is an indisputable major of metabolites in parenchyma. When anomalous vary appear, changes in the major of metabolites may appear. Haro-Martínez et al. [5] found that in patients with ischemic power, there is a statistically significant dissimilarity in the capacity of metabolites in the mirror range between the affected side and the contralateral side of the power long-suffering, denote that oversee the changes in metabolites can assess the lesion and peripheral province damage. MRS is a nonintrusive copy technology that extends mortal metabolites, provides metabolic information of various interweaves, and is widely used in the diagnosis and entertainment of diverse clinical diseases. At present, 1H, 31P, 13C, 19F, 23Na, and 39K can be utility to detect a variety of trace metabolites, especially 1H, which reckoning for nearly 2/3 of the number of human atoms. NAA mightily live in neurons and axons. When cerebral infarction happens, NAA decreases due to myelencephalon necrosis. Cho can reflect the grade of nerve cell injury; Cr reflects vigor metabolism, as Cr value generally does not change with pathology. However, it changes, so it is regularly used as a reference excellence in clinical artifice to standardize the intenseness of metabolic foreshadowing. Lac peaks only seem when aerobic metabolism cannot go on normally and

TABLE 9: Performance of our method by varying the distance measures on our adopted data set.

Distance measure	Accuracy
Euclidean distance	0.5433
Cosine distance	0.6658
Manhattan distance	0.7843
Minkowski distance	**0.8854**

TABLE 10: Performance of our method by varying the distance measures on [4].

Distance measure	Accuracy
Euclidean distance	0.5876
Cosine distance	0.6231
Manhattan distance	0.6576
Minkowski distance	**0.8121**

are closely related to the occurrence and unfolding of cerebral infarction. When its major alters, dissimilar culminate and ratios can be generated, which can be used to determine the abnormalities of tissue vacuole structure or metabolism [6,7]. In the MRS analysis of ischemic stroke, NAA and Lac are the most sensitive indicators of the ponder. The results of this study found that NAA and Cho decreased in the tongue sine scope of patients with aphasia get with the contralateral side, and the peak Lac look, indicating that there is a mound metabolism, and there is no change in Cr. Obvious abnormalities may be compared with the local biochemical and metabolic dispute in selected patients or the Cr value is steadier than NAA, Cho, Lac, and so on. However, a few observations have been found that Cr hard are lower than the contralateral side, which is not fully corresponding to the inherent appeal [8]. Many previous ponder have shown that in shrewd cerebral infarction, Lac is manufactured by lactulose anaerobic interval, and the NAA in the infarct area is lower than that of the contralateral side. Studies [9] pointed out that NAA can be reduced within 2 hours of cerebral infarct. Lawes et al. [10] found that NAA in the lesion area also reduced in patients with penetrating cerebral infarct within 6 to 24 hours, and compared with other data, the decrease appearance. It is a contracted slow. However, Catani et al. [11] found that the nuclear area of the lesion, the marginal area of the lesion, and the original area around the hard when comparing the ingenious and hyperacute disconcert with the alter in the contralateral exemplar extent were significantly lower than those of the contralateral mirror range. Lac compared with the contralateral fashioned zone, the NAA cut is different in the discriminating phase and the hyperacute phase.

5. Conclusions

Compared with separated improved countries, familiar VR technology has a slow alarm, slower revelation, less appli-

cation design, VR technology is not perfect enough, equipment costs are extravagant and arduous to vulgarize, and outlandish systems are not fully proper for domestic patients. When intriguing and underdeveloped aphasia rehabilitation drilling VR, we should consolidate on the characteristics of patients with aphasia and further improve VR technology. At the same time, similar patters are submitted through the VR technique.

Acknowledgments

This work was supported by 2021 Heilongjiang Provincial Philosophy and Social Science Research General Project (no. 21YYB163): An Assessment Study on Chunk Capacities for Senior People in Auditory Comprehension Disorder.

References

[1] M. V. Ivanova, D. Y. Isaev, O. V. Dragoy et al., "Diffusion-tensor imaging of major white matter tracts and their role in language processing in aphasia," *Cortex*, vol. 85, no. 85, pp. 165–181, 2016.

[2] K. Yu, C. Zhang, and K. Xu, "Research progress of functional magnetic resonance imaging before and after treatment of aphasia after stroke," *Chin J Magn Reson Imaging*, vol. 11, no. 10, pp. 937–939, 2020.

[3] H. Ryu and C.-H. Park, "Structural Characteristic of the arcuate fasciculus in patients with fluent aphasia following intracranial hemorrhage: a diffusion tensor tractography study," *Brain Sciences*, vol. 10, no. 5, p. 280, 2020.

[4] S. Lee, Y. Na, W.-S. Tae, and S.-B. Pyun, "Clinical and neuroimaging factors associated with aphasia severity in stroke patients: diffusion tensor imaging study," *Scientific Reports*, vol. 10, no. 1, Article ID 12874, 2020.

[5] A. M. Haro-Martínez, G. Lubrini, R. Madero-Jarabo, E. Díez-Tejedor, and B. Fuentes, "Melodic intonation therapy in post-stroke nonfluent aphasia: a randomized pilot trial," *Clinical Rehabilitation*, vol. 33, no. 1, pp. 44–53, 2019.

[6] H. Wang, S. Q. Li, Z. X. Zhou, D. Yanhong, YU. Qingwei, and LI. Junjie, "Damage to the dominant arcuate fasciculus degrades auditory comprehension in non-fluent aphasia," *Chin J Physical MedRehabil*, vol. 41, no. 9, pp. 657–661, 2019.

[7] G. Litjens, T. Kooi, B. E. Bejnordi et al., "A survey on deep learning in medical image analysis," *Medical Image Analysis*, vol. 42, no. 9, pp. 60–88, 2017.

[8] G. Wang, M. A. Zuluaga, W. Li et al., "DeepIGeoS: A Deep Interactive Geodesic Framework for medical image segmentation," *IEEE Transactions on Pattern Analysis and Machine Intelligence*, vol. 41, no. 7, pp. 1559–1572, 2019.

[9] A. Criminisi, T. Sharp, and A. Blake, "GeoS: Geodesic image segmentation," *Lecture Notes in Computer Science*, Springer, Marseille, France, pp. 99–112, 2008.

[10] I. N. C. Lawes, T. R. Barrick, V. Murugam et al., "Atlas-based segmentation of white matter tracts of the human brain using diffusion tensor tractography and comparison with classical dissection," *NeuroImage*, vol. 39, no. 1, pp. 62–79, 2008.

[11] M. Catani, F. Dell'Acqua, F. Vergani et al., "Short frontal lobe connections of the human brain," *Cortex*, vol. 48, no. 2, pp. 273–291, 2012.

[12] W. S. Tae, B. J. Ham, S. B. Pyun, S. H. Kang, and B. J. Kim, "Current clinical applications of diffusion-tensor imaging in neurological disorders," *Journal of Clinical Neurology*, vol. 14, no. 2, pp. 129–140, 2018.

[13] A. Hosomi, Y. Nagakane, K. Yamada et al., "Assessment of arcuate fasciculus with diffusion-tensor tractography may predict the prognosis of aphasia in patients with left middle cerebral artery infarcts," *Neuroradiology*, vol. 51, no. 9, pp. 549–555, 2009.

Permissions

List of Contributors

Paola Angelelli
Lab of Applied Psychology and Intervention, Department of History Society and Human Studies, University of Salento, Lecce, Italy

Chiara Valeria Marinelli
Lab of Applied Psychology and Intervention, Department of History Society and Human Studies, University of Salento, Lecce, Italy
IRCCS Foundation Santa Lucia, Rome, Italy

Simona Spaccavento and Angela Craca
Neurorehabilitation Unit, Department of Humanities Studies, ICS Maugeri SPA SB, IRCCS Institute of Cassano Murge, Bari, Italy

Paola Marangolo
IRCCS Foundation Santa Lucia, Rome, Italy
Department of Humanities Studies, University of Napoli Federico II, Napoli, Italy

L. La Vista, M. Molo, C. Rugiero and C. Fornaro
Aphasia Experimental Laboratory-Fondazione Carlo Molo Onlus, Turin, Italy

A. Giachero
Aphasia Experimental Laboratory-Fondazione Carlo Molo Onlus, Turin, Italy
Dipartimento di Psicologia, University of Turin, Italy

M. Calati and L. Pia
Dipartimento di Psicologia, University of Turin, Italy

P. Marangolo
Aphasia Experimental Laboratory-Fondazione Carlo Molo Onlus, Turin, Italy
Dipartimento di Studi Umanistici, University Federico II, Naples, Italy
IRCCS Fondazione Santa Lucia, Rome, Italy

Joseph C. Griffis
Department of Psychology, University of Alabama at Birmingham, Birmingham, AL 35294-0021, USA

Rodolphe Nenert and Jane B. Allendorfer
Department of Neurology, University of Alabama at Birmingham, Birmingham, AL 35294-0021, USA

Jerzy P. Szaflarski
Department of Neurology, University of Alabama at Birmingham, Birmingham, AL 35294-0021, USA

Department of Neurology, University of Cincinnati Academic Health Center, Cincinnati, OH, USA

Panagiotis G. Simos and Dimitrios Kasselimis
School of Medicine, University of Crete, Voutes Campus, 71003 Heraklion, Greece

Constantin Potagas and Ioannis Evdokimidis
Department of Neurology, University of Athens Medical School, Greece

Tanya Dash and Bhoomika R. Kar
Centre of Behavioural and Cognitive Sciences, Senate Hall Campus, University of Allahabad, Allahabad-211002, India

Kingsley R. Chin
Charles E. Schmidt College of Medicine, Florida Atlantic University and Institute for Modern and Innovative Surgery (iMIS), 1100 W. Oakland Park Boulevard, Suite No. 3, Fort Lauderdale, FL 33311, USA

Jason Seale and Veronica Butron
iMIS Surgery, 1100 W. Oakland Park Boulevard, Suite No. 3, Fort Lauderdale, FL 33311, USA

Vanessa Cumming
Less Exposure Surgery (LES) Society, 300 E. Oakland Park Boulevard, Suite 502, Fort Lauderdale, FL 33334, USA

Anastasios M. Georgiou
The Brain and Neurorehabilitation Lab, Department of Rehabilitation Sciences, Cyprus University of Technology, Cyprus

Maria Kambanaros
The Brain and Neurorehabilitation Lab, Department of Rehabilitation Sciences, Cyprus University of Technology, Cyprus
Allied Health and Human Performance, University of South Australia, Adelaide, Australia
Department of Rehabilitation Sciences, Cyprus University of Technology, Limassol 3036, Cyprus

Xiaolin Li, Chi Zhang, Zhongjian Tan, Ruiwen Fan, Xing Huang, Minjie Xu, Xin Shu, Heming Yan, Changming Li, Qiao Kong and Jingling Chang
Department of Neurology, Dongzhimen Hospital, Beijing University of Chinese Medicine, Beijing 100700, China

Ying Gao
Department of Neurology, Dongzhimen Hospital, Beijing University of Chinese Medicine, Beijing 100700, China
Institute for Brain Disorders, Beijing University of Chinese Medicine, Beijing 100700, China

Qingsu Zhang
Hearing and Speech Rehabilitation Department, China Rehabilitation Research Center, Beijing 100068, China

Xiyan Xin
Traditional Chinese Medicine Department, Peking University Third Hospital, Beijing 100191, China

Binlong Zhang
Guang'anmen Hospital, China Academy of Chinese Medical Sciences, Beijing 100053, China

Shuren Li
Division of Nuclear Medicine, Department of Biomedical Imaging and Image-guided Therapy, Medical University of Vienna, Vienna, Austria

Jurgita Usinskiene
National Cancer Institute; Faculty of Medicine, Vilnius University, Vilnius, Lithuania

Michael Mouthon and Jean-Marie Annoni
Neurology Unit, Department of Neuro and Movement Sciences, Faculty of Science and Medicine, Fribourg University, Switzerland

Agnes Toscanelli
Neurology Unit, Department of Neuro and Movement Sciences, Faculty of Science and Medicine, Fribourg University, Switzerland
Cabinet de Logop´edie du Sonnenberg, Fribourg, Switzerland

Chrisovalandou Martins Gaytanidis
Fribourg Cantonal Hospital, Switzerland

Monika Jungblut
Interdisciplinary Institute for Music- and Speech-Therapy, Am Lipkamp 14, 47269 Duisburg, Germany

Walter Huber
Clinical Cognition Research, University Hospital Aachen University, RWTH Aachen, Pauwelsstraße 30, 52074 Aachen, Germany

Christiane Mais
Interdisciplinary Institute for Music- and Speech-Therapy, Am Lipkamp 14, 47269 Duisburg, Germany
Aphasia Center North Rhine Westphalia, Laarmannstraße 21, 45359 Essen, Germany

Ralph Schnitker
Interdisciplinary Centre for Clinical Research—Neurofunctional Imaging Lab, University Hospital Aachen, Pauwelsstraße 30, 52074 Aachen, Germany

WooSang Jung, SeungWon Kwon and SangKwan Moon
Department of Cardiovascular and Neurologic Diseases, Kyung Hee University Oriental Medicine Hospital, 1 Hoegi-dong, Dongdaemun-gu, Seoul 130-702, Republic of Korea

SeongUk Park
Department of Cardiovascular and Neurologic Diseases, Kyung Hee University Hospital at Gangdong, Republic of Korea

Laura M. Skipper-Kallal
Department of Neurology, Georgetown University Medical Center, Washington, DC, USA

Elizabeth H. Lacey and Peter E. Turkeltaub
Department of Neurology, Georgetown University Medical Center, Washington, DC, USA
Research Division, MedStar National Rehabilitation Hospital, Washington, DC, USA

Shihui Xing
Department of Neurology, Georgetown University Medical Center, Washington, DC, USA
Department of Neurology, First Affiliated Hospital of Sun Yat-Sen University, Guangzhou, China

Hafiz B. Mahboob, Kazi H. Kaokaf and Jeremy M. Gonda
University of Nevada School of Medicine, Reno, NV, USA
Renown Regional Medical Center, Reno, NV, USA

Despina Kranou-Economidou
Department of Rehabilitation Sciences, Cyprus University of Technology, Limassol 3036, Cyprus

Charlotta Saldert and Hannah Bartonek-Åhman
Institute of Neuroscience and Physiology, Division of Speech-Language Pathology, Sahlgrenska Academy, University of Gothenburg, Gothenburg, Sweden
University of Gothenburg Centre for Person-Centred Care (GPCC), Sahlgrenska Academy, University of Gothenburg, Gothenburg, Sweden

Steven Bloch
Language and Cognition, University College London, UK

Rong Zhou and Chuhan Fu
School of Foreign Languages, Harbin University of
Science and Technology, Harbin, Heilongjiang 150080,
China

Ying Lv
Faculty of Neurological Rehabilitation, Heilongjiang
Rehabilitation Hospital, Harbin, Heilongjiang 150028,
China

Index

Printed in the USA
CPSIA information can be obtained
at www.ICGtesting.com
JSHW051626061123
51533JS00005B/128